BROWN BEAUTY

Brown Beauty

*Color, Sex, and Race from
the Harlem Renaissance
to World War II*

Laila Haidarali

NEW YORK UNIVERSITY PRESS
New York

NEW YORK UNIVERSITY PRESS
New York
www.nyupress.org

© 2018 by New York University
All rights reserved

The publisher wishes to thank the Crisis Publishing Co., Inc., the publisher of the magazine of the National Association for the Advancement of Colored People, for the use of the images and material first published in issues of Crisis.

References to Internet websites (URLs) were accurate at the time of writing. Neither the author nor New York University Press is responsible for URLs that may have expired or changed since the manuscript was prepared.

Library of Congress Cataloging-in-Publication Data
Names: Haidarali, Laila, author.
Title: Brown beauty : color, sex, and race from the Harlem Renaissance to World War II / Laila Haidarali.
Other titles: Color, sex, and race from the Harlem Renaissance to World War II
Description: New York : New York University Press, 2018. | Includes bibliographical references and index.
Identifiers: LCCN 2017045026| ISBN 978-1-4798-7510-8 (cl : alk. paper) | ISBN 978-1-4798-0208-1 (pb : alk. paper)
Subjects: LCSH: African American women—Race identity—20th century. | African American women—Social conditions—20th century. | Beauty, Personal—Social aspects—United States—20th century.
Classification: LCC E185.86 .H225 2018 | DDC 305.48/896073—dc23
LC record available at https://lccn.loc.gov/2017045026

New York University Press books are printed on acid-free paper, and their binding materials are chosen for strength and durability. We strive to use environmentally responsible suppliers and materials to the greatest extent possible in publishing our books.

Manufactured in the United States of America

10 9 8 7 6 5 4 3 2 1

For my mother, Anisa Grace Haidarali,
who taught me of beauty's true meanings

CONTENTS

List of Figures and Color Plates	ix
Introduction	1
1. Brown Beginnings: Imaging the New Negro Woman in 1920s Literary Print Culture	31
2. Beautiful Brown Skin: Advertising New Negro Womanhood	62
3. "Of the Brown-Skin Type": Madonnas, Mulattas, and Modern Women in Literary Print Culture	104
4. To a Brown Girl: The Poetic Discourse of Brown	153
5. Browning the *Dark Princess*: Asian Indian Embodiment of New Negro Womanhood	193
6. Sociological Discourses on Color, Class, and Gender, from Depression to World War II	225
Epilogue	261
Acknowledgments	263
Notes	267
Bibliography	295
Index	317
About the Author	335

LIST OF FIGURES AND COLOR PLATES

FIGURES

Figure 2.1. Advertisement for O.K. Colored Doll Company, 1923	63
Figure 2.2. Josephine Baker doll, 1927	76
Figure 2.3. Bell Manufacturing advertisement for Brown Skin Dolls, 1923	81
Figure 2.4. Bethel Manufacturing advertisement for Colored Dolls and Novelties, 1927	81
Figure 2.5. S. D. Lyons advertisement for India Hair Grower, 1930	93
Figure 2.6. Kashmir advertisement, 1916	98
Figure 2.7. S. D. Lyons advertisement for India Hair Grower, circa 1926 and Duncan's Business School advertisement for Training, 1926	99
Figure 3.1. Winold Reiss, *Type Study, I* (Ancestral), c. 1924	109
Figure 3.2. "A Master of Arts," *Crisis* cover, July 1924	130
Figure 3.3. Ermine Casey Bush, *Crisis* cover, October 1925	134
Figure 3.4. "Photograph from Life," *Crisis* cover, November 1928	136
Figure 3.5. "Study of a Negro Girl," *Crisis* cover, July 1925	137
Figure 3.6. "Photographic Study of the Head of a Negro Woman," *Crisis* cover, November 1925	138
Figure 3.7. "Drawing from Life," *Crisis* cover, July 1927	139
Figure 3.8. "A North African Cousin of Ours," *Crisis* cover, May 1926	141
Figure 3.9. Manila's "Queen of Carnival," *Crisis* cover, March 1925	143
Figure 3.10. "A Colored Graduate of the Philippine Normal School," *Crisis* cover, July 1926	145
Figure 3.11. Clarissa Mae Scott, *Crisis* cover, July 1923	147

Figure 3.12. "Bachelor of Philosophy," *Crisis* cover, August 1924 — 148

Figure 3.13. "A Bachelor of Music from Oberlin," *Crisis* cover, August 1926 — 149

Figure 3.14. "A Salutatorian," *Crisis* cover, August 1930 — 150

Figure 3.15. "A Western School Teacher," *Crisis* cover, September 1930 — 151

COLOR PLATES

Color images are gathered as an insert following page 86.

Plate 1.1: Winold Reiss, *Miss Hurston* (Zora Neale Hurston), c. 1925

Plate 1.2: Winold Reiss, *Elise J. McDougald*, 1924

Plate 1.3: Winold Reiss, *Harlem Girl 1*, 1925

Plate 1.4: Winold Reiss, *Type Study, II* (Two Public School Teachers), c. 1925

Plate 1.5: Winold Reiss, *Brown Madonna*, circa 1925

Introduction

I remember the very day I became colored. Up to my thirteenth year, I lived in a little Negro town of Eatonville, Florida. It is exclusively a colored town. The only white people I knew passed through the town going in or coming from Orlando. . . .

But changes came in the family when I was thirteen, and I was sent to school in Jacksonville. I left Eatonville, the town of the oleanders, as Zora. When I disembarked from the river-boat at Jacksonville, she was no more. It seemed that I had suffered a sea change. I was not Zora of Orange County any more, I was now a little colored girl. I found it out in certain ways. In my heart as well as in my mirror, *I became a fast brown*—warranted not to rub or run.

. . . in the main, *I feel like a brown bag of miscellany* propped against a wall. Against a wall in company with other bags, white, red and yellow. Pour out the contents, and there is discovered a jumble of small things priceless and worthless . . . a bit of colored glass more or less would not matter. Perhaps that is how the Great Stuffer of bags filled them in the first place—who knows?
—Zora Neale Hurston, "How It Feels to Be Colored Me" (1928; my italics)

In 1928 the nonfiction essay "How It Feels to Be Colored Me," Zora Neale Hurston pinpointed the moment she first perceived herself as racially different. On that day, she envisioned herself as brown in complexion and identity. In her account of migration from Eatonville, Florida—a rural all-black town—to Jacksonville, Florida, a fast-growing center of Southern urbanism, the Harlem Renaissance writer used brown as the color to enunciate this coming of racial age as the "very day" she "became colored." Published in *World Tomorrow*, Hurston's essay describes this movement as pivotal in shifting her identity from "Zora of Orange County" to a "little colored girl." In this account, the rapidity of Hurston's racialization, and the accompanying sense of loss of individuality that is not only connected but also defined by place, is dramatic and striking. Still, the author signaled a layering to this understanding of self—brown was an entity both felt and seen; it was "found . . . out in certain ways," Hurston explained, alluding to the ongoing capacity of antiblack racism in the Jim Crow South to shape this new identity. As she pinpointed the origin of this racialized identity, Hurston found that, on the one hand, her becoming "a fast brown" was forged in enhanced proximity to white Southerners; on the other, she bolstered the "little colored girl" who suddenly appeared in her mirror by reinforcing brownness through her vision and feeling of self. At once subject and object in identifying herself as a "fast brown," Hurston's brown complexion appears to first function as a psychological defense against white hostilities. Second, "brown" operates as a permanent claim to a racial identity that, while self-determined, was not altogether autonomously defined. Hurston observed, "I became a fast brown—warranted not to rub or run."[1]

Hurston's assessment on what it feels like to be her and "colored" underscores a view of brownness as both relative and malleable despite its fixed hue. Weighing out her range of responses, Hurston concludes: "In the main, I feel like a brown bag of miscellany propped against a wall. Against a wall in company with other bags, white, red and yellow." The bags are objects—different only in their color. Hurston, a trained anthropologist, questions the motivation of the "Great Stuffer of Bags," a God-like figure, in creating these differences. Studying the superficial assortment of "small things priceless and worthless" that constitute and mark those differences, Hurston concludes that "a little bit of colo[r] . . . more or less would not matter." In this instance, color shows through in the material form of glass, which not only refracts light, but, in its mirrored form, also reflects imagery. With this view, the racial identity of the bag (or "subject" presented as "object") emerges as one that has been constructed, internalized, and enacted; the subject too appears passive, willing, and open to reinvention at the hands of an omniscient power that endows its body with first meaning. Yet, there is happenstance in this view of brown and other color notions of race, or "bags" that are constituted by a series of not-so-readily understood, or fixed, "jumble" of things.[2] It is this jumble of things, this making of brown skin as a real and representational identity that interests me. It leads to my study of brown beauty as a discourse and cultural product fueled by diverse and at times competing forces rising in the urban interwar setting. This book interrogates the multiple meanings of brown as reference to physical complexion in the representation of African American womanhood during the interwar years. It questions how and why color in general and brownness in particular came to intimate race, class, gender, and sex identity as one prominent response to modernity and urbanization. Indeed, as this book shows, Hurston was not alone in her use of color: throughout the interwar years, diverse sets of African American women and men, all of whom can be defined as middle-class within this constituency's widely varying class membership, privileged brown complexions in their reworking of ideas, images, and expressions to identify the representative bodies of women as modern "New Negro" women.

Hurston's deployment of color highlights the relativity of color's meanings to people, places, and things. In particular, proximity to whites figures prominently as Hurston explains her feeling "most colored" when thrown up against a "stark white background"; color is felt in both relative and oppositional ways: Hurston appears brown next to a male figure, "so pale with his whiteness." Indeed, Hurston's use of brown as a racial descriptor is clearly connected to place and nearness to whites—it is the movement between and among African Americans, and integrated spaces, that calls heightened attention to color. Hurston, like many thousand more African Americans, travelled from Eatonville, Florida, to Harlem, New York City, through a process of chain migration.

Born in 1891, Hurston's movement was precipitated by "changes in the family" following her mother's death when she was only thirteen years old. Her father's swift remarriage to a young woman with whom Zora physically sparred signaled her break with the family and her beginning movement out of the South. Traveling as a maid with a Gilbert and Sullivan touring group, Hurston eventually made her way to Baltimore, Maryland. There she enrolled in school, dating her birth to 1901 to do so; in 1918, when she completed her high school education, Hurston continued on to Washington, D.C., eventually entering Howard University where she studied until 1924. When she arrived in Harlem in 1925, Hurston was already a published writer and a cause célèbre on the Columbia campus. Yet, graduating at the age of thirty-seven, her status as a migrant woman who made her way independently to the North showcases the variances in the life cycles of racialized Americans and emphasizes the historic attainment gap in women's education. Hurston was proud; she hid her age as she moved among younger women and men, working closely with young poets, radicals, and the *avant garde* of Harlem's literati (plate I.1).[3]

In 1925, when she arrived in Manhattan to continue her studies in anthropology at Barnard College at Columbia University, Hurston did so by transferring from Howard University in Washington, D.C., where between 1919 and 1924 she pursued her undergraduate degree. Famed for her ability to command white patronage and support, Hurston's entrance and tuition fees at Barnard were funded by the college's cofounder and longtime trustee, Annie Nathan Meyer. Still, Hurston remained practical about living in the city. In her "Record of Freshman Interest," Hurston, already a published short story writer, noted her plan to earn her living expenses while at college by working as "a manicurist, social worker or waitress [or] perhaps sell a manuscript or two."[4] In 1928, when she graduated, she did so as the college's first African American graduate. Famed for her sardonic nature, critical stance to the movement's more conservative factions, and contradictory race politics, Hurston had no formal complaint of discrimination on the college campus; still, when she recalled the degree of attention she attracted from the "Social Register crowd," she likened herself to the college's "sacred black cow."[5] This use of color, and its connection to Hindu beliefs about the cow, captured the stark exoticism of her difference: Hurston was an African American woman on a northern, urban, and elite university campus.

In other places, color's distinction was felt most acutely within one's own community. Hurston, among the most radical of Harlem's literati, wrote openly about the taboo topic of colorism, a long-standing and troublesome practice among some African American communities. Her award-winning play, "Color Struck" (1926), cast its main characters by color, race, and gender: John appears as "a light brown-skinned man"; Emmaline, a "black woman," and Effie "a mulatto girl." Set in the first decade of the twentieth century, the play begins in a southern city and follows the train journey of its trio to the North. As the play unfolds, color or complexion emerges as a site of conflict, jealousy, and marginalization with the "black woman," Emmaline, as the loser. She has internalized the judgment of dark complexions as inferior and undesirable to the point where she cannot accept the love of John, a "good man," whose light brown complexion does not occlude his long-standing love for Emmaline. Although "Color Struck" underlines the personal insecurity of the "black woman," it also showcases the shared experience of race in America: like hundreds of thousands, the characters in "Color Struck" make the hopeful train journey northward; like countless others, they take pleasure in dance. Indeed, when Emmaline rejects John at the Cakewalk for dancing with a light-skinned "mulatto" named Effie, the action symbolizes her rejection of self, her partner, and her race.[6] Still, Hurston's play does not leave the fault with the "black woman." Indeed, "Color Struck" exposes the complex problematic of race, color, class, and womanhood as issues that resonate far beyond the intimate and the individual.

A long taboo topic, colorism was a contentious issue in the era of the New Negro. Some African Americans critiqued intraracial colorism. They called attention to a system that not only privileged lighter complexions over darker tones but also engaged diverse sets of ritualistic exclusionary practices that hierarchized complexion by color. Some considered it an outdated practice, while others found its resonant influence within their own communities and within white dominant culture. Though Hurston was among the very group to claim the range of African American complexions as a proud index of the New Negro, she was among those members of Harlem's literati to denounce colorism as an ongoing practice. Apparently, Hurston herself was on the "right" side of the color scale but, as Mary Helen Washington explains, depending on which one of Hurston's contemporaries you relied on, descriptions cast the author as "light yellow," "black as coal," and "reddish light brown."[7] Clearly, any judgment of complexion remains subjective and relative, and as one may wonder, how meaningful is it? Ultimately, Hurston's perception of self and reliance on a *feeling* of color matters most, and her writings intimate rather than tell about any "real" color or complexion. Hurston's use of brown as a racial identifier shows how the meanings associated with color elicit different interpretations that remain contingent on place, space, and time.

For various reasons I draw on Hurston's essay "How It Feels to Be Colored Me" to introduce this study of the interwar discourse on brownness and beauty. No doubt today Zora Neale Hurston is one of the best-known and most celebrated authors of the literary and intellectual movement of the Harlem Renaissance. Her expression also affects some of the temperament of the political identity of the New Negro, albeit remaining more complicated in its embrace of "race pride" and "race progress" as key goals of African American migration and modernization. Hurston's references to brown as identity and color are important not because of their rarity but, rather, because they reflect the common use of color and brown during the years when modernization and urbanization were well underway. Her allusions to brown, then, exemplify one of the many ways that Harlem Renaissance writers signaled and used color to produce an ideology of race pride that developed across the decades. Hurston's use of color in this essay and other works is also instructive because it further emphasizes the importance of time and place to the author's adjectival use of color. "How It Feels" invokes the bag as a metaphor to signify the racialized body: its purposeful imaging foregrounds a lack of aspiration to modern displays of beauty and fashion, and to shape or relative form; the bag is an everyday object, a conveyance, utilitarian and changeable in its haul. Furthermore, the metaphor bypasses any connection of brown complexions with beauty that featured prominently in other representations of the period suggesting that color's use was individualistic, varied, and changeable.

How does one historicize color and beauty—two dimensions of human judgment so acutely subjective that, despite their physical manifestations, they remain abstract, inexact, and malleable? *Brown Beauty* considers the use of color as filtered through a nexus of discourses on race, sex, class, and womanhood that emerged and shifted in its meanings throughout the interwar years to underscore the inexact determinations of color as a feature of culture. In addition to time and place, color is a phenomenon experienced by the senses. Color relies on light to manifest its appearance as hue and tone; it requires the seer to envision color, although the other four senses also compensate when people lack the ability of sight. Ultimately, the classification of human complexion by color relies on imprecise and changing cultural values and standards; on sensory interpretations that differ according to time, place, and subject; on language that, despite its growing expansive range, remains finite in its ability to "fix" color.[8] Above all, assessments of color remain subjective and individualistic. Consequently, abstract and tangible notions of color shape this historical study of brown-skin womanhood. Here, brown, brownness, or brown skin, refers to physical color as a discursive ideal and as a historic reference to the real tones of complexion; at the same time, when picturing a body constituted as brown, a broad range of brown tones likely emerge. In recognizing the subjective and relative assessment of "brown" as a descriptor of complexion, this book studies brownness as a performative ideal that was not always bound to physical color, despite remaining within its intimate boundary.

As with any category, the exclusionary parameters of brown as a racial descriptor must be noted. By virtue of their dark skin tones, some African American girls and women would never be considered "brown" in complexion. Cultural producers in this study engaged a diverse set of color names, including those that accented hues other than brown; for example, those considered—"blue black," "ashy gray," and "inky black"—could not be described as brown no matter how broad a range of tones brown covered. No doubt, for some, these exclusions were painful, particularly because these boundaries emanated from places of racial belonging.[9] A contestatory politics of inclusion/exclusion occurs with this othering. On the one hand, people with very dark complexions could not be described as brown; on the other, African Americans who fell within the fairly broad spectrum of brown complexions could not be considered as anything other than "black," where black is cast as oppositional to whiteness and upholds a binarized view of racial difference.

To understand why interwar middle-class African Americans turned to color as a rhetorical device and shorthand maker as they worked to reconstruct modern representations of people, we need to outline a larger historical and analytical context. Thus, the rest of this introduction will consider four points. First, it will discuss the importance of modernization in prompting the development of brown beauty as both a process of modernization and a modernizing discourse. The key events of the Great Migration and urbanization bolstered the mass mobilization and politicization of African Americans and spurred a diverse New Negro movement. New Negroes formed political organizations, forged new cultural expressions, and negotiated the political economy in innovative ways. Second, it will trace the changing discourse on respectability to find among its shifting values the rise of beauty as an important signifier of modernity. It shows how the discourse on brown beauty was formulated as one strategy to advance integration, economic justice, and enhanced employment in the industrial urban setting. To be precise, it draws attention to the growing ethos around consumption as among the modernizing forces that help set in motion the use of brown as a racial identifier that carried particular meanings for women. Third, it will outline the fundamental shifts in intellectualizing on race during the interwar years, and show how new conceptualizations yielded space for the advance of alternate interpretations—brown became useful to signify difference in more favorable terms and ways less associated with biological views of the "raced" body. Fourth, it positions the interwar discourse on brown beauty along the trajectory understanding of the long civil rights movement by showing the origins of a liberal black politics that put women at the center of the equation. Finally, it situates African American interwar print and visual culture as a dynamic set of sources and a rich matrix to study beauty's gendered connection to color during the interwar years. This examination of a range of representations produced by diverse groups foregrounds the question: how and why, as a racial discourse and public identity, did brown beauty emerge during the interwar years to forge an intermediary middle ground for asserting and negotiating racial pride?

The Great Migration, Modernization, and Harlem's New Negro

The movement of African Americans fueled the interwar discourse on brown complexions. Hurston recalls "the day [she] became brown" through the process of migration: she was one of the near three million migrants who, between 1914 and 1940, abandoned rural spaces to settle, and often resettle, in a chain of urban locales predominantly in the Northeast and Midwest. Migration fueled the mass modernization of a people whose historical denial of freedoms and rights met no full redress in the progressive urban promised land.[10] Historians underscore the push and pull factors that compelled the movement of men and women, as individuals and families, to new industrial centers. At the same time, some point to the intimate and personal dimensions that compelled movement out of the Jim Crow South. Darlene Clarke

Hine shows how rape and the threat of rape was an important impetus for black women's migration in the first several decades of the twentieth century. Not dismissing the importance of economic motivations, Hine underscores women's vulnerability to a system of sexual terrorism in the South.[11] Other tenuous life conditions also propelled the movement of everyday people like Hurston whose migration from the South to the North followed a pattern of "secondary migration" rather than the single complete journey that "as a rule" marked the movement of single African American women.[12]

During World War I, the migration of African Americans from the rural South to the urban North and Midwest accelerated moving from an earlier modest trickle out of the South three decades earlier to an energetic flow that came to be known as the "first" phase of the Great migration (1916-40). Rural Southerners most often embarked on the migratory process to escape the horrors of Jim Crow. Between 1890 and 1920, a period characterized by Rayford Logan as the "nadir" or low point in African American history, economic stagnation, underemployment, disenfranchisement, and violence characterized the lives of rural Southerners.[13] Curtailed movements during wartime stemmed the flow of immigrant labor from southern and eastern Europe, creating a labor shortage in the new industrial centers in the North and Midwest, and parts of the urban South. New opportunities for employment included work in steel, oil, and auto production; manufacturing plants, factories, and mail-order enterprises; and the services and retail trades. These economic opportunities beckoned African American men, women, and families. Ultimately however, the migrant experience of the harsh realities of urban living belied the view that north of the Mason-Dixon Line lay the promised land. Still, African Americans forged communities, maintained cultural ties, and found new pleasures and freedom in urban town and cities.[14]

Between 1910 and 1920, eight cities—New York, Chicago, Pittsburgh, Detroit, Norfolk, Cleveland, Indianapolis, Cincinnati—experienced massive growth rates, with the first three experiencing the greatest expansion. For example, between 1910 and 1930, the black population in New York City rose from 91,709 to 327,706. Between 1920 and 1930, that city's African-descended population increased by 115 percent.[15] Women as well as men traveled to these places, but as Darlene Clarke Hine shows, fewer women than men migrated to the urban Midwest whereas in "most eastern and southern cities" women formed the migrating majority. Limited economic opportunities for women's work in midwestern cities explain some of the gender differential in settlement, but as Hine makes clear, migration's complexities demand closer scrutiny to fully explicate differences in gender patterns of migration.[16]

By the second decade of the twentieth century African Americans, like other Americans, were becoming increasingly urbanized. In 1920 the U.S. Federal Census noted the historic moment: for the first time the majority of Americans resided in urban areas, defined by the U.S. federal government as areas populated by 2,500 or more people. By 1930, 46 percent of African Americans lived in urban centers.[17] Urbanization brought African Americans and African-descended people of different classes, religions, languages, and cultural backgrounds to closer proximity with one another. It also decreased the spatial distance between whites, African Americans, and other ethnicized people. This modernizing effect reoriented the vision of urban dwellers who caught new sights of racial difference in rapidly expanding industrial centers. Cities took on colorful hues, prompting descriptions of spaces as ethnic and racialized people by color.

The late-nineteenth-century influx of new immigrants prompted Jacob Riis, Progressive reformer and journalist, to describe "The Color Line in New York" by enumerating its changing composition by color. In 1890, Riis wrote, "A map of the city, colored to designate nationalities, would show more stripes than on the skin of a zebra, more colors than any rainbow." He went on to describe ethnic enclaves by color, associating Jewish people with "dull gray," Italians with "red," while Chinatown formed a "sharp streak of yellow." Riis seemed displeased that the "blacks" or "colored" were being pushed uptown by the foreign-born "red" Italians who "occupied his home, his church, his trade and all, with merciless impartiality."[18] This "push" uptown eventually facilitated the development of Harlem as a dynamic and important space for the development of African American culture, community, and political expression. "Black Manhattan," as prominent African American writer James Weldon Johnson dubbed Harlem in 1925, was home to a vast and diverse number of African-descended people who, regardless of color or complexion, found a home in Harlem. As Johnson celebrated Harlem's unique character, he underlined its difference from other modern cities in the United States, finding that really there was "no change, . . . in the appearance of the people, except in their color."[19]

Another influential editor and writer, Charles S. Johnson, assessed Harlem by demography, judging its population as "one part native, one part West Indian, and about three parts Southern." After forty years of migrations and intermingling between these and other groups, Johnson found that "imperceptible gradations have changed the whole complexion and outlook of the New Yorker."[20] Between 1920 and 1930, Harlem's population grew from 84,000 to 190,000, absorbing large numbers of migrants from the rural South. Other immigrants, namely African-descended Caribbeans and Africans, many of whom were from Ethiopia, were also drawn to this Black Mecca.[21] According to Jeffrey Ogbar, Harlem became "the largest black urban centre in North America and mecca of black culture and the arts."[22]

No doubt African American urban life existed well beyond Harlem, and recent scholarship cautions against the reification of Harlem as the only site of cultural expression, culture building, and the New Negro movement.[23] Important studies showcase the dynamic range of activism and cultural production across the nation. Still, Harlem played a unique role in shaping the cultural expression of brown beauty in this era of mass modernization. Indeed, in "Black Manhattan" brownness abounded as *New York Age* columnist Vere Johns noted with displeasure. In 1934, Johns found the terminology around brown complexions in persistent use by African Americans in Harlem. Johns wrote, "In Harlem we love to speak of brownskin girls, and I hate the term. Everybody is some kind of brown, nobody is ever 'black.' There is light brown, olive brown, chocolate brown, teasing brown, medium brown, mahogany brown, Egyptian brown, bronze, and a dozen others. Everytime I hear dark brownskin, I look for ebony black."[24]

By the first decade of the twentieth century, the new urban character of African Americans spurred a new identity and a modern New Negro movement that encompassed a broad and diverse range of goals and strategies in the struggle for racial equality. The momentous events of World War I, the Bolshevik Revolution, and the Red Scare that followed, fueled a starker divide between white and African America. African American soldiers returned home to meet violence, segregation, and little improvement in status or opportunity.[25] Claude McKay articulates the disillusion of returning veterans who found they had not truly met "the common foe" in trenches abroad or in the service labor positions for which the majority of the 380,000 African American male troops were used. Rather, wartime participation proved another white American "mock[ery] of our accursed lot."[26] The angry despair of McKay's 1919 poem "If We Must Die" reverberated during the Red Summer of 1919, when, after a decade of sporadic race riots, over forty violent confrontations erupted throughout the nation.[27] During that summer, urban race riots fueled the more radical tones adopted by New Negroes as injustices around employment, housing, and segregated public services showed the denial of civil rights was not simply a southern affair.[28]

The New Negro movement of the interwar years signals the mass politicization of urban African Americans and their agitation for change. Diverse and varied strategies developed at the grass-roots, community, and individual level.[29] At the same time, powerful organizations like the National Association for the Advancement of Colored People (NAACP, 1909) and the National Urban League (1910), both based in Harlem, directed attention to employment training, social reform, racial uplift, and, in the case of the NAACP, legislative change. The Pan-Africanist organization, the Universal Negro Improvement Association (UNIA) founded in 1914 also had headquarters in Harlem. Founded by Jamaican-born Marcus Garvey, the UNIA espoused a platform of economic nationalism and called for separatism from white Western dominance. Commanding a significant following among working-class Harlemites, Garvey endorsed antimiscegenation platforms as he exalted the dark complexions of African Americans as a sign of racial purity; darker toned people were characterized honorably as "true Negroes."[30] In Harlem, Garvey's New Negro conflicted with intellectuals and race leaders of middle-class standing who viewed integration as the main avenue for racial progress. The 1925 publication of the *New Negro*, an anthology of writing and artwork, introduced white readers to Harlem's New Negro and, in doing so, asserted a middle-class vision and voice to its expression. Regardless of these, and other vital differences, diverse groups of urban African Americans claimed the New Negro identity as a badge of racial pride and commitment to racial equality.

The modern New Negro movement responded to the period's clear denial of civil rights. The isolationist and reactionary political character that defined white America stood in stark tension with the growing creative expression, global outlook, and sharpening political foci. Across the nation, different groups of African Americans engaged with this modernizing racial identity, incorporating diverse and sometimes radical political stances to do so. Between the late 1910s and 1920s, New Negroes were urban, modern, and internationalist in outlook; as Davarain Baldwin explains, they paid attention to the concerns of the proletariat.[31] The quelling of the more radical energies of the New Negro occurred between the mid-1920s and the mid-1930s. Indeed, between these years a moderate, middle-class, and integrationist strategy premised on the key tenets of education, consumption, and social mobility moved to a more central positioning.[32]

Yet, no matter how radical, conservative, or in-between these positions may appear, the modern discourse on the New Negro remained overwhelmingly masculinist in character, temper, and expectation. As Deborah Gray White clarifies, "the proponents of New Negro ideology made race progress dependent on virile masculinity."[33] No doubt, women participated in the production, performance, and politicization of the New Negro identity; many did so by negotiating the demands of the racial collective that were frequently determined on patriarchal terms. Amid the climate of New Negro racial politics, the discourse of brown beauty emerged.

Respectability, Beauty, and New Negro Women

The New Negro woman of the 1920s might be assumed as an ideological formation that meshed the race proud militancy of the New Negro with the political autonomy of the New Woman, but reality reveals a much more tenuous and complicated portrait of womanhood in modern America. Both figures, the New Woman and the New Negro, date to the 1890s, and modern womanhood struggled between a series of traditional and conservative values associated with Victorian propriety to offset both older and newer threats in the urban environment. The status of women as new migrants, native-born urbanites, or earlier settlers from the more recent wave of migration shaped the experiences of modern African American women. In addition to other markers of status that included marriage and motherhood, women's socioeconomic status held an explicit material impact on their negotiations as modern subjects in urban America. Among the key changes, the Nineteenth Amendment granted the franchise to American women in 1920. African American women in the North, unlike their southern sisters and brothers, were now able to vote, but pervasive barriers in education, housing, and employment presented daunting obstacles to progress. In the industrialized North and Midwest, women's work was curtailed by both race and gender, and work was often segregated along racial lines. Industrial employment was gendered as male labor and African American women made little headway in industrial work, although some brokered a foothold in jobs that called upon skills traditionally gendered as "woman's work."

At the same time, a greater number of women entered higher education during the interwar years. Between 1917 and 1927, enrollment in colleges and universities sextupled, burgeoning from 2,132 to 13,500.[34] These years also witnessed a growth in African American educators at institutions of higher learning.[35] While de facto and Jim Crow segregation limited educational opportunities, some liberal white institutions, such as Oberlin, Cornell, and Radcliffe played prominent roles in matriculating women. Historically black colleges and universities (HBCUs) such as Howard, Fisk, and Spelman offered the physical and intellectual space for higher education.[36] Jeanne Noble's important study of women's education found that by the eve of World War II more African American women earned undergraduate degrees than did their male counterparts, noting the significant change during the interwar years.[37] As members of the growing urban middle class, women predominantly worked as teachers, social workers, and nurses; like their working-class sisters, many women, though certainly not all, balanced these waged-labor roles with marriage and motherhood.

The greater visibility of young African American women on the urban landscape elicited varied responses from those individuals and organizations working to reconstitute the view of New Negro women as modern, progress-oriented, politicized subjects. The discourse on brown beauty modernized the older practice of respectability that developed between the late nineteenth and early twentieth century. In her pathbreaking study, Evelyn Brooks Higginbotham shows how elite and middle-class women in the black Baptist church engaged a "politics of respectability" as a practice of racial uplift. Higginbotham demonstrates how respectability politics engaged the gendered tenets of good grooming and demure presentation to regulate and reform the behaviors of working-class women. Reforming women, drawn from the ranks for the elite and middle class, also "led by example" by displaying genteel manners, thrifty living, and purposeful work. The politics of respectability emphasized domesticity and chaste living as key principles of respectable "race womanhood."[38] Concerns over the public image of women foregrounded good grooming and demure self-presentation as important strategies to overturn the oversexualization of African American women as a vicious legacy of slavery.[39]

Historians, building on Higginbotham's pioneering scholarship, emphasize respectability's broader reach and meanings by showing its less top-down applicability between African American working-class and middle-class women. Stephanie Shaw explores the role of respectability in the quest for the social mobility of many young African American women whose middle-class footing was tenuous at best.[40] Working-class women also embraced respectability, and often for their own reasons: Tera Hunter demonstrates how migrant women appropriated standards of respectability by interpreting them in ways that provided meaning into their lives as workers, wives, mothers, community members, and individuals.[41]

Respectability remained a key concept and practice for middle-class and elite urban women, many of whom played a crucial role in organizing and providing support for their communities. In 1896, the founding of the National Association of Colored Women (NACW) formalized on a national scale the work performed by thousands of African American women in voluntary associations, and in doing so, the NACW unmoored community work from its local roots and directives. The NACW's motto, "Lifting as We Climb," advocated reform of individual behavior through self-help methods directed toward progress. The discourse on "race womanhood" was so powerful during these years that clubwoman Josephine St. Pierre Ruffin claimed the period the "Woman's Era"; Ruffin founded the *Woman's Era* magazine in 1894; it was one of the "earliest known periodicals published for and by African American women."[42] Embracing the premise of women's greater morality, the NACW emphasized women's domesticity as the path to race progress. Women's watchful care over the home, the family, and the moralism of the community supported domesticity as an especially important trait and skill among African American women. By the dawn of the new century, clubwomen ran day-care programs, old-age homes, and community houses for migrant women. As much as they were concerned about the dangers lurking ready to prey on young, migrant women, clubwomen and other African American moral reformers "understood the consequences of all such work in terms of improving conditions for the race."[43]

Racial uplift persisted as one cornerstone of reform. With focus on interwar Detroit, Victoria Wolcott demonstrates how the ideology of racial uplift was geared toward showing off "evolutionary progress of the African American masses only a generation after slavery." Wolcott shows how reformers worked to uplift and reform the dress, deportment, and behavior of working-class migrants. Similar to other reform-based organizations of the period, the efforts of the Detroit Urban League were framed by their middle-class desire to hide what they felt were shameful displays that let down the race and belied the view of African Americans as a modern people. Such displays, as Wolcott explains, included women who "wandered down to the business district . . . in calico 'Mother Hubbards'" compelling the attempts of reformers to make women hide their "boudoir caps . . . modest and unassuming attire." Deemed unsuitable when not at work in domestic labor, the long, loose dress and the headwear were viewed as items of clothing that pronounced the servility of African American women as they grew more visible in the public urban realm. For the vast majority of migrating women, opportunities for waged labor remained relegated to domestic work while other fields, namely industrial work and white-collar labor, expanded as fields for the employment of women. Wolcott shows how many working-class migrant women adopted this and other advice without blindly complying to the demands of reformers. Rather, their attention to changes of clothing reflected the effort to "forge a new identity for themselves in the urban North that combined aspects of southern culture with norms of respectability shared across class lines." As a platform for reform, Wolcott finds that respectability declined during the 1930s as it failed to enact real change in the lives of women; wartime exigencies helped shift concerns from the racial uplift of women to a heightened advocacy for the employment of men. The historian notes, "by World War II, racial leaders did not cite domesticity, chastity, and self-restraint as the primary goals of respectable citizens, but [i]nstead focused on civil rights, unionization and self-determination."[44]

The declension narrative on respectability during the Depression years showcases the intensifying focus on male employment, trade unionism, and citizenship rights. These shifting priorities might well explain the declining importance of respectability as a woman-initiated/woman-oriented reform strategy, but it does not fully elucidate what happened to the ideal of respectability. Indeed, Wolcott insists that respectability did not disappear; rather, by 1930 these classed dictates were less policing of African American women.[45] Closer scrutiny shows respectability's changing rather than declining meanings, prompting questions. Did respectability truly decline as an elite and middle-class ideal of womanhood, or was it channeled differently? To what extent did respectability continue to bolster the position of men, and if it continued to do so, had those grounds shifted? To answer these and other questions, we must consider more closely how modernization and various modernizing apparatuses fueled the modern discourse and ideal of respectable brown beauty.

The Changing Composition of the African American Middle Class

The history of brown beauty during the interwar years reveals the centrality of class status in shaping this ideal. As modernization brought greater access to goods, education, and class mobility, clearer divides between African Americans, along class lines, became apparent. Urbanization buoyed the development of a new African American middle class. By 1920, this new cohort of the upwardly mobile had supplanted the social authority of the old "mulatto elite," a group described by historian Willard Gatewood as "aristocrats of color." Gatewood shows how their elite position relied not on color alone but rather a combination of factors assured their status position during the antebellum era. These were the fortunate few who benefited from white ancestry "by gaining access to education, wealth, or opportunities unavailable ... even to free blacks."[46] Small but distinct, this mulatto elite faced sharp criticism from other African Americans who blamed them for "the existence of a scale of color among Negroes that perverted the whole system of social stratification."[47] In their defense, this group of elites insisted that "character, not color" determined entry into their ranks, yet they remained "unwilling to admit to their ranks anyone, including those of light-skin, who failed to measure up to their standards or culture, gentility, refinement, and character."[48] By the first decade of the twentieth century, this mulatto elite was losing its foothold as Jim Crow's sharper division between the races eradicated their role as an intermediary between whites and African Americans. Despite these changes, societies of the mulatto elite endured in Boston, Charleston, Philadelphia, and

Washington, D.C., though criticism against them gained wider support and its "ranks were thinning and its power as social arbiter were waning."[49]

Not only did the social status of the mulatto elite decline, but its very categorization of difference ceased to exist. In 1920, "mulatto" appeared for the last time in the U.S. Census. As it disappeared from official terminology if not from the vernacular, color descriptive names garnered greater significance. Historian Joel Williamson underlines how the brokering category disappeared, and, propelled by a "rising awareness that blacks and mulattoes were melting together physically," generations of mulattoes became America's "new people." Williamson concludes not only was the New Negro a modern construction but "he was Brown."[50] Despite his important findings, Williamson's language, like that of the period he studies, assumed the male character of the New Negro. Elisions like these presume a genderless nature to this modern racial identity and obscure the interplay of race, sex, color, and gender in the making of the African American middle class.

The growing urban middle class comprised women and men of all complexions who worked in a number of professions. Though conditions varied by region, middle-class people were often employed as skilled artisans, "civil servants, teachers, Pullman porters of good family background, domestic servants in the most elite white families, the more eminent and better educated ministers, a few doctors and an occasional lawyer." Two groups emerged among the ranks of the urban middle class: the first included writers, poets, intellectuals, artists, and scholars whose cultural production of the New Negro circulated in various forms of print culture; the second were entrepreneurs whose small and sizable businesses focused on catering to African Americans rather than servicing white needs, as did the older mulatto elite.[51] Urbanization was essential for the success of the new middle class who relied on the patronage and support of New Negroes to sustain their creative and commercial enterprises.[52] Between 1920 and 1940, this middle class remained relatively small compared to the mass of urban working-class African American people, but as historian Bart Landry tells us, "these men and women formed the core of a rising new black elite that would eventually form a bridge from status groups to classes with the black community."[53]

Across the interwar years, among other forces, New Negro print culture, namely newspapers and magazines, played a crucial role in shoring up the ties of mass consumption to social mobility, middle-class status, and race progress. Nationally circulating newspapers like the *Pittsburgh Courier* and widely read, more specialized magazines like the *Crisis* helped enshrine a view of consumption as a practice of economic, cultural, and political value for African Americans. Particularly gendered dimensions shaped advertising messages. Throughout the 1920s, a range of products and services for brown complexions was commodified as identities for sale, purchase, and performance. These materials offer one way to bridge the interstice in understanding the modern African American woman during the era when respectability itself underwent significant modernization. To a considerable extent, the participation of New Negro women in the modern consumer economy was writ large as an index of modernity.

Consumer culture industries helped forge the identity of the politicized New Negro. In his study of Chicago's New Negroes, Davarian Baldwin examines the role of "consumer-based control over black labor and leisure" and demonstrates how "race papers, race records, race films, and race entrepreneurship were essential spheres . . . to rethink the established parameters of community, progress, and freedom." Baldwin finds that interwar culture industries not only "transformed the marketplace into a public sphere of dialogue and debate over competing visions of the New Negro world," but also did so via intersections of "high" and "low" culture as reproduced in a variety of forms.[54] Certainly, cultural expressions on brown complexions erupted in multiple and diverse spaces, with different shape, intent, scope, and meanings. Popular cultural expressive forms describing brown women, brown beauty, and brownness abounded throughout these years as urbanization facilitated the growth of recorded music and commercial leisure venues including nightclubs, cabarets, and stage shows. In Manhattan, Broadway and off-Broadway stages, nightclub performances, and cabaret shows featured brown-skinned women who performed for white, mixed-sex, elite audiences.[55] On the opposite end of the socioeconomic commercialized spectrum, "nightclub spaces on the margins of the margins," colloquially dubbed "black and tans" encouraged interracial sociability and other sexually transgressive encounters, including those among people of the same sex.[56]

Furthermore, an expansive range of color-inflected language developed during the 1920s in popular urban culture, with varied meanings in their respective realms. Brown's transgressive, playful, and "other" meanings can be found in the classic blues of the 1920s, when African American women arose to cultural prominence as recording artists of "race records" and performers of the rough-and-ready music that made little apology for southern rhythms or for their own maltreatment at the hands of men. In "Young Woman Blues," Bessie Smith, the Empress of the Blues, celebrated the sexual freedom of youth, mobility, and womanhood by intoning color as formative to her pleasurable roaming:

> Nobody knows my name, nobody knows what I've done
> I'm as good as any woman in your town
> I ain't no high yeller, I'm a deep killer of brown
> I ain't gonna marry, ain't gonna settle down
> I'm gonna drink good moonshine and rub these browns down
> See that long lonesome road
> Lawd, you know it's gotta and I'm a good woman and I can get plenty men.[57]

Focused on print culture intended for the middle-class New Negro aspirant, as well as for a larger global audience, this study stays attuned to the influence of popular culture and working-class discourses in shaping cultural views of women's brown complexion. Representations of women's brown-skin beauty erupted in recorded music, on the printed page, in works of art, and on stage well beyond Harlem's borders and throughout the interwar years. Ideals around brownness and beauty might be understood as a "trickle up" phenomenon in their effects on middle-class views. At the same time, what distinguished middle-class proponents of the discourse of brown beauty was their formulation of brown beauty as being fundamentally connected with racial progress and social mobility. Across three decades, these middle-class views grew to idealize brownness of skin as the real, representational, and respectable complexion of African American women. By exploring multiple voices and the multiplicity of ways that brown seeped into popular parlance and visual culture, this book recognizes the broader scope of New Negro cultural production and signals some of the multifarious meanings captured in the descriptor of "brown" across these years. At the same time, it recognizes that some beauty ideals escaped the historic effort of middle-class cultural producers to categorize and streamline women by complexions envisioned as brown. Recognizing these parameters, this book studies the social values accorded to brown complexions and finds them narrowing across the interwar decades into a single standard.

This book studies brown beauty as a consumerist discourse that held powerful sway over the public imaging of African American women. It examines the interwar years when significant changes in ideologies of race in the United States were underway. Watershed events, the New Negro movement, the onset of the Great Depression, and World War II demarcate this as an important period in America's race relations. Over these years, scientific racism and its dogma of biological explanations of race declined, then witnessed a precipitous drop with the rise of the Third Reich in Germany. By the late 1930s, liberal ideologies increasingly shaped New Deal policies that adapted to broad changes at home and abroad, and in doing so, race and ethnicity grew more central to the liberal agenda. New Deal liberalism maintained some tenets central to Progressive era beliefs: progress, rational reform, and government action. In 1944, *An American Dilemma: The Negro Problem and Modern Democracy* was published as the most comprehensive social science study on race relations to date, and white liberal thinkers could no longer ignore what the Swedish sociologist Gunnar Myrdal described as the "moral dilemma" in the United States. In his comprehensive study that provided a blueprint for many racial liberals, Myrdal denounced racial discrimination as the moral failing of whites. Commandeering new attention to race relations, Myrdal underscored the role of the federal government in securing equality of economic opportunity as a redress and mode for change.[58]

By the end of World War II, when this study ends, the discourse on brown beauty was supporting a racial liberal position that viewed integration, antidiscrimination, and legalistic rights as the primary goals and main correctives to the racial dilemma. Education and interracial activism played a crucial role here, too. Less concerned with morality as being pathological and biological, racial liberals pointed to the accessibility of goods, services, and products as a means to equality. Revisionist historians identify the long civil rights movement and signal the importance of African American labor organizing and consumer activism as important actions between the Depression era and World War II.[59] Historians also point to the growth of "media apparatus" as increasingly important during the years between 1954 and 1965, a time Peniel Joseph defines as a "heroic period" of the modern struggle for civil rights that foregrounded its key goals on legalistic and legislative change as activists fought for integration, antidiscrimination, and voting rights; a defense of these positions necessitated the leavening out of racial difference as just cause for denials of rights and protections under the U.S. Constitution.[60] *Brown Beauty* shows how this effort was long in the making and points to the central role of color, class, and sex in shoring up the mainstream alternative line of African American liberal politics.

The connection between brown beauty and civil rights activism is partly premised on the growing ethos of consumer empowerment during the Depression era. As Lizbeth Cohen explains, African American activism during this period was vital for the brokerage of a "consumers' republic." During these years, greater numbers of African Americans were keen to distinguish themselves as participants in mass consumer society, viewing such an avenue as a bridge to the political. No doubt, pleasure and profit remained central to the interests and activities of consumers, yet, at same time, many urban African Americans were cognizant that their value as consumers failed to parallel their broader social value in American society. Those who recognized consumption as a form of racial oppression under America's capitalist system initiated a range of activist responses, particularly by the postwar years. By highlighting their exclusions from the political economy on bases that were increasingly debunked by social science, African Americans provided to their government and to private enterprise a clear image of their anticipation in postwar America.[61] Earlier community and organizational responses ranged from the woman-centered to the nationalist to the integrationist. Some, such as the Housewives' League, which was first formed in 1930 in Harlem, highlighted women's gendered role as consumers to encourage fairer prices as participants in the capitalist consumer economy.[62] Others underscored the disconnect between their value as consumers and their suitability for white-collar work. During the Depression years, some African Americans made salient the connection between collective labor and purchasing power through boycotts and cooperative campaigns that "brought together local institutions with various political orientations."[63] As movements of mass protest that mobilized cross sections of African Americans in urban centers, these campaigns drew on the rhetoric of democracy that linked the identity of African Americans as U.S. citizens to their identity as consumers and workers.

Newspapers initiated boycott tactics against a number of enterprises. Beginning in 1929, this consumer activism targeted shops on Chicago's South Side, including Woolworth's, a hugely popular budget-priced chain store. Between 1929 and 1932, the *Chicago Whip*'s "Spend Your Money Where You Can Work" gained wider momentum and success in cities across the country in Los Angeles, Cleveland, Baltimore, Newark, Washington, D.C., and Detroit.[64] In Harlem, poor, and working-class African Americans were least likely to reap the benefits of these campaigns since middle-class members were poised as those most likely to gain—or rather to regain positions lost to whites in the shade of the Depression. Still, when the "Don't Buy Where You Can't Work" movement finally reached Harlem in the spring of 1934, it helped coalesce the energies, concerns, and motivations of Harlem's diverse community. At the end of 1934, "Don't Buy" was ruled illegal because it was not a formal labor dispute.[65]

African American purchasing power and employment in local neighborhoods were central aims of these protests; color or complexion manifested as an index of change. For example, Lizbeth Cohen points to the militancy of Chicago's Black Belt. The campaign, led by the radical newspaper the *Chicago Whip*, "not only demanded that African-American salesclerks be hired, but that their skin be dark enough for their racial identity to be unmistakable."[66] In Harlem, complexion also seemed to matter. The conservative *New*

York Age, a long-standing publication, reported on women's employment and found that particularly in frontline positions and integrated workspaces, racist attitudes supported a hierarchical ranking of color, with preference toward lighter tones. Columnist Vere Johns mused, "I have no doubt that the black girl will come into her own eventually, but if we can gain a toe-hold with a light-colored girl, let us do so. Eventually we will get a foothold with the browngirl and actually go in and sit down with the black girl." Conciliatory and conservative, Johns presented the brown-skin woman as a safe intermediary in a slow step-up approach to antidiscriminatory hiring practices.[67]

It is wrong to glean too much from a single account or to suggest that interwar urban African Americans rejected black as a color of racial identification, but it is true that until the mid-1960s the term was not widely embraced or pressed into broad and official use. Some African Americans long embraced "black"; very likely, that usage was as nuanced and varied as I suggest "brown" was during the interwar period. Between the 1910s and 1930s, "Negro" came into most common usage among African Americans, but that did not prevent people from proudly claiming the term and espousing "black" as racial identity. Among the most famous are radicals like Marcus Garvey and Adam Clayton Powell, but so-called moderates employed the term as well.[68] For example, in 1920, W. E. B. Du Bois proclaimed in the *Crisis*, "Let us train ourselves to see beauty in black."[69] Still, as this study shows, a steady stream of visual and textual descriptions foregrounded brownness in shaping beauty. All of this would change by the late 1960s and 1970s as black consciousness inspired the mass embrace of black as a powerful claim to beauty and to African-descended identity. Indeed, as Ariela J. Gross shows in her study of legal trials over race, "the creation of 'black' and 'white' was a slow, gradual and vexed process."[70] By focusing on the rise of brownness as gendered shorthand for race during the interwar years, *Brown Beauty* moves into the vexed process to trace its emergence as an intermediary middle ground for negotiating and asserting race pride.

Print Culture, Public Imaging, and Brown Beauty

In the realm of culture, the public discourse on women's physical beauty endorsed its cultivation as an important strategy in the struggle for civil rights. This book explores African American print culture to study the renegotiation of middle-class respectability along lines that celebrated beauty as the modern marker and central terrain of respectable New Negro womanhood. It studies the racial discourse on brown beauty that circulated widely in African American print culture between the Harlem Renaissance and World

War II. Newspapers, magazines, novels, anthologies, and other print material produced and consumed by African Americans featured a range of textual and visual information and news on race matters. Modernization buoyed these changes: rising literacy rates, urbanization, and modernized technologies created the wider availability and mass distribution of print materials among African Americans nationwide, marking the interwar years as the golden age of the "black press."[71] Furthermore, advances in printing, namely halftone technologies, improved upon in the 1880s, "made it possible and more common to reproduce photographs and written text on the same page." Shawn Smith explains that many though not all magazines and newspapers embraced this modern presentation of news and opinions; African American publications were among these innovators.[72]

Throughout the interwar year, African American newspapers, magazines, and other print materials foregrounded words and pictures to assail long decades of pictorial depictions of crude racist caricatures, denigrating stereotypes, and disfigured, lynched bodies. Representations of the New Negro buoyed the mass mobilization of African Americans as American citizens. Its bolster to the racial psyche came from casting a vision of collective racial progress, one generation after slavery. By the turn of the century, photography played an increasingly important role in disseminating that vision to a broad public.

bell hooks underscores how photography both held historic "access and appeal" for African Americans and it was a crucial form in crafting "an oppositional black aesthetic."[73] As a medium of mass production, photographic imaging developed into an important tool for representing the New Negro in realist and prideful form. Paula Giddings's astute reminder that African Americans "did not have the luxury of broadcasting more than one message to White society" reinforces our understanding of the heightened importance these representations held for interwar African Americans.[74] Henry Louis Gates Jr. explains that the New Negro was "only a metaphor" but it was a powerful one. Dating the "era of the myth of the New Negro" between 1895 and 1925, Gates explains how race intellectuals who spearheaded remaking the "Public Negro Self" embraced integration as a key goal as they debated strategies for social, political, and economic inclusion in Jim Crow America.[75]

Among the most prominent of these intellectuals was W. E. B. Du Bois who, at the dawn of the new century, worked to showcase New Negroes in realist form. In 1900, in Paris, the Exhibit of American Negroes featured in 363 photographic portraits of African Americans as a diverse group of individuals who were clean, healthy, well dressed, and respectable. Curated by W. E. B. Du Bois, a Harvard-trained sociologist, race leader, and intellectual whose influence burgeoned throughout the first decade of the twentieth century, the exhibit showcased an "honest, straight-forward exhibit of a small nation of people, picturing their life and development without apology or gloss."[76] Defining identity in terms of nation rather than race, Du Bois used the vast display of unidentified portraits to challenge racial stereotypes. By showcasing the diversity of African American people, he emphasized how these "typical Negro faces, . . . hardly square with conventional ideas."[77] These typical faces presented a range of people who, Deborah Willis explains, were introduced to readers as a range of "types." Taken by photographers whose names are largely unknown, the portraits depict hundreds of unidentified people, the majority of whom were drawn from the ranks of the Atlanta elite. Willis describes the "types" to include "the scholar, minister, entrepreneur, mother, father, brother, sister, nursemaid, student, musician, homeowner, surrey driver, and even the femme fatale," representing the "different characteristics of these lived experiences of the New Negro."[78]

The portraits complemented maps, charts, and graphs that evidenced population growth, economic development, and rising literacy among African Americans in Georgia; other photographic evidence of racial progress materialized in pictures of homes, businesses, and churches, denying any view of poverty, immorality, ill health, or squalor as defining African American life, society, and culture. The portraits provided a visual testimony to the physical and moral fitness of African Americans as citizens of the United States.[79] Color mattered in Du Bois's selection of portraits, although color itself remains subjective in scholarly assessments. For example, David Levering Lewis finds the selection showed "a decided preference for African Americans of lighter hue."[80] Deborah Willis finds that a diversity of skin tones appeared.[81] In 1906, many of these portraits were published in Du Bois's study, *The Health and Physique of the Negro American*. In this work, Du Bois worked to provide a scientific view of different types of people rather than to sustain the view of race as an inherited, stable, biological identity. The study engaged anthropological methods to measure skin color, hair texture, and features to describe racial composition. Citing academic findings, Du Bois further connected climate to complexion, finding brown complexions common among a vast range of people.[82]

As he categorized the complexions of the photographic coterie of clean, healthy, well-dressed, respectable African Americans, Du Bois frequently described the complexions of his subjects as "brown." An extensive "description of types" enumerated each individual image through measures of physical traits; brown complexions ranged from "very dark brown," "dark brown," "brown," "light brown," and "smooth brown color." "Yellow," "white," and "cream" also occurred with less frequency. Du Bois appeared cognizant of his use of brown as a commonsense judgment on color; he explained this usage: "The color we usually denominate black, although it is really a series of browns varying between black and yellow as limits."[83] By proclaiming these bodies as brown, Du Bois opposed the period's racist science in the biological nature of race by showing the diversity and mutability of racial characteristics that included color. As an alternative understanding about "race," "brown" emerged as a new taxonomizing device to identify complexions as one variable in the equation of race.

To grasp more fully the multiple significations of brown beauty as racial discourse constructed around a language of color, we must unravel more carefully a series of transformative changes in the intellectualizing about race that erupted throughout the interwar era. As they reframed understandings of race, these modernizing shifts granted the space for fresh methods, languages, and devices to organize and understand the diversity of the human experience.

Shifts in Intellectualizing about Race

At first glance, the use of color as a visual language to signify characteristics of literary, poetic, and ordinary human subjects may appear deterministic in its connection between race and color; yet, the modern discourse of brownness worked to dispel narrow categorizations of race as rooted in the biologized body. Indeed, throughout the 1920s the rise of color and brown as a descriptor of race was a modern invention that connoted a departure from both whiteness and darkness of complexion. Its social usage continued to gain and change currency, refracting the critical changes in conceptualizations of race. Lee D. Baker explains that, within the U.S. context, race is best understood as both an "utter illusion and material reality, a fiction and a 'scientific fact.'"[84] In this view, race is understood as both a lived and shared experience among people, and as a category of difference that has been artificially and repeatedly produced and reproduced to create and sustain a "commonsense" view of race. Always in flux, this commonsense understanding of race responds to different forms of cultural knowledge; historically, it relies on a set of readily accessible categories to determine human identity by race designation. In addition to "common sense," the law and science play powerful roles in creating and sustaining racial categories, giving both meaning and structure to race. The interwar era witnessed important changes in the legal, scientific, and popular ideas of race in the United States.

By the late nineteenth century, legal interpretations of race lost much of the fluidity that characterized its construction during the antebellum period when the status of "free" and "unfree" asserted a hierarchy of racial difference between whites and African-descended people. By the mid-1800s, science and the performance of race accrued heightened importance in determinations of racial status. Assessing the illogic of racial categories, historian Ariela J. Gross explains how the "law gave meaning and content to a racial 'common sense' created by experts at every level."[85] Examining freedom suits, miscegenation trials, and naturalization cases that came before the courts, Gross shows how trials to determine racial identity drew upon local law and culture rather than quantification of "blood line"—or hereditary ancestry—alone to render these judgments.[86] Ultimately, these commonsense rulings denied civil rights and constitutional equality to American residents by upholding hierarchal rankings of people into discrete racial categories.

This study of brown beauty begins during the 1920s, a decade when antimiscegenation fears were at their height. Laws against miscegenation emerged as a measure of Jim Crow, spreading across the nation during the first decades of the twentieth century to severely curtail the viability of multiracial identities. Peggy Pascoe explores the development of miscegenation as a concept and practice and shows how between 1860 and 1960 the U.S. legal system played a crucial role in rendering interracial marriages between different groups of ethnic people unnatural and illegal. Pascoe shows how, despite their existence since the colonial period, miscegenation laws that developed between 1880 and 1930 upheld the racial project of white supremacy as they sought to protect the racial purity of native-born white American people or "stock." Spurred on by modern anxieties over the influx of Progressive-era "new" immigrants, and compounded with the movement of African Americans into industrializing urban centers, nativist fears that interracial sexual couplings would result in offspring of mixed ancestry accelerated the passage of laws that denied interracial marriage. Yet, as courts across the nation updated or initiated antimiscegenation laws, tightening legal definitions of whiteness to highlight racial purity, organizations and individuals challenged these legal classifications of race, achieving the greatest success on the West Coast.[87] Antimiscegenation laws worked to deny mixed ancestry as legal and "natural," thereby encouraging alternative practices of racial identification.

In 1900, the U.S. Census for the first time dropped all classifications of racial intermixture. Terms including "mulatto," "quadroon," and "octoroon" appeared and reappeared between 1870 and 1900. In 1910 and 1920, only one term—"mulatto"—reappeared: derived in the antebellum South to define people of African and white ancestry, the terminology disappeared for good after 1920. By 1930, people were defined as "White," "Negro," "Mexican," "Indian," and "Chinese." So assumed was whiteness as the color of U.S. citizens that the term itself never appeared in the federal census until 1870. After 1920, the disappearance of the legal classification of "mulatto" left open the negotiation of color as a popular cultural reference to identify a broad assortment of African-descended people. One century later, African-descended people could be defined as "Negro" or "Black."[88] Though "Brown" never materialized as official terminology, this changing notion of race during these interceding decades facilitated its popular usage.

As "animating fictions," the law, science, and popularly held beliefs bolstered the legality of white superiority, but they were not unchallenged.[89] Throughout the 1920s, NAACP lawyers and lobbyists continually challenged the courts on miscegenation laws to the point where such defense became rote among its local membership.[90] Other people also resisted reductionist classifications of color by challenging the meanings of "white" as a legal condition of naturalization. In 1923, Bhagat Singh Thind, an Asian Indian, appealed to the courts after his citizenship was revoked on the basis of being a nonwhite person. The case for Thind argued that the classification of Caucasian, a taxonomy legitimized and accepted in the science of the period, included Asian Indians. In *United States v. Thind*, the U.S. Supreme Court ruled against the Asian Indian, contending that the 1790 Naturalization Law "does not employ the word 'Caucasian' but the words 'white persons.'"[91]

The ruling on *Thind* directly contradicted another judgment made just one year earlier when Takao Ozawa, a Japanese immigrant of fair complexion, challenged the determination of whiteness as based on racial designation. Though very fair in complexion, Ozawa would not be judged as "white" by the court on account of his non-Caucasian status, although Caucasian status proved insufficient grounds to assure Thind's right to citizenship. The cases of *Ozawa* and *Thind* demonstrate how race and color were contested classifications during the 1920s and that the correlation between the two remained even more inexact. Whiteness, as opposed to any other classification, remained the central tenet around which citizenship was endowed. In his study of these and fifty other court cases concerning race-based naturalization, Ian Haney-Lopez finds "the court's eventual embrace of common knowledge confirms the falsity of natural notions of race, exposing race instead as a social product measurable only in terms of what people believe."[92]

By the turn of the century, racist science ascended to its zenith, upholding views of race as structured on biological difference to whiteness.[93] Through the middle decades of the nineteenth century, physical anthropology and ethnology advanced these views by rendering physical measures of difference as indices of race that were rooted in the biological body. A broad acceptance of social Darwinism propelled the cultivation of early-twentieth-century eugenics as a popularly accepted science. Eugenics championed a biologically determined divide between people viewed as "fit" and "unfit." Eugenics endorsed a clear directive against intermixture between these two groups. Discouraging propagation of the "unfit" and championing racial purity in the name of social improvement, eugenicist views gained broad support. Throughout the 1920s, racist science encountered serious challenges as a lack of scientific proof. As well, larger social changes, including the enhanced participation of ethnic scholars, and the development of new disciplines to investigate race, resulted in the further demise of these scientific views before World War II. They were eventually repudiated as the horrors of the Holocaust made clear the odious and false premises such science relied upon.

The interwar years witnessed the rise of new fields of genetics, social and cultural anthropology, sociology, and psychology; while these disciplines did not fully dismantle views of innate physical difference among people as the cornerstone understanding of race, a competitive paradigm emerged in the social sciences. In particular, cultural anthropology rejected the eugenicist belief in several dozen races but maintained the "grand divisions of mankind—white, red, yellow, brown, and black."[94] Color emerged as a descriptor of race that denied biologized views of race while at the same time upholding the general acceptance of categorization.

Precipitating the slow decline of biological understandings of race was the twentieth century turn to the study of culture and social environment to explain human actions.[95] Between the 1920s and 1930s, cultural relativism, a theory advanced by anthropologist and Columbia University professor Franz Boas, overturned biological essentialism as the exclusive way of explaining racial difference. Cultural relativism challenged the acceptance of racist evolutionary discourse; it maintained the equality of different cultural forms while detaching them from the category of race: race and culture were conceptually different. Race, by Boasian definition, defined biological form alone and could not be equated with mental, emotional, or intellectual attributes and capacities. Furthermore, Boas showed the mutability of physical typologies to underscore the fluidity of race as a biologically defined category. Culture remained somewhat less defined, but it encompassed the realm of social institutions, attitudes, and practices while understanding that culture itself was relative and particular. During the interwar years, the Boasian theory of cultural relativism won intellectual endorsement, influencing new critiques of race and racism in the United States.[96] Increasingly, associations of race by color shifted "common sense" understandings of race that in the modern age of commercialized sight and sound relied on a visual association of color as new marker of racial identity.

* * *

With this framework, *Brown Beauty* studies how diverse groups of cultural producers used a language and visual of brown to craft a politicized racial discourse on race, gender, and modernity. It explores the diffuse ways that brownness impinged on socially mobile New Negro women in the urban environment during the interval years, and shows how the discourse was constructed as a self-regulating guide directed at an aspiring middle class. *Brown Beauty* discovers how brownness of complexion and feminized beauty first became aligned with middle-class values during the 1920s; over the next two decades, the public discourse encouraged women's cultivation of beauty along modern consumerist standards, helping to uphold a representational ideal of beautiful brown-skin womanhood as a salve to a host of problems encountered by urbanized New Negro women. By tracing brown's changing meanings and showing how a visual language of brown grew into a dynamic racial shorthand used to denote modern African American womanhood, *Brown Beauty* works to unpack a set of intertwined values and judgments, compromises and contradictions, adjustments and resistances, that were fused into social valuations of women.

By studying how women's enhanced public status stimulated a modern discourse on middle-class respectability through the lens of brownness, this book explores the changing concept that relied on some older notions, but recast beauty as a modern value and women's central aim. I argue that beauty eclipsed chastity and demure self-presentation as central tenets in cultivating the image of respectable middle-class African American womanhood. I study brown beauty as a modernizing strategy and show how the discourse on brown complexions celebrated rather than repudiated the sexual as the domain of respectable New Negro women. This book demonstrates how the interwar discourse on sex, gender, and race revised and rejected older class-bound tenets of respectability—namely, domesticity, sexual purity, and frugality—and how it did so by embracing modern values of consumerism, sexual pleasure, and individual self-expression. At the same time, brown beauty was defined within narrow middle-class parameters that maintained the view of race and gender progress by conservative standards of social mobility, heterosexual appeal, and marriageability.

Throughout the interwar years, urban African Americans rallied against a seemingly permanent tide of racial injustices, including violent threats, discrimination in housing and hiring, residential segregation, and other new encounters and pressures of urban living. At the same time, the growth of a new African American middle class created fresh divisions among urban people. By World War II, social mobility and the acquisition of middle-class status as an index of American citizenship was seen to rely on a set of values that were channeled through the discourse of brown beauty. This ideology upheld the values of African American participation in mass consumption, women's performance of conservative sex and gender norms, and activism that was interracial in cooperation and integrationist in direction as central to the struggle for African American civil rights.

The racial discourse on brown complexions sought to invalidate understandings of race as based on difference to ones that touted race pride by disseminating new representations of African American identity and culture in an egalitarian framework. Against the backdrop of continuous migration from the rural South, a reconstituted public imagery of African American women, forged by a diverse set of cultural producers, increasingly encouraged women's beautification along commercialized trends, holding up beauty's cultivation as a measure of racial progress, social mobility, and modern womanhood. References to brown, brown skin, and brownness circulated broadly and aplenty across a range of outlets to increasingly underwrite a public discourse on African American women's beauty that, across the interwar years, grew in middle-class meanings and integrationist intent to solidify by the end of World War II.

The following chapters interrogate how views of womanhood came to idealize brownness of skin as the real, representational, and respectable complexion of African American middle-class women and accrued significant currency in urban, middle-class determinations of the New Negro identity in the three decades leading up to the civil rights movement. It studies the changing meanings of brownness by examining a series of print-based expressions, including essays, poetry, fiction, artwork, advertising text, and other imagery that circulated widely in interwar print culture. Exploring a diverse set of representations and teasing out the changing meanings of brownness, this book shows how, by the mid 1940s, brown-skin beauty endorsed values that upheld mass consumption, interracial activism, and conservative gender norms as strategies directed at integration as an ultimate goal.

Chapter 1 explores the life of Elise Johnson McDougald, a Harlem educator, essayist, and social investigator. It studies her public and private writings, including a scrapbook she maintained as a record of her accomplishments. As a prominent educator and as a middle-aged woman, McDougald was a figure transitioning between the "woman's era" and that of the "new woman." For this and other reasons that emerge in the chapter, I question why she came to embody the "brown beauty" of the New Negro woman. Chapter 2 studies the rise of consumer advertising with a focus on two products geared toward girls and women. I examine advertisements for dolls and cosmetics that circulated broadly throughout the 1920s in mass media newspapers and literary magazines. Such analysis finds the rise of a consumer-based discourse on brown beauty that linked displays of brown beauty with the New Negro ideology of "race progress." Chapters 3, 4, and 5 offer close readings of photography, poetry, and literature in Harlem Renaissance magazine and book culture. These chapters tease out the growing transnationalism of New Negro ideologies and explore the different ways that African American women and men crafted representations of New Negro women by relying on varying tropes of brown-skin beauty. Chapter 6 extends its study of print culture by examining three sociological studies produced by prominent African American male scholars. These racial liberals offered critical assessments of the rising idealization of brown complexions among African American youth coming of age during the Great Depression.

Ultimately, the shifting gendered ideal of African American womanhood centers my study and compels my examination of beauty as a historical index of brown's changing meanings within the era of African American modernization. By locating sites, spaces, and ways that language, images, and ideals of brownness impinged on women's negotiations with the modern, and by interrogating the nuanced meanings of color, this study seeks to dismantle historical understandings of race and color as fixed, genderless, and collapsible. In the six chapters to follow, I explain why notions of brownness arose to influence new formulations on African American womanhood and how, by World War II, this interwar discourse claimed brown-skin beauty to set the coordinates for integration of African Americans into the democratic, capitalist nation. In a state of ongoing change, categorizations of race, class, and gender identity connecting women's power to beauty provided an important public terrain for reinventing race representations. In doing so, across three decades, multiple groups and individuals recast a view of women through brown beauty as a positive protest against race and sex discrimination that held particular sway among the processes of modernization and urbanization in the North, Midwest, and parts of the South. This book concludes that brown beauty was a powerful but double-edged sword in women's arsenal against the "multiple jeopardies" they faced as greater numbers attained visibility, voice, and public status on the urban landscape.

1

Brown Beginnings

Imaging the New Negro Woman in 1920s Literary Print Culture

Woman has been the weather-vane, the indicator, showing in which direction the wind of destiny blows. Her status and development have augured now calm and stability, now swift currents of progress. What then is to be said of the Negro woman of to-day, whose problems are of such import to her race?

There is . . . an advantage in focusing upon the women of Harlem—modern city in the world's metropolis. Here, more than anywhere else, the Negro woman is free from the cruder handicaps of primitive household hardships and the grosser forms of sex and race subjugation. Here, she has considerable opportunity to measure her powers in the intellectual and industrial fields of the great city. The questions naturally arise: "What are her difficulties?" and, "How is she solving them?"

To answer these questions, one must have in mind not any one Negro woman, but rather a colorful pageant of individuals, each differently endowed. Like the red and yellow of the tiger-lily, the skin of one is brilliant against the star-lit darkness of a racial sister. From grace to strength, they vary in infinite degree, with traces of the race's history left in the physical and mental outline on each. With a discerning mind, one catches the multiform charm, beauty and character of Negro women, and grasps the fact that their problems cannot be thought of in mass.
—Elise Johnson McDougald, "The Task of Negro Womanhood"

In 1925, Elise Johnson McDougald, an African American educator, social investigator, and vocational guidance counselor, reflected on the problems facing the "Negro woman of to-day" in an essay she titled "The Task of Negro Womanhood."[1] The essay was featured that year in the critical anthology *The New Negro* and showcased the view of African American women on the modern urban landscape of Harlem. McDougald, a native New Yorker, wrote how the city's more expansive freedoms buoyed the progress of "Negro women" doing so not only "amidst rapid and continuing change" but also by "inculcat[ing] a calm and stability" among them. Addressing the interracial, middle-class, and liberal-minded reading audience of *The New Negro*, McDougald emphasized their need to grasp the diversity of modern urban women, who by virtue of the anthology's focus on the "New Negro" was presented to readers as such.

To underline these differences among women, McDougald relied on descriptors of color, light, and tone to trouble the pejorative stereotypes of African American women that circulated widely in modern culture; she coaxed readers: "have in mind not any one Negro woman, but rather a colourful pageant of individuals, each differently endowed." A complementarity among and between women appeared in McDougald's foregrounding of diverse skin tones. Color-filled imagery such as "the red and yellow of the tiger-lily" posed a metaphoric comparative to darker tones, and in doing so underlined the diversity among women in positive and egalitarian terms, reasoning that "the skin of one is brilliant against the star-lit darkness of a racial sister." Regardless of these differences and others, African American women, McDougald argued, shared a considerable burden on the modern urban-scape of Harlem. Though free from "cruder handicaps" and "grosser forms of sex and race subjugation," Harlem's women confronted "the less tangible and measurable impediments" and when assessed by dominant white standards, they fared poorly. McDougald explained how "ideals of beauty, built up in the fine arts," crafted a beauty aesthetic that not only "exclude[d] [New Negro women] entirely," but further rendered invisible the "multiform charm, beauty and character of Negro women."[2]

Image in the modern metropolis mattered in ways that affected women's economic, social, and sexual lives. The most acute affront to the progress of New Negro women appeared in the commercialized imagery that moved, with New Yorkers and other modern urbanites, through public space. Representations of "grotesque Aunt Jemimas" abounded in pictorial form; its celebration of the "pitiful black mammy of slavery days" reinforced notions that service and servility were the sole capacities of African American women. Other representations subjected women to further "ridicule" and "mirthless laugh(ter)." McDougald explained how dramatic portrayals engaged in representations of women's "feminine viciousness or vulgarity," although she clarified that these behaviors were "not particular to Negroes." These distorted images no doubt affected the "general attitude of mind" of white Americans, but McDougald underlined even broader concerns: she noted how these misrepresentations worked to justify discriminatory hiring practices, thereby curtailing the already-limited opportunities in industrial work. In pointing to racial discrimination as a systemic feature in modern hiring practices, Mc-

Dougald argued that these denials traded on stereotypes of women's bodies, behaviors, and beauty that circulated widely and with broad effect. In "Black Mecca" of Harlem, McDougald found the New Negro woman of the mid-1920s, "struck in the face daily by contempt from the world about her," as she worked to "maintai[n] her natural beauty and charm and improv[e] her mind and opportunity."[3]

McDougald highlighted the need for a new public imaging of African American women, clearly defining the parameters for women's self-presentation in the urban political economy around beauty, charm, and education. In her essay, these attributes materialize to offset, oppose, and eventually overturn pejorative stereotyping that bound women to a racist past. While not altogether new to the 1920s, this strategy departed from older and longer-standing practices that were also directed at recasting the self-presentation of African American women. The best known of these efforts emanated from organizations geared toward racial uplift and reform. For example, members of the National Association of Colored Women (NACW), established in 1896, and the Urban League, founded in 1910, engaged in a gendered practice of racial uplift. These moral reformers and clubwomen, drawn from the ranks of elite and middle-class African Americans, set out to reform the presentation, behavior, and public representation of women of lesser socioeconomic means and status. This top-down, reform-based approach emphasized traits of public displays and behaviors to showcase women's morality, chastity, hygiene, temperance, domesticity, and motherhood; as prescriptions of respectability, this public image was seen to offset crude stereotypes that envisioned all African American women as sexual, servile, and depraved. At the same time, other women developed their own displays of respectability, but as a middle-class ideology and practice, respectability remained linked to collective "race pride and progress." McDougald's focus on women's beauty, charm, and education rather than chastity, self-control, virtue, and domesticity hints at an important shift in the values underlying middle-class respectability that occurred throughout the interwar years.

Indeed, McDougald's emphasis on the need to reorder the public view of women as concretely tied to employment opportunities reflected broader changes in reformist efforts. By the early 1920s, the declining influence of moral reform in women's organizations encountered rising concerns over economic issues. For example, in 1924, when Mary McLeod Bethune, an experienced educator, clubwoman, and organizer, became president of the NACW, she worked to realign the group's focus more clearly around economic issues rather than women's individual behaviors and morality.[4] McDougald, herself a clubwoman, made an alternate connection: she exposed the link between popular stereotypes and the economic exclusion of women from employment across almost all fields that were opening to white working-class women throughout the late 1910s and 1920s. The distorted imagery fueled ideas of race, class, and gender difference that sustained discrimination, particularly in industrial labor in the North.

McDougald's essay "The Task of Negro Womanhood" broke with older reformist traditions by foregrounding a scholarly and social scientific approach to define the problems facing modern women; it relied on investigations, firsthand observations, and data collected on women's industrial, domestic, and professional employment. Though not without critique, McDougald's essay appeared to fulfill the goal of *The New Negro* anthology—its editor, Alain Locke, presented the collection as "ample evidence of a New Negro in the latest phases of social change and progress." Locke decried that the vast degree of public knowledge "is about the Negro rather than of him, so that it is the Negro problem rather than the Negro that is known and mooted in the general mind."[5] McDougald sanctioned this view with a focus on women. She reframed longer-standing justifications for challenging stereotypes by positioning claims to beauty rather than morality as necessary to this remaking; in doing so, the Harlem educator accentuated the political, social, and economic realities of women in the urban environment. "The Task of Negro Womanhood" argued for the increasing weight of employment, occupational status, and physical appearance as primary forces that shaped women's negotiations with modernity, modernization, and the class aspirations of New Negro womanhood.

Writing in a decade characterized by the politically autonomous "New Woman," race-proud "New Negroes," and an energized youth culture, McDougald, born in 1884, was already middle-aged. Her lifelong commitment to service and respectability upheld middle-class tenets of racial uplift that characterized reform in the "Woman's Era" of the late nineteenth century. At the same time, McDougald's education and growing understanding of inequality as rooted in administrative mechanisms and institutions rather than solely in perceptions of individual behavior acknowledged the systemic working of discrimination based on race and sex. In this view, age alone cannot render McDougald as a transitional figure who studied, wrote, and reflected on the employment issues of modern or New Negro women: her role as a professional educator underscores the continuity and disconnect of middle-class women's activism between these two time periods.

By the 1920s, New Negro women were many things. Some like McDougald were transitioning figures who were already tired in an era characterized by a vibrant youth culture energized by jazz, automobiles, flapperdom, and the mass consumption of cosmetics, clothing, records, books, and magazines. Others, also like McDougald, held to an older race politics of respectability and service, while at the same time pioneering new fields in African American women's professionalized labor. Formal and higher education grew increasingly important for women younger than McDougald as women's waged work took on enhanced importance in urban living. Others still, like McDougald, found their careers punctuated by marriage and motherhood; they were compelled to negotiate those breaks and reenter the workforce to support middle-class lifestyles and advance their ambitions. Finally, New Negro women like McDougald were also concerned about beauty. Technically "middle-aged" at the time of *The New Negro*'s publication, McDougald's concern with the "multiform charm, beauty and character of Negro women" showcases beauty as not merely a youthful concern or matter of superficial vanity among modern middle-class women who were seen to emblematize New Negro womanhood of this decade.[6]

This chapter undertakes a twofold approach to study the emergence of brown beauty as a development in Harlem Renaissance literary print culture. First, it examines the relatively obscure life of Gertrude Elise Johnson McDougald Ayer. By tracing McDougald's biography and exploring her professional development in social scientific work, labor organizing, vocational guidance, and education, this chapter highlights the connections between women's public image and women's labor. It further questions how McDougald's physical image came to embody the "brown beauty" featured in Locke's *New Negro* by examining a series of portraits created by Winold Reiss, a white German-born male artist whose prefiguration of brown complexions emerged as central to his artistic rendering of Harlem's New Negroes. Reiss's portraits provide one window into understanding how beauty grew to be represented through brown complexions and how the trope of color developed to form one primary means to communicate race collectivizing ideas and gendered ideals among middle-class and aspiring New Negroes.

By the 1920s, beauty and brownness, two physical determinations that were modern and malleable in meaning, emerged as modern characteristics with the potential power to offset racist views of African American women. In explaining how these stereotypes impinged on the lives of New Negro women, McDougald described how this "shadow over [women]" perpetuated feelings of "self-doubt" and "personal inferiority." Although McDougald's essay foregrounded empirical data to support her presentation of "The Task of Negro Women" on beauty's effect, she underscored that the "potent and detrimental influences" over New Negro women were not always easy to recognize "because they are in the realm of the mental and spiritual."[7]

Gertrude Elise Johnson McDougald Ayer

Gertrude Elise Johnson McDougald Ayer offers a compelling portrait of one modern African American woman about whom still much is left to know. Obscured from the view of contemporary scholars, Ayer was a public figure whose professional accomplishments were widely reported in local newspapers, national magazines, and in the African American press. A substantial portion of the Gertrude Elise Ayer Papers, a small, largely unmined archival collection acquired by auction in 1985 and donated to the Schomburg Center, consists of scrapbooks kept by McDougald. Spanning a period of thirty years (1931–66), the scrapbooks document her professional and prominent career as the first African American principal in the New York City school system. The scrapbook is filled with newspaper clippings and other documents recording the accolades McDougald received for her work as an educator. In their microfilmed format, many news clippings show signs of material wear and tear; the originals, destroyed after filming due to their degraded condition, cannot be consulted. It is not impossible to trace some of the better-preserved news clippings to the source of their original publication, but the scrapbook is most extraordinary in underscoring the important role of African American print culture, namely newspapers and periodicals and magazines, in documenting the lives of ordinary women who maintained records of their extraordinary success.

McDougald's two different first and last names have resulted in McDougald's relative invisibility in scholarship on the Harlem Renaissance. Francille Rusan Wilson explains, "historians . . . separate her life as if she were three different people."[8] Born Gertrude Elise Johnson in New York City in 1884, the "prominent figure in Gotham educational circles" assumed the McDougald surname upon marriage to Attorney Neal McDougald in 1911.[9] The union resulted in two children, but it was an unhappy one that ended in divorce. In 1934, McDougald married physician Vernon A. Ayer, precipitating a name change to Gertrude Elise Ayer. Between 1934 and 1954, the period marking her appointment as first African American woman to the role of principal in a New York City public school to her retirement at the age of seventy, she was professionally known as Gertrude Elise Ayer.[10] Throughout this work, I refer to Gertrude Elise Johnson McDougald Ayer as Elise Johnson McDougald; despite divorcing her husband in 1925, she used this name when publishing "The Task of Negro Womanhood" in *The New Negro* that same year. In addition, the portrait that provides the first view of the educator as a woman of brown-skinned beauty bore, in caption, the name Gertrude J. McDougald.

In addition to this confusion surrounding her name, Gertrude Elise Johnson McDougald Ayer has escaped serious scrutiny by historians partly because she has not been seen as part of the "mainstream" Harlem Renaissance movement.¹¹ In 1990, biographers Lorraine Elena Roses and Ruth Elizabeth Randolph predicted that McDougald's "advanced" feminist ideas would attract the interest of scholars although no such bonanza has yet occurred.¹² Readers familiar with the writings and visuals of the Harlem Renaissance have likely encountered Reiss's portrait of McDougald. Roses and Randolph argue that this image not only "made famous" McDougald's beauty but further skewed attention away from her critical voice as "her looks attracted more attention than her ideas."¹³ Then and now, Elise Johnson McDougald has peered out at readers accruing some judgment of light-skinned privilege and "bougey" social standing. At closer scrutiny, McDougald's personal history exposes the complicated life of a committed "race woman" of mixed ancestry whose personal and professional life was punctuated with disappointment, struggle, sacrifice, and success.¹⁴

McDougald's undated, unpublished memoir appears to be crafted specifically for her daughter, Elizabeth J. McDougald, or "Bessie." In the twenty-five-page handwritten document, McDougald focused on the role of women, but this time on her own mother, her daughter Bessie's namesake. In an undated letter to her adult daughter, McDougald advised Bessie on the problems of sex and men; her counsel reflected modern, middle-class values around marriage that championed the companionate role of partners within a marital union.¹⁵ She warned her daughter against "loneliness now and fear of loneliness in . . . later life" as leading to the "most serious mistake"—"seeking a person to ease this loneliness." The mother worried most about her daughter's attraction to men with "a selfish egotism—incapable of love (beyond . . . sexual desire)." "Watch out," she warned, "there are more of them about than generous and kind men." McDougald further cautioned Bessie to stay away from "the intellectuals who unfortunately always attracted me." As she admitted her own "serious mistakes" that no doubt included marriage to Bessie's father, McDougald described marriage to these types of men as "disastrous." A woman's unfortunate find was a man who "cared only about himself."¹⁶

McDougald's frank advice to her daughter seems to have been precipitated by a falling-out between the two—one McDougald seemed eager to move past. The letter greeted Bessie with a casual cheerfulness; the mother enquired on the purchase of her daughter's new coat and wished her enjoyment of the item. She ended her letter by referencing the histories of Bessie's great grandmother and grandmother that her child appeared eager to know. Before asking, "Won't you come and see me?," McDougald enticed Bessie to visit her using the rationale that she would rather relate this family history in person rather than write it.[17] In the end, for whatever reason, McDougald produced a lengthy, handwritten document that detailed the lives of Bessie's maternal ancestors that in part emphasized the "compelling emotional makeup" that drove two generations of women "head-long into [ill-fated] love affairs."[18]

Whiteness, rather than brownness, appeared the race-color dyad most salient in McDougald's account of her young life. "The Women of the White Strain" recounts the story of her mother, Elizabeth Johnson, a white English seamstress who emigrated to New York City as a "lady's maid." In New York, the young immigrant met her future husband, an African American man who, at the time of their courtship, was studying to be a physician. As "Woman of the White Strain" continues, it describes the growing unhappiness of McDougald's white mother as she endured not only societal rebuff but suffered personal neglect and little material comfort from a man who "wore his marriage lightly and went on living without much sacrifice on his part." As a young woman, McDougald also acquired the "strain" of her mother's gendered burden, assuming waged labor to assist with household expenses and her brother's training as a medical doctor.[19]

With unveiled disappointment, McDougald recounts the failures of Peter Augustus Johnson as a husband and father. Johnson was a founding member of the New York Urban League; he was also a physician whose education was brokered through the "immensely rich New York family" for whom his mother—a woman described in the story as "clearly of mostly American Indian blood"—"had been the expert cook for various branches of that family for years." One obituary for Mary Elizabeth Johnson, McDougald's white English-born mother, applauded "her devotion to her family and adopted race [as] a worthy contribution to the life of this community" as it recounted a life of sacrifice, Christian piety, and "devoted service to her husband."[20] Unlike her mother, McDougald, who was born, raised, and educated in New York City, was party to the dissolution of her unhappy marriage; McDougald's second marriage did not appear to offer greater joy or fulfillment. Her resignation to stay in a less-than-happy marriage emerges in the last lines of the unpublished memoir; she comments that her second husband's "kind attitude, at least, to my children has been a source of comfort."[21]

News coverage underscored McDougald's elite class background by proudly introducing her as the "daughter of the first Negro physician in the city and sister of the first Negro to enter the College of Physicians and Surgeons";[22] yet, evidence depicts a woman who attained great success despite not having received the same opportunity at formal education as did her brother whom she helped to support. Although McDougald took courses at the New York Training School for Teachers, at Columbia University, and at City College of New York, and conducted important social work surveys for the Department of Labor during the war, she was not a college graduate. Years later, when she was well into retirement, McDougald expressed little regret about not obtaining an academic degree. In 1954, she explained to *Newsweek* magazine her view that "Too many people with B.A.'s only know their subject matter and don't know how to teach."²³ Indeed, McDougald accumulated vast hands-on experience. In 1905, she began work as a public school teacher, as did many other women "resign[ed] for marriage" in 1911.²⁴ In 1916, when she returned to paid employment, McDougald worked with the Women's Trade Union League, the YWCA, and the Urban League in various capacities, including labor activist and vocational guidance counselor. The lack of a formal degree did not diminish her sense of herself as a professional. In 1931, McDougald celebrated the traditional role of domesticity as instructive to her professional knowledge and expertise; to *New York News* reporter Nell Occomy, she explained that her "social service career" began "after the years spent at home training my children."²⁵

Though a committed "race woman," McDougald also dreamed of less service-oriented work. A 1935 news report touted the "varied career" of the new school principal of P.S. 24, judging her a "pioneer in labor work" due to her labor organizing and social science survey work. At the same time, the news countered these endeavors with McDougald's recent admission of a once-held "consuming desire to be a singer."²⁶ Another dream deferred appeared in the field of creative writing. In an apparent response to McDougald's request for information on their editing and publishing services, the U.S. Literacy Agency in New York City wrote explaining their services and inviting submission for "free examination."²⁷ No evidence appears to help determine if McDougald followed up on this interest for publishing her creative work, possibly her memoir, by any other avenue. Still, the fact that she kept this letter in her scrapbook among many news clippings that covered her professional career, suggests it was a dream of some significance to her.

Throughout the decades, news coverage of the respected "teacher, social investigator and vocational guidance expert" foregrounded McDougald's professional accomplishments, yet from the very beginning McDougald's physical body attracted specific attention.²⁸ In 1903, one assumedly "white" mainstream newspaper reported on the graduating class of the Girls' Technical High School, the first and only girls' high school in Manhattan at that time. Its headline announced the controversial decision: "Quadroon Girl Class President." As the article reported on the graduation of twenty-nine students, it underscored the racial difference of its class president, Elise Gertrude McDougald, as it reported on the "Quadroon's" clever wordplay quip in her presentation. Dr. William Maxwell, the city superintendent who attended the ceremony, found the rundown building such a "shame and disgrace" that he promised "a modern building" in the near future. In his address to the 1903 graduating class, Maxwell reflected on the needs of students, finding that the cultivation of the "feminine characteristic of curiosity" was a necessary component of education for girls.[29]

Though the news report offered little else to describe McDougald's physique, its sensational headline, and subheading, "Gertrude Elise Johnson Conspicuous at Graduation," was not subtle in highlighting a view of difference that was based on race. From McDougald's perspective, color dominated this vision as seen years later in the *Sunday Coloroto Magazine* that reported on McDougald's successes as an educator. The magazine provided readers with a biographical overview of her achievement, describing McDougald as a native New Yorker who was born "opposite the area where Gimbels Department Store is now." The article related the "flare-up" caused by McDougald's graduation as the "first Negro" from the Girls' Technical High School, renamed Washington Irving High School in 1913. McDougald was reported as explaining—"with a smile"—how "one paper, went to pains to say that I was a quadroon, quite black."[30] The report itself did not reference race by complexion or color—it quantified measures of "Negro blood" to define racial identity. Still, McDougald's recollection of the designation of "quadroon" as "quite black" reveals the complex layers structuring views of racial self, racial other, and racial passing; for example, a "quite black" quadroon would never "pass" for white. Ultimately, McDougald rejected the quadroon identity as one that presented a derisive and oppositional view of race as defined by color, and that color was defined by blackness. The sting of the label, felt long after the formal existence of these categories, also illuminates some of the modern energies at work during the Harlem Renaissance that tacitly disassociated black from progress-oriented, socially mobile, urban womanhood. In 1903, news coverage of McDougald as class president of the first high school for girls in the modern metropolis made conspicuous the young woman's racialized body.

In 1900, for the first time, the U.S. Census did not enumerate by measures of racial intermixing. As a native-born New Yorker, the young McDougald would have been counted among 60,066 African Americans in the city, making up a mere 1.8 percent of the urban population.[31] Preceding the first Great Migration (pre-1914), small numbers of African American women traveled mostly from Virginia and Carolinas to Philadelphia, New York, and Boston; often young, single, separated, and widowed, they migrated to take up job offers in domestic service. Their migration contributed to an imbalance in urban sex ratios. For example, in 1900, New York City hosted 124 women to 100 men; in 1905, one-quarter of all adult African American female migrants lived alone or lodged in houses.[32] As a young African American woman in New York City, McDougald was conspicuous not only because of her race but because of her gender. As a young woman graduating from high school, McDougald represented a small class of educated urban elites. As migration accelerated in the subsequent decades, education became a defining characteristic of African American womanhood as "daughters of black migrant parents attained educational parity not only with second-generation immigrant women but also with native white women of native parentage."[33]

Education alone did not facilitate employment. The majority of occupational fields were battlegrounds for African American women seeking entry or advancement in them. For example, in Boston Addie W. Hunter, a high school graduate holding certification requirements for clerical work and civil service employment, found these opportunities "closed to the Negro girl." Hunter filed a lawsuit that charged private employers and the civil service with racial discrimination. When she lost her case, Hunter was forced to take up factory work. Writing in the *Crisis* in 1916, Hunter reported: "it is useless to have the requirements. Color—the reason nobody will give, the reason nobody is required to give, will always be in the way."[34]

Like Hunter, McDougald encountered obstacles in her attempt to ascend to a higher position in teaching and identified discrimination as the cause. When she took a licensing exam to become a principal, her application was turned down, but the rationale was suspicious: she was expected to "repeat certain tests, excepting the written exam."[35] Her failure was based on "less than generous" ratings by the white male principal under whom McDougald had served as assistant principal between 1924 and 1927. McDougald appealed to the Board of Education to rectify the discrepancy between these ratings and the "excellent" ones received, from the same principal, on her semiannual review. She won her appointment four years later when the Board of Education ruled, "when the teachers are candidates for higher licenses," principals must justify discrepancies between rating sheets and reports.[36]

McDougald's appointment as the first African American high school principal in New York City was indeed a rare achievement: African American teachers comprised a mere 2–3 percent of the city's teaching staff. Some taught in white and racially mixed schools, but many were assigned to schools where African American students predominated. McDougald was made principal of P.S. 24 in Harlem where 95 percent of the student body was African American, and the majority of the twenty-five teachers on staff were white.[37] Based on her study of hearings conducted to study the conditions that gave rise to Harlem Riot of 1935, Lauri Johnson finds how some white teachers viewed their assignments to Harlem schools as "punishment." When an African American principal was appointed to head the school where they worked, some white teachers felt little effect, but fifteen others felt so threatened that they requested transfers to other schools. The Board of Education denied these requests.[38]

In the decades to follow, McDougald's looks continued to attract attention from journalists who celebrated her appointment as a "Harle[m] First." *Time* magazine, a popular and widely circulating news publication, described the "tall" and "scholarly" Mrs. Gertrude Elise Johnson McDougald Ayer as "one of Harlem's handsomest women." The news report went on to annotate the native New Yorker's "creamy complexion, set off by kinkless grey hair with a streak of black running straight back from the forehead"; it used these same descriptors to caption the photograph of McDougald that ran in its feature. In this image, the fifty-year-old McDougald appears somewhat matronly, surrounded by children identified as "friends."[39] Looks aside, this connection with children reflected the educator's long-held view that "the Negro woman teacher needs be mother and guide, as well as class-room instructor." In 1925, in an essay published in the Harlem-based journal the *Messenger*, McDougald blamed the complexities of modern life for adding "much that was taught formerly in even the humblest home . . . to the scope of the teachers' duty." McDougald did not denounce the "Negro mother [who] must work outside of the home to supplement the Negro father's earnings" for the new onus put onto African American teachers, finding this shifting of parental-to-educator responsibility a reality among all racial groups.[40]

In Harlem, teachers were also tasked with creating harmony among increasingly diverse communities. In 1910, Harlem's African American population more than doubled; by 1920, that number increased by 66 percent; by 1930, it expanded further at 115 percent. In 1920, the African-descended population in Harlem stood at 152,467; 24 percent of this number was foreign-born, marking the height of the foreign-born influx of African-descended people into Harlem in that year.[41] While "Black Manhattan" conjured a melting pot image of Africa-descended people, conflicts also existed.[42] When fractious relations between native-born African Americans and African Caribbean students became evident to McDougald, she introduced a social studies unit on Caribbean life and culture.[43] As an act of cultural exchange, a visit to the Schomburg Center in Harlem was arranged to expose students to history and literature as produced by African American intellectuals and writers.[44] Recalling this "experiment in [teaching] methods" three decades later in an essay that assessed "Education in Harlem," McDougald judged that "after that cooperative venture, there was no more friction due to ignorance." Though "approved and recommended for city-wide use" by the State Education Department of New York, McDougald's experimental teaching method "fell into disuse" due to opposition from teachers on professional and religious grounds. "And so," McDougald surmised, "history repeated itself." Writing at a "crucial time in race relations," McDougald assessed the current state of education in Harlem in 1963. She charged the current superintendent of three Harlem schools of ignoring the long decades of work and innovative methods devised to educate urban children, described by Superintendent Dr. Charles M. Schapp as "underprivileged."[45]

Other news reports avowed the beauty of the prominent educator. Reporting on McDougald's "blue book marriage" to her second husband, Dr. Vernon A. Ayer, the journalist assured readers that the somewhat overused adjective "charming" was "one term which more intimately and accurately describes [McDougald] than any other." This assessment was qualified in descriptions of "fetching gray hair outlining her fine features, and her stately physique ma[de] her a woman of unusual comeliness."[46] As beautiful as she may have appeared to this reporter, McDougald's looks did not escape critique: the columnist expressed "great concern, with attendant surprise, over the reticence with which this distinguished pair chose to clothe their nuptials." Clearly, the wedding wardrobe looked so inadequate, understated, or unsuitable for a "blue book wedding" that the journalist did not spare time to provide even a brief description of the garb. McDougald's personality and professional conduct appeared to taint her appearance; the wedding outfit was judged as reflecting "the manner that has characterized . . . [McDougald's] aggressive climb from grade teacher to . . . Assistant Principal of P.S. 90."[47] The writer's connection between poor clothing choices and "aggressive" careerism not only underscores the unfavorable view of women who did not keep up with fashionable trends deemed suitable to their station, but it further connects such disregard with ambition, implicitly cast as a masculinized pursuit.

Color, clothing, and McDougald's "love of beauty" appear throughout the collected news coverage and assert McDougald's feminized characteristics through her hobbies of "reading, dressmaking, writing, music, theatre [and] travel."[48] One article in the *New York Amsterdam News* evoked color as it reported on McDougald's life as one that denied any "pastel experience." The article described McDougald's home, her work in labor organizing, and her 1919 published survey, "A New Day for the Colored Woman Worker," prefacing its account of McDougald as someone who "meets life militantly and surrounds herself with splashes of brilliant colour."[49] As the *New York Amsterdam News* recalled the "vivid shades of green" that decorated McDougald's home, another news article captured a much older McDougald and attributed the "Indian in [her]" as responsible for "bring[ing] out a love for flashing colours" that included "deep blues and reds in her clothes." The busy educator reported little time for socializing and identified "her own home" as the "only other major concern of her life." Readers learned that McDougald not only "did all her marketing," but she also "ma[de] all her own clothes." The gendered labor of sewing and its long and historical connections to enslaved women's labor demands fuller treatment that remains outside the purview of this study. Here, it is worth noting how this work was not presented as entirely utilitarian in purpose; in her busy life, McDougald found "sewing restful."[50]

Ayer's scrapbook collection also presents a fascinating glimpse into the cultural and classed values surrounding age, aging, and the generational divide between women. Another undated article shares the Harlem educator's prizewinning recipe for custard. The photograph displayed an older woman at work in the kitchen while she provided readers with the "secret" to her custard's success as "stirring constantly" until the point of thickening.[51] While this article seemingly trivializes the accomplishments of a professional educator, it foreshadows the media coverage of domesticity that arose alongside glamour to dominate in postwar representations of women. For our present purposes, the news report celebrated McDougald's talent in attaining a seemingly not-small accomplishment; happily, the article declared, "Whole Family Likes Custard."

When read together with other coverage that traces her development between high school graduation and the firm establishment as respected high school principal, McDougald's representation in mass media print culture illuminates how domesticity, dress, and beauty appeared as key, positive characteristics in shaping the public image of modern middle-class African American women. It also shows how age and aging also affected these gendered portrayals; the younger McDougald won accolades for her daring use of color in interior design; as an older woman, McDougald's domestic cooking skills won particular acclaim. One crucial difference that existed between representations of African American domesticity appears in this latter depiction. Unlike the servile and domestic mammy stereotype against which McDougald railed, the depiction of an apron-clad McDougald stirring custard on the stovetop defies this representation. Her ability to cook for and please *her* whole family, rather than someone else's, remains key to the narrative.

McDougald's scrapbooks provide a collage overview of one woman's life captured through news print culture. Certainly, generational change was neither linear nor tidy. Women who transitioned from Progressive politics of the "Woman's Era" to the decade of the modern New Negro brokered sets of demands that were born from modern sensibilities, from conservative needs surrounding race collectivizing, and from an older reform-based activism that had long defined the public role of middle-class women in service of their communities. McDougald's public leadership role and dedication to the advancement of students in the Harlem school systems characterize important aspects of women's activism during the interwar years.

McDougald provides a fitting metaphoric reflection on the challenges facing African American women who worked to fulfill these competing demands. In 1931, a journalist interviewed McDougald to explore her "two-fold service" as a teacher and social worker. Conducted while she was "summering in Jersey and resting comfortably within her screened porch," the writer gained a degree of intimacy into the educator's life. The journalist explained McDougald's work to complete an "old fashioned cross stitch . . . intended for use as a chair back covering" as an assignment that had been "left unfinished by her mother." The article recalled the educator's "hands, which are seldom idle," as ones then keenly at work on "the exquisite pattern of a landscape." The journalist recalled McDougald's wry and practical musing on her mother's incomplete task: "It's so hard to match these colors now."[52] As McDougald puzzled over matching up the colors of the past she appeared so very different from her contemporary and peer Zora Neale Hurston, whose bold creative expressions on the changing landscape of race, color, and womanhood won critical acclaim. Though less well known to contemporary audiences, McDougald's contribution to the Harlem Renaissance deserves attention.

The Task of Negro Womanhood

In March 1925, "The Double Task: The Struggle of Negro Women for Sex and Race Emancipation," appeared in *Survey Graphic*'s special issue, "Harlem: Mecca of the New Negro." Sociological in focus, the magazine was geared to an audience of lay readers, the majority of whom were white; in the Harlem issue, they learned that "Harlem represents the Negro's latest thrust towards Democracy." The issue was edited by Alain Locke, a prominent philosopher professor at Howard University in Washington, D.C., and illustrated by white German-born artist Winold Reiss. Filled with essays, fiction, poetry, graphs, charts, illustrations, and photographs, *Survey Graphic*'s Harlem edition described a "new order" of race pride and race consciousness. In his introduction, Locke highlighted the "present tone and temper of the Negro press" and the "shift in popular support from officially recognized and orthodox spokesmen to independent, popular, and often radical types" as "unmistakable symptoms of the new order." Emphasizing the centrality of Harlem to this "stage of the pageant of contemporary Negro life," Locke also motioned to "kindred centres in the Northern and Mid-Western cities" as sites for the rise of the New Negro. Still, Locke argued, one "may dramatically glimpse the New Negro" in Harlem.[53]

The Harlem issue was a critical success. In two print runs, it sold over forty thousand copies, winning for Paul Underwood Kellogg, *Survey Graphic's* white publisher, six hundred new subscribers.[54] African American students received free copies of the issue when bibliophiles and philanthropists, most notably Joel and Amy Spingarn, sponsored a second print run of the issue.[55] For McDougald, the magazine provided the first venue for her exposé on the myriad burdens and obstacles confronting the modern woman in Harlem. When the essay was republished in *The New Negro*, she attracted an even greater audience, but the rhetoric of conflict and struggle was minimized in the essay's title. Although the original title claimed the "double task" facing women and framed women's "struggle" for "emancipation" from "sex and race," when it appeared in *The New Negro*, the essay was titled simply, "The Task of Negro Womanhood."

McDougald based her assessment of the "Task of Negro Womanhood" on survey research she conducted during and after World War I. Women's work in industrial and wartime work, though viewed as temporary, stimulated a "sudden demand" for research on women workers. With reluctance, organizations ranging from the American Federation of Labor (AFL) to the U.S. federal government established committees and subcommittees to attend to women's working conditions. Yet, as David M. Kennedy tells us, "even agencies like the Women in Industry Service—mandated to protect women workers, and run by a no-nonsense woman like Mary Van Kleeck—accomplished little." The agency managed by Van Kleeck could not protect existing workplace standards for women because "those standards simply did not exist, . . . no women had ever before worked in the industry."[56] For African American women, economic need facilitated their entry into jobs in heavy industry and mechanics. As migration accelerated throughout the war years, women's waged labor became even more crucial to the maintenance of families who struggled to contend with wage differentials and the chronic insecurity of men's work. The trend continued after the war. By 1920, the percentage of African American wives engaged in waged labor outside the home was five times greater than any other group of women. These numbers varied according to the city as the types of employment that characterized male-female patterns of work, but in New York in 1920, 46.4 percent of married women worked.[57]

When the "sudden" interest in women workers emerged during the war, McDougald was prepared for the task. Her ability to assume this paid role can be traced to the commitment of "black clubwomen and college graduates" who embraced social science to assist their communities. McDougald's role as a social investigator marks one important transition from the activities and practices of the late-nineteenth- and early-twentieth-century middle-class clubwomen whose reform work emerged and operated primarily within voluntary associations. Historian Francille Rusan Wilson shows how McDougald's social scientific investigation forms a "bridge" between "unpaid social investigations" generated from women's voluntarism and community service work and the work performed by professionally trained African American social scientists in the age of the New Negro. Involved in a growing number of "local social reform projects," the "research-oriented social welfare activities" of early-twentieth-century clubwomen were "based on the best practices of social work and community surveys." Indeed, the founding of various community service agencies was based on "social scientific methods and theories gained through women's participation at the Atlanta University conferences, directives of the NACW, and [women's] own self-study." By 1920, more than seven hundred black women were employed as social workers; their training in the social sciences and understanding of survey research methods and goals augmented the initiatives of clubwomen. Studying this era's "lost generation of black women social scientists," Wilson concludes that their work was essentially "short-lived, lacking advancement possibilities, and abruptly terminated after World War I."[58]

McDougald was the principal investigator of the labor market conditions on women's industrial employment between July and November 1918. She worked on a study on the conditions of African American women's work in industrial jobs that was commissioned by a joint committee that represented "labor, social work, and black organizations," including the Consumers League of the City of New York. From more extensive lists of women workers across 242 factories in Manhattan and Brooklyn, McDougald gathered over 400 names of women workers and conducted in-depth interviews with 175 women. The study's white co-investigator, Jessie Clark, interviewed 300 employers; together, the data described McDougald's research and compilation of "detailed data on black women's previous work history and wages, education, family, and housing costs" that was published in 1919. Entitled *A New Day for the Colored Woman*, the report was overly optimistic in signaling a significant change regarding race and gender in the labor market.[59] Still, women's work in industrial jobs offered higher pay and greater freedom from servile service positions in domestic work that continued to dominate as African American women's work.

McDougald retained this focus on labor as she took charge of the vocational guidance bureau of P.S. 119 in Manhattan, holding this position between 1919 and 1924. During these years, she proposed an important study that polled four thousand employers to assess the job opportunities available to African American students.[60] McDougald also worked on behalf of a citizen's group in North Harlem and brokered the cosponsorship of a study from the New York Board of Education and the U.S. Department of Labor. When the 1921 study encountered a serious delay through the loss of its supervisor, McDougald's protest to the U.S. Congress finally moved it along to completion; the North Harlem citizens' group used the study's findings for educational activist ends.[61]

Drawing on this social scientific research background, data, and knowledge, McDougald outlined "The Double Task" of New York's New Negro women for *Survey Graphic* readers; with some modifications to the original essay, she offered a mostly similar overview to readers of *The New Negro*. Equivocating against the public imaging of New Negro women "in mass," McDougald examined the status of New Negro women in "groups on the basis of activity."[62] As she identified four different groups of women, ranking them hierarchically by their economic station, social status, and laboring roles, McDougald pinpointed problems particular to each group; in a variety of ways, she found resonant a cultural acceptance of potentially harmful notions of sex and race as they moved through the modern, urban environment.

Organized by socioeconomic status, McDougald identified groups of women who ranged from the "very small leisure group" "picked for outward beauty by Negro men" to the "le[ast] fortunate fringe of causal workers," urban African American women who also included those "active and progressive" in business and the professions as well as "many" who labored "in the trades and industry." Women in this group, slowly but surely, were beginning to organize in industries that included the flower and feather workers' union and the garment industry.[63] McDougald, who appears in the nonfiction essay as an "anonymous unpaid labor organizer," concludes that the "alienated or unintelligent attitude of Negro worker[s]" necessitated "sincerity and understanding" and "education in union principles."[64] Indeed, McDougald remains an unclaimed hero in the history of labor organizing: she helped establish the Trade Union Committee for Organizing Negro Workers and she also worked with Rose Schneiderman to organize laundry workers.[65]

When she expanded her discussion to engage more intimate views of women's lives, McDougald expressed views that were both feminist and elitist.

While arguing that the "Negro" woman had been "singled out and advertised as having lower sex standards," McDougald insisted that "the Negro woman does not maintain any moral standard assigned chiefly to the qualities of the race any more than a white woman does." In doing so, McDougald chastised whites as "superficial critics" for not seeing the same failings in white women of a particular class. McDougald did not claim equality between white and African American working-class women, but she did signal their "similar" grounds on emotional and sexual matters.[66] Furthermore, when considering the plight of the unmarried mother, McDougald described how women kin rallied around young mothers; if possible, families maintained secrecy as mothers and married aunts took charge of children born to unmarried women. This banding together of family members meant that "the foundling asylum is never sought." Unmarried mothers did not escape sanction as "stigma does fall upon [them]," but McDougald found that "schooled in this kind of suffering in the days of slavery, the Negro woman often tempered scorn with sympathy for weakness." The "Negro's attitude," McDougald mused, "is nearer the modern enlightened ideal for the social treatment of the unfortunate"; she queried, "May not this, too, be considered another contribution to America?"[67]

In 1920, almost 40 percent of African American women were "gainfully employed." While working-class women encountered multiple subjugations, middle-class and upwardly mobile women labored under somewhat less crude but no less burdensome conditions. Businesswomen, professionals, and skilled and semiskilled workers formed the two middling groups in McDougald's hierarchical ranking of New Negro women. She identified a small but growing number of women working as teachers, librarians, nurses, and writers. By the early twentieth century, the feminization of teaching as a profession bode well for African American women who outnumbered men at a ratio that approximated five to one.[68] Still, the most substantial increase in women's employment occurred between 1900 and 1930 in the professional and technical sector. Between 1900 and 1930, the increase of African American women's employment in these fields from .2 percent to 1.2 percent represented a sixfold rise in employment that was not at all insignificant.[69] Other jobs included clerical work, but employers were particularly hostile to New Negro women on the basis of their appearance and many places barred their inclusion in offices, department stores, and other frontline sales or service positions. In places such as Harlem, where African Americans owned less than 20 percent of businesses, clerical jobs were given to men. In Harlem and other cities with sizable African American populations, white stores and companies, though welcoming African Americans as customers, continued to employ white staff.[70]

As clerical work became increasingly gendered and racialized as white female labor, it grew more closely tied to class-bound notions of respectability.[71] Judged as lacking middle-class morals and manners deemed necessary for white-collar work, African American women were largely excluded from these jobs but, when hired, many endured segregation in the workplace. White employees and customers were kept "safe" by slotting African American women and men into positions that restricted interracial contact.[72] African American women workers formed a mere 1.2 percent of the clerical and sales workforce despite being fast-growing sectors during the post–World War I era. Jacqueline Jones explains this total exclusion of women from the clerical and sales workforce as underscoring the "complicated ways in which racial prejudice could shape the hiring policies of industrial and commercial capitalists." As tasks were assigned according to physical and cultural characteristics rather than ability, Jones raises the crucial point that "discrimination proved to be good business in terms of employee and customer relations."[73] In light of these limitations and obstacles, McDougald underscored women's greater successes in positions that demanded little interaction with white coworkers or a white public. In the tonal spirit of racial uplift, McDougald celebrated the "one Negro woman, beginning as a uniformed maid, [who] has pulled herself up to the position of 'head of stock.'"[74]

Discrimination in hiring practices was particularly odious. McDougald admonished the federal government and the civil service of New York City for relying on the "tenacious and retrogressive practice" of the "casual personal interview."[75] Introduced during the presidency of Woodrow Wilson, the increasing segregation of federal administrative jobs employed various methods to bar African Americans from steady employment in white-collar positions. By May 1914, candidates were required to submit photographs with applications for employment in the civil service.[76] This discriminatory measure met protest from groups and individuals throughout the interwar era. For example, as late as 1935, under Mary McLeod Bethune, the newly formed National Council of Negro Women included in their platform the elimination of photographs from applications.[77] Photographic images readily helped filter out African American applicants, but the personal interview brought women who possibly looked less African American by early twentieth-century racialized standards under even closer scrutiny. McDougald recounted the case of one woman who passed her written exam, but "three times [was] 'turned down' as undesirable on the basis of the personal interview." These rejections, combined with public images that conveyed the view of "Negro" women as servile, grotesque, and targets for ridicule concerned McDougald, who worried about the "self-doubt" and "sense of personal inferiority" accruing in women because of racist and sexist stereotyping.[78]

Respectable work demanded women display respectability in cleanliness, dress, deportment, and behavior. When combined with education or training, respectability was seen to heighten a woman's access to respectable work that ranged from white-collar jobs as clerks and salespersons to professional positions as librarians and teachers. Color or complexion persisted as a marker of respectability that was not easily overturned. Indeed, as Victoria Wolcott finds, "during and after World War I, skin color and job status became intricately linked for African American women." With a focus on interwar Detroit, Wolcott shows how African American reformers "sought to present the black community in the most 'attractive' way possible." In their efforts to facilitate the employment of migrant women and to fulfill the expectations of what white employers defined as "attractive," these reformers angled to place the "most 'respectable' women in public view." For example, in department stores where African American women were almost entirely excluded as frontline sales staff, when hired, employers favored "light-skinned, well-educated African American women" in these public roles.[79] In other jobs, complexion mattered: "It was well known that most coveted jobs, in department stores, factories (other than laundries), and theatres were assigned based on skin color."[80] Between the wars, African American southern migrant women met further exclusion in garment and laundry work in New York City; there, specialized sewing skills among Caribbean immigrant women increased their employability in "responsible jobs as dress-makers in factories." As Rosalyn Terborg-Penn explains, at times these women were "forced to reject their heritage on the job site" by passing for white.[81]

Reformers encouraged employers to hire according to "intelligence and graciousness" rather than on "surface beauty." For example, when John Dancy of the Detroit Urban League encouraged Hudsons, a large department store, to hire African Americans as elevator operators, he assembled a group of good-looking women, many of whom "had gone to good schools in the South; some were college graduates." Dancy defended one applicant; he admitted that she was "very dark ... not as good looking as the others," but he encouraged Hudsons to consider how "a good education and manners could overcome the deficit of skin color."[82] Brown complexions seemed to have less "deficit" to overcome. References to brown skin appeared as a brokering language use to advertise one's own labor or to advocate for someone else's employment. One letter from the executive secretary of the St. Paul Urban League to John Dancy in Detroit described a woman, who was seeking employment as a chemist, as "a fine looking brownskin girl." The letter went on to describe "a very pleasant face and pleasing manner. She is attractive, dresses neatly but not gaudily."⁸³

* * *

In other communiqués, African Americans appropriated the description of brown-skin complexion to denote their suitability for respectable work. Letters from migrants written to the *Chicago Defender* during and after World War I also show how some women and men self-described their complexions as brown in efforts to enhance their prospects for employment. In some cases, letter writers emphasized health and cleanliness in descriptions of their physical bodies. For example, one writer from Natchez, Mississippi, who one might assume was a woman, solicited the newspaper's help "to put my application in the papers." "I am a body servant or nice house maid," wrote the hopeful migrant. "My hair is black and my eyes are black and smooth skin and clear and brown."⁸⁴ Describing her weight, "good teeth," and "strong and good health," the migrant presented herself as brown in packaging her value as a worker in 1917 in the industrial Midwest. Another woman explained to the *Defender* her "wish to go North" and her willingness to "do any kind of housework," including laundering, nursing, and cooking. At twenty-seven years of age, the letter writer assured the newspaper that, unburdened by family, it was "just myself." Soliciting "a job with some rich white people who would send me a ticket and I pay them back," she appeals to the potential white employers by ending this request for employment in polite and conciliatory terms: "please help me. I am brown skin just meaden size."⁸⁵

In 1925, "The Task of Negro Womanhood" offered little salve for the problematic of women's dual subjugation. Having laid bare the complex tangle of socioeconomic forces that withheld progress for New Negro women, McDougald championed women's individual striving on behalf of "family, community, and race." "Women's feminist efforts," McDougald concluded, "were chiefly geared toward the realization of the equality of the races, rather than equality of the sexes," and educated, middle-class women were specially tasked as a "progressive and privileged" group to "express their community and race consciousness." This was a particularly important role, for despite the vast differences that existed among and between New Negro women in Harlem, many white Americans appeared unable to see beyond the racist imagery that featured broadly in advertising, theater, newspapers, and other print venues. Indeed, save the most elite group, "Negro women" were "figuratively struck in the face daily by contempt from the world around her."⁸⁶ So, in 1925, when McDougald's portrait appeared in the Harlem issue of *Survey*

Graphic and Locke's *The New Negro*, the image clearly upset the common view of African American women as grotesque, servile, and unrefined; in doing so, it sought to provide an inspirational view of the modern New Negro woman, showcasing McDougald's beauty and brown complexion.

From Stereotype to Type

In 1925, a portrait "sketch" of decidedly brown-complexioned "teacher, social investigator and vocational guidance expert"[87] Elise Johnson McDougald appeared in the critical anthology *The New Negro* (see plate I.2). The portrait of the assistant principal of a Harlem high school captured something of the burden of New Negro women as one long held, doing so in the representative form of a gendered body that is both beautiful and brown. McDougald's large dark eyes appear determined and focused in their forward-looking gaze, but her body, clad in a shapeless, almost matronly garment, is sedate. Despite a youthful countenance, McDougald's maturity appears through long strokes of gray that highlight her black hair; although worn unfashionably (presumably in a bun), this same swoop of gray skims her forehead as tendrils of black and gray softly frame and feminize her face. The subject's mixed-race difference comes through in her straight hair that also intimates McDougald's age, class status, and retention of femininity despite her growing departure from youth. Consistent with all other bodies as they appeared in the color-print versions of *The New Negro* (1925 and 1927), McDougald not only appears brown in complexion, but she is rendered beautiful in this brown skin. The portrait accompanied McDougald's essay "The Task of Negro Womanhood." The essay critiqued the vicious stereotyping of women in advertising images as a pernicious cultural phenomenon that infiltrated broader views of New Negro women: McDougald's portrait appeared to embody the very qualities that were routinely denied to African American women: beauty, educated accomplishment, and middle-class status.

McDougald appears a somewhat lighter brown color than other women depicted in Locke's edited collection, either as unnamed or representative types. The only other view of a New Negro woman as a known persona showcased a less-feminized portrait of Mary McLeod Bethune, who appears as an older woman, slightly unkempt and dark brown in complexion. Unlike McDougald, Bethune made no written contribution to the anthology. In this way, McDougald is pointedly presented as a New Negro woman. In addition, her image accompanies the only woman-authored, non-arts-based essay published in the anthology; it offers the only focused statement on women's issues. Contrasting with the abundant celebration of men's voices and visuals featured throughout *The New Negro*, this depiction of McDougald offered readers the only view of the New Negro woman as a contributor to the volume. Rendered not only by a man but a white, German-born artist, the portraits of New Negro women and men met intense criticism from some Harlemites, but McDougald herself was a fan of the artist, Winold Reiss. Indeed, there appeared little to dislike about the portrait, which depicted a brown-complexioned woman of middle-class composure, serious intellect, and pleasing beauty.

Edited by Alain Locke and illustrated by Reiss, *Survey Graphic*'s Harlem issue was a precursor to *The New Negro*. In color, Reiss's original portraits of sixteen notable New Negroes appeared as a key visual feature in the anthology, which was seen to mark the rise of the Harlem Renaissance. Reiss, who emigrated to the United States in 1913, settled in New York City where he worked as a commercial artist gaining renown for his bold use of color and his modern, graphic designs. In addition to advertising, design, and commercial artwork, Reiss was a portrait artist. His almost singular attention to nonwhite subjects diminished the importance of his work within the U.S. art establishment.[88] Reiss's compelling portraits of the Blackfeet and Blood Indians of the American Northwest and Canada, Aztec revolutionaries in Mexico, European peasants, Asian Americans, and Harlem's "New Negroes" reveal a modernist artist of great skill and sensitivity who, according to Jeffery Stewart, used color in bold and nuanced ways and who painted people not only as he saw them but also "painted people as contemporaries."[89]

So when Alain Locke commissioned Reiss, Locke asked not only for graphic and abstract designs to illustrate the text but also sought Reiss's specific skills to capture Harlem residents and prominent New Negroes in portraiture. As Stewart explains, Reiss and his brother, Hans, searched Harlem daily looking for willing subjects whom they paid to pose for Reiss in his Greenwich Village studio.[90] Certainly the pitfalls of ethnographic fieldwork in rendering the subject as "real" must be considered when assessing the motivations and actions of these two white, Western, foreign-born men who sought out those subjects; indeed, as James Clifford argues, "ethnographic truths are . . . inherently partial—committed and incomplete."[91] With this view, Reiss's portraits of Harlem residents and well-known New Negroes cannot be assumed to be all-encompassing representations of women, men, and children in Harlem during the 1920s. Reiss's "Type" sketches of ordinary Harlemites were complemented by images of prominent New Negroes, including writer Zora Neale Hurston, poet Jean Toomer, opera singer Roland Hayes, and *Crisis* editor W. E. B. Du Bois, who all sat for sketches and portraits. Reiss was assisted by Alain Locke and editor Charles S. Johnson, who facilitated the involvement of important New Negroes.⁹² McDougald also brokered these sittings; considering her work as a survey researcher, union organizer, vocational guidance officer, and educator, McDougald very likely assisted in securing middle-class, educated schoolteachers, librarians, and other "ordinary" women to sit for the white, foreign-born artist.

Little is known about the non-elite African Americans whose names do not caption their portraits, but it is likely that McDougald facilitated the portrait sitting of young girls and boys who might well have been students familiar to her in her role as educator and vocational guidance counselor. "Harlem Girl 1" (plate I.3) is the most stunning of these portraits of younger New Negroes. Her simple white dress with laced-capped sleeves offsets her dark brown complexion; she looks un-self-consciously to the right to show off an edgy bob that has an Afro-modern vibe as it picks up on multiple influences of the era, including changing sensibilities in women's fashion and hairstyling, pan-African celebrations of diasporic society and culture, and white fascination with the "civilization" of ancient Egypt.

Ethiopia, more so than Egypt, was first celebrated by New Negroes as a site of ancestral heritage; among the most vocal of these pan-African proponents was the working-class organization, the Universal Negro Improvement Association (UNIA). Its founder, the Jamaican-born Marcus Garvey, found symbolic promise in Ethiopia. Citing Psalm 68, Garvey urged African diasporic people to "Look to Africa . . . Princes shall come out of Egypt; Ethiopia shall soon stretch out her hand unto God."⁹³ The physical Ethiopia evolved into a symbol for Africa as a whole and as a promise for self-governance. Garvey contrasted the imagined "purity" of both the Ethiopian land and people, with the second-class citizenship and growing ghettoizing of African people in the West. As a shorthand reference for Africa, Ethiopia represented the unconquered land, the undiluted African spirit, and the unmixed African body. In real physical terms, the pure African, according to Garvey's ideology, existed within a dark-skinned body. In this doctrine of racial purity, the black body was more closely connected to the ancestral and spiritual center of Africa.⁹⁴

Egypt also held important sway as Amy Helene Kirschke shows in her study of artwork that appeared in the *Crisis*. In the NAACP magazine that was clearly oriented toward an interracial, middle-class audience, Egypt regularly featured in its connection to Africa.⁹⁵ With the founding of King Tutankhamen's tomb in 1922, mainstream white culture, inclusive of fashion and style, appropriated interest in all things Egyptian. As the chapter that follows shows, the bob was a fashionable woman's hairstyle that attracted critique from older, elite, and middle-class African Americans; many women bobbed their hair nonetheless. The Harlem Girl's crowning glory—a so-called "Tut cut"—

reflected the many concomitant energies surrounding New Negro youthful womanhood of the 1920s; at the same time, Reiss's portrait of the girl conveyed a distinctly individualistic young female subject as "native" to Harlem. This portrait underscores that a range of expressive styles and beauty politics constituted the New Negro of Harlem's Renaissance.

"Harlem Girl 1" was not among the thirteen portraits selected by Locke to appear in *Survey Graphic*, and it was not published in *The New Negro*. However, on the day of the magazine's publication, all thirty-seven of Reiss's portraits were exhibited at the New York Public Library in Harlem.[96] These portraits, which combined pencil, charcoal, pastel, and conté crayon on board were all designed for reproduction using modern print techniques and materials.[97] The exhibition was likely the first time the portraits were viewed in full color as the magazine images did not run color images. According to McDougald, these color portraits created a "furore" when featured at the exhibition in Harlem.[98]

In her undated letter to Alain Locke, circa March 1925, McDougald reported that "many interesting episodes have centred around the appearance of the Harlem issue," and that Reiss's artwork had created "lively discussion."[99] McDougald wrote to Locke explaining how "one Mr. Williams" was deeply troubled by Reiss's portrait "Type Study, II (Two Public School Teachers)" (plate I.4). She reported that Mr. Williams stated that if he had a chance encounter with these women "in the street, he would be afraid of them." One of those schoolteachers, Miss Price, just so happened to have arrived late from another meeting with McDougald. She recalled how Miss Price, not afraid to voice her opinion, "stood to express her regret that she would frighten him but claimed the portrait as a 'pretty good likeness.'"[100]

The pastel on board depicted two young women, seated with a book, looking directly at their viewer; fixed and focused, the eyes of one hold the viewer in a scrutinizing, unapologetic gaze, while the other, somewhat less animated in fortitude, looks wearily on. Shoulders touching, the two women lean into each other, almost offering support in the demanding job of public schoolteaching. Dressed simply, both women are young; they approximate nothing of the cosmeticized, modern beauty associated with the era. As Stewart notes, both women wear sorority keys portraying their respectable, educated, middle-class associations;[101] as well, the exhibition title of the portrait assured viewers of the women's service-oriented vocations. So what then did Mr. Williams find in the image to frighten him? Stewart comments that both women were dark-skinned; this judgment is not difficult to make when compared to the shades of brown that Reiss used to depict McDougald. The portrait's power emerges in the strength embodied in their dark-brown complexions. Both women hold a forthright gaze, and one teacher props up her chin as if sizing up but not caring about the viewer. Neither are passive posers; neither avert their eyes; neither appears deferential to the viewer.

The portrait of "Two Public School Teachers" was not the only dimension of the exhibition to cause offense. A considered critique was lobbied against Reiss's depictions of African Americans, particularly as a white man who rendered portraits of dark brown women and men from Harlem's varied social classes to an audience of largely middle-class New Negroes. As well, Locke bore criticism not only for choosing a white artist but also for editing the Harlem issue when Locke "lived elsewhere."[102] In his defense of Reiss, Locke reinforced the need for new images to counter "caricature conventions" while noting that these prevailing representations caused the development of "touchy reactions." Writing in *Opportunity* in May 1925, Locke argued that, in rendering a view of African Americans in modern society, painting as portraiture was "most untouched of all." He considered how this deficiency might partly be accrued due to its technical challenge. Locke judged this form "the most difficult because of the variety of pigmentation and subtlety of values" called upon to represent the African American body and spirit. As he underscored the need to "break through stereotypes" and "flout the conventions," Locke found New Negro art to be a form vital to representing the contemporary characteristics of Harlem's New Negro.[103]

Clearly a fan of Reiss, McDougald sympathized with him. In a letter to Locke, she reported on the response of community members to the Harlem issue of *Survey Graphic* that included favorable feedback on her essay. She also granted space in her letter to consider the German artist. She related to Locke a conversation held earlier with Reiss, in which he confided that he mostly heard "'cons' about his work." Readily, McDougald "had a few 'pros' to tell him." She bolstered the artist by telling him that the "best" of these pros came from Tuskegee, "where the types selected and the work met with general approval." This reference to "types" included the sketches in *Survey Graphic*, namely "Congo," "Mother and Child," "Young America: Native-Born," "A Boy Scout," "A Woman Lawyer," "Girl in the White Blouse," and "A College Lad." Each image provided view of a particular "type" found in Harlem. One community member, as McDougald reported, contemplated the "whole art side of the [Harlem] issue"; Mr. Williams questioned if Reiss's artwork was a "piece of subtle propaganda to prejudice the white reader?"[104]

Types, rather than stereotypes, appeared aplenty in *Survey Graphic*. Geared toward white readers that included the lay educated, philanthropists, social workers, and professionals, the magazine intended its "social exploration of the New World" to be geared toward collective social progress.[105] By the 1920s, *Survey Graphic* reflected important changes in academic understandings of race and ethnic difference as witness to the demise of biological interpretations of race and the rise of new academic approaches. Franz Boas, a German-born scholar, was hugely influential on the development of American social science; based at Columbia University in New York City, Boas assisted in a crucial paradigmatic shift in the study of race and culture through his concept of cultural relativism. In 1911, at an address to the First Universal Race Congress in London, Boas challenged the view of the "stability of race-types," arguing how "detailed study of the phenomena of growth" defied the static, unchanging character of race as a classification of difference. Boas pointed to "the phenomena of growth" as an example of mutable bodies, minds, and psyches. Underscoring the influence of the "social and geographical environment" on mental development, Boas roundly rejected essentialized views of difference, embracing the idea of the "decided plasticity of human types" instead.[106] Other social scientists provided more details on understanding racial typologies. In *Survey Graphic* in 1926, Robert E. Park, an influential white sociologist of the Chicago school explained: "When strangers meet it is not the individual that they see in one another first, but the type." As he argued for understanding "race prejudice" as a "function of visibility," Park found that individuals from a "race of high visibility" turned out to be "the natural and inevitable objects of race prejudice." The pronouncement of "racial characteristics" and enhanced social distance was foregrounded as crucial factors leading to the "conceal[ment] of the individual man."[107]

The representation of Harlem people as native types presents a challenging view of Reiss's portraits as studies of Harlem's New Negroes. Type studies date to the mid-1800s in Europe and the United States, and as Ann Elizabeth Carroll tells us, treated subjects as "specimens." Type studies provided visual evidence of "identifying features" as distinct markers of character with particular emphasis on social deviants, including the criminal and the insane. Carroll views Reiss's "type studies" as ones crafted with greater sensitivity, nuance, and less ignoble purpose, finding nonetheless an "implicit othering" in place. Carroll also points to Locke's problematic defense of this "material" as the subject for social scrutiny rather than as representations of individual human subjects who helped compose everyday Harlem. Indeed, *Survey Graphic*'s broad mission to represent to its white readers the social communities and cultural groups judged most in need of financial, reform, or political support very likely skewed the vision of unnamed Harlem people as individuals. As well, few if any biographical details help complicate this view of types as material evidence or showcase the heterogeneity of African Americans as modern people. Finally, these type studies seem to uphold the middle-class practice of racial uplift. As Carroll argues, "class rather than race becomes the factor that divides readers and subjects."[108]

Color connected the reader to the raced subject by presenting a bold view of brown bodies that looked and felt modern, introspective, and engaged. Reiss was well-known for his use of color, which was innovative at the time, yet the majority of portraits that appeared in *The New Negro* relied on a few colors—namely black, white, and brown—to render the image of the New Negro. The studied portraits of known persona, such as McDougald, Bethune, Locke, and sociologist Charles S. Johnson were set against diminished backgrounds, and the finer details of clothing were crafted mainly in black and white to showcase the faces of African American women and men. In Reiss's type sketches, two of the four are rendered to different effect in color. Both portrait sketches depict African American women simulating particular aspects of cultural retention and bodily renewal of the New Negro. The first appeared as the frontispiece to the anthology. Chapter 3 attends to this Madonna image in fuller detail (plate I.5). The second, "Type Study I (Ancestral)" (fig. 3.1) shows a young African American woman ensconced in and surrounded by vibrant colors. The portrait signifies and acknowledges Native American heritage in the display of American raced identities.

The powerful image celebrated indigenous culture in U.S. history as it suggested Afro-Indian ties binding New Negroes to a more complex ancestral rooting in North America. Partly due to the bold use of color in the background tapestry of Native American design, the image of the brown-skinned young woman asserted distance from progress-oriented modernity as the only way forward. Her straightened hair, parted in the middle, bears no allusion to whiteness or emulation of white women's hair: it forms a part of her distinct heritage. As well, the sitter holds one of the few full smiles on brown faces as they appeared in *The New Negro*, suggesting at once both Reiss's joyful interpretation of Afro–Native American culture and the sitter's pleasure in holding this pose.

In *Survey Graphic*, color is absent. However, Reiss's second series of "types" unfolded a photo narrative on class mobility among Harlem's African-descended community. Nestled between two women-authored essays, the series "Four Portraits of Negro Women" offered full-page images of four women. The first portrait depicted "A Woman from the Virgin Islands" who sat somewhat slumped in her chair in a white dress. In profile, she faces Eunice Roberta Hunton's essay "Breaking Through." In this piece, the sociologist describes Harlem as "a riot of personality, a canvas of browns and golds and flaming reds," and a "modern ghetto." She describes sets of divided and differently ordered communities, including youth who revolt and older people who submit. Hunton depicts an insular-looking working class and a more expansive middle class who, in the spirit of racial uplift, needs to help break "the bonds linked together by ignorance and misunderstanding."[109]

Reiss's sketch, "A Woman from the Virgin Islands," appears to be intimately connected to the urban "ghetto." Her body, inanimate and passive, seems filtered through an elitist lens that saw West Indian immigrants in Harlem needing particular direction from U.S.-born New Negroes. Black-and-white shading render "A Woman from the Virgin Islands" dark brown in complexion, and her clothes seem slightly disheveled. Three portraits that follow the image of the African Caribbean immigrant imply a hierarchical ordering of women's social class as dictated by dress, style, employment position, and physical beauty. Second is "The Librarian," dressed in a fur-lined coat and large-brimmed hat. She is steadfast in her sideways stare as she nestles a book close to her body. The detailed rendering of her clothing sets this image apart from Reiss's other work. For the most part, the artist depicted the clothing of New Negroes simply, often leaving garments white and unadorned, thereby heightening focus on the human subject. No doubt this technique made color print reproductions possible, but it also produced a powerful effect as faces and skin tones command the viewer's attention. The clothing of the subject in "The Librarian" comes to the fore in this type study to suggest its inappropriate look for a bookish professional woman. The third sketch, "Two Public School Teachers" (plate I.4) shows women also posing with a book; these young women appear more sedately dressed than the stylish librarian. The last image introduced "The Double Task." Here readers found the portrait of McDougald as the only woman named in the entire issue. Clearly, a narrative of upward social mobility through migration, employment, appropriate dress, and educated commitment emerges when viewing these four portraits.

Through black-and-white print images, the notion of brownness first became apparent. In stark visual terms, the binary color scheme may have helped to differentiate lighter- and darker-skinned tones. The simple charcoal drawings also provided key visual markers of progressive development from Afro-Caribbean immigrant to the named beauty as the true New Negro woman. *The New Negro* did not repeat this use of "types"; rather, it relied on the portraits of prominent New Negroes, including McDougald, the only person both seen and heard in *Survey Graphic*'s Harlem issue.[110]

Conclusion

The life, work, and visual representation of Elise Johnson McDougald underline the intertwining realities that increasingly impinged on the public identities of New Negro women as respectable in the mid-1920s. Locke's *The New Negro* and *Survey Graphic*'s Harlem issue presented McDougald as a New Negro Harlem educator, yet, as a woman transitioning between two periods—and doing so during the 1920s when the status of American women climbed to a symbolic apex—her reality was more complex and nuanced. As a social investigator, vocational guidance counselor, educator, and activist, McDougald worked to uphold a set of gender values that were in flux. These efforts illuminate some of the distinct changes that occurred as middle-class ideals of womanhood in the process of African American modernization oscillated between older values connected with race woman of the "Woman's Era" and the increasingly public New Negro woman.

Though not young, McDougald worked at the heart of youthful Harlem in her role as an educator where she designed innovative teaching methods to accommodate an increasingly diverse student body. Her beauty, captured in brown tones, showcased a modern yet modest display that shored up the respectable image of African American women for public consumption and respectable employment. At the same time, tenets of service and racial activism imbued McDougald's work as a social investigator, vocational guidance counselor, and educator. In this sense, McDougald maintained older traditions of clubwomen's service to race, but by relying on social scientific and discriminatory patterns in industrial waged labor, McDougald made central the unique sets of issues encountered by different groups of African American women. Frequently viewed as the quintessential representation of the respectable, bourgeois New Negro woman, the portrait of McDougald depicts a woman whose life reveals an activism long eclipsed by a narrow focus on her beauty.

Still, this image remains relevant. Showcased in the portrait were gendered characteristics that came to forge and define an ideal of brown beauty. This representation of New Negro women's beauty as being brown in complexion developed powerfully in print culture and extended far beyond interracial groups of intellectuals, scholars, and artists. At the same time that newspapers and magazines enjoyed great popularity and print culture more readily incorporated visual images to accompany news stories and editorial roundups, representations of beautiful brown-complexioned women abounded throughout the decade. As migrants and other urban settlers acclimated themselves to the urban environment, they encountered powerful advertising text and imagery that lured them to consume modern goods and services. The following chapter examines how beauty featured prominently in this advertising that increasingly embedded brown complexions as a modern standard of beauty for New Negro women.

2

Beautiful Brown Skin

Advertising New Negro Womanhood

"This Doll has beautiful brown skin," intoned an advertisement for the "Negro Crying and Walking Doll" that appeared in the *Crisis Advertiser* in December 1923. In the approximately ten-page section that closed each month's issue of the official magazine of the NAACP, the O.K. Colored Doll Company at Seventh Avenue, New York City, plied its trade as one of a handful of companies engaged in this era's growing large-scale manufacture and sale of "Negro dolls" (fig. 2.1). Like its competitors who also advertised in the *Crisis* and in other major African American journals and newspapers, the O.K. Colored Doll Company pitched its sale of the "Colored" doll through the verbal descriptor of "brown skin." At the set price of $2.49, the fourteen-inch doll was sold "As Shown." Clad in a white bonnet to match the toy's simple child's dress, the doll's baby face and body appeared "white" and made little visual impact as a "Negro doll."[1] Neither unique among their competitors in promoting the child's toy through the descriptor of brown, nor in advertising a doll that clearly was not brown in color as brown-skinned, the O.K. Colored Doll Company signaled the beauty of brown skin as a crucial selling feature, as did other companies that sold differently "Colored" dolls as "Negro" ones.

By the 1920s, doll companies increasingly relied on the association of brown skin with beauty as a marketing tool to target African Americans as modern, New Negro consumers. Between the 1910s and 1920s, advertisements for "Negro" or "Colored" dolls supported the cultural currency of brown beauty as it first emerged on the modern scene. Dolls described as brown in complexion provided important gendered cues to young girls and women. In the marketing and access of consumer goods, this association of beauty with brownness played a dominant role, making femininity central to the project of modernizing the New Negro woman.

By the 1920s, upwardly mobile advertising featured broadly in black magazines, newspapers, and journals to provide a sharp vision of African American modernization, and a guide to success through the access of certain consumer products. Often advertisements for dolls alongside those that featured other goods, such as wigs, cosmetics, and hair preparations were

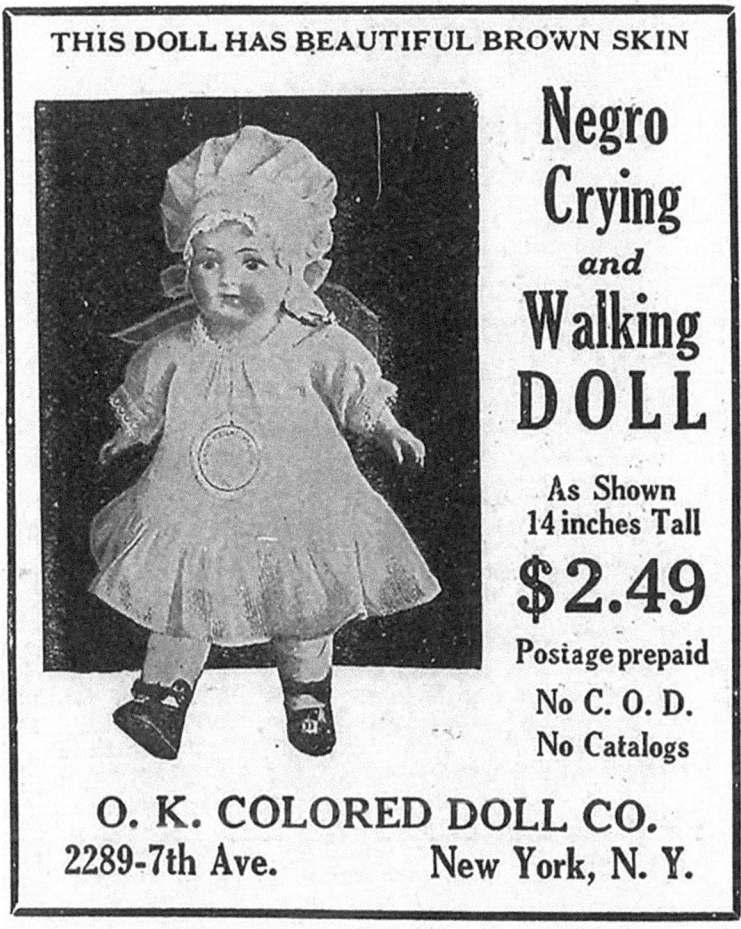

Figure 2.1. Advertisement for O.K. Colored Doll Company, 1923 (*Crisis Advertiser*).

clearly marketed at women. Listings also included job opportunities, services for hire, and training courses in white-collar clerical work and beauty. In addition to large nationals like the *Chicago Defender*, specialized magazines also drew on advertising as a source of revenue in the spirit of racial uplift. For example, between 1910 and January 1928, at the end of each month's issue of the *Crisis*, an advertising section appeared; after this date, advertisements were integrated into the magazine's front and final pages. The *Crisis Advertiser*, as the section was known, offered a view of goods and services as tools that promised to help embody norms, practices, and values associated with respectable, urban, middle-class, public identities. An exploration into the marketing of consumerist goods geared toward women and girls exposes some of the social meanings embedded in the view of brown complexions as an increasingly popular and politicized metaphor for middle-class status and aspirations to such standing in the age of the modern New Negro.

Throughout the 1920s, "brown" and "brown skin" captioned other equally incongruent messages on race, color, and gender when advertising to New Negro consumers. On a regular basis, the appearance of these advertisements in the *Crisis* and other important print venues helped to cultivate a set of class-based ideas of New Negro womanhood that made clear the importance of beauty in defining modern identities. The virtue of the beautiful brown-skin doll, personal hair-grooming practices that celebrated femininity, and at-home cosmetic use emerged as key tools for urban women to attain respectability. By the middle of the 1920s, amid the growing swing of the New Negro renaissance, modernity, not morality, shaped brown beauty's respectability. Businesses cast the sale of brown beauty through a range of products that were advertised in important national newspapers, in consumer-oriented magazines, and in New Negro literary journals; in "Black Manhattan," these publications included the "little magazines" associated with the Harlem Renaissance that framed the discourse on brown beauty through a gendered rhetoric of women's racial pride. Advertisements connecting beauty with brown skin signaled the growth of a new culture of beauty as an ideal of womanhood; these advertisements appealed to women as New Negroes, as American citizens, and as gendered consumers. The relatively reasonable cost of personal grooming items and availability of postal order services assisted the greater access of products among a wider spectrum of African Americans. Consistent with the long-standing obligation among elite, middle-class, and professional women to enact and uphold middle-class standards of respectability, modern New Negro women were encouraged to display middle-class urbanism through the cultivation of beauty. These advertisements signaled women's willingness and unencumbered capacity to do so through purchase and use of consumer products.

This chapter studies a select series of advertisements that appeared in African American newspapers, magazines, and journals throughout the 1910s and 1920s, and traces the development of brown-skin beauty as a rising consumerist ideal. It analyzes an advertising discourse that presumed a central focus on personal beauty in the lives of modern African American women, emitting important cues to girls and women on the enactment of middle-class respectability in the urban environment. The cultivation of beauty was presented as a private pursuit geared and directed toward three intersecting goals: social mobility through employment in respectable waged labor; cultivation of personal happiness through appeal to the other sex; and the display of race pride as an ultimate challenge to white cultural beliefs in the physical inferiority of African American people. By considering the ways editors, entrepreneurs, and advertisers underscored particular products and services as essential to women's socioeconomic success in urban spaces, this chapter indicates the rise of brown-skin beauty as a consumerist idealization beginning in the late 1910s and rising to greater prominence throughout the decade that followed.

Advertising Brown Beauty in the Black Press

Newspapers and magazines provided advertising space to companies that brokered in the emerging ideal of brown-skin beauty. Harlem-based journals including the *Messenger*, the *Crisis*, and *Negro World* ran some of the same advertising, as did the Chicago-based women's magazine, *Half-Century*. Nationally circulating weekly newspapers such as the *New York Age* and the *Pittsburgh Courier* also sold space to advertisers for similar, if not the same, products. Beyond the feature of "novelties" like dolls and cosmetics as "beauty preparations," other "reputable businesses" also advertised in periodicals and newspapers, explains historian Robert E. Weems Jr. African American–owned businesses included "grocers, insurance companies, clothiers, real estate brokers, and educational institutions" and provided much of the "respectable advertising found in African American newspapers in the 1920s."[2]

Advertising dollars provided much needed revenue for early-twentieth-century African American print publications. Some publishers made clear the outlay of their endeavor. For example, readers of *Half-Century* magazine learned all about fees from the magazine's owner and editor-in-chief. Katherine Williams made clear to readers "the costs, the costs!" of publishing a quality magazine as she reproached those who relied on the subscriptions of friends. Williams reasoned: "It costs to print the magazine on the very highest grade of paper that can be secured. It costs to get the brown-skin color scheme on the Cover. It costs to make the Fashion Page attractive to 'mi-lady'—It costs to settle the Printer's monthly bill." Williams reasoned with readers, "If the magazine is worth reading, it is also worth paying for. . . . So why not pay for it?"[3]

Whether she knew it or not, Williams described a fairly common trend among African American readers. More than a decade later, Paul K. Edwards, a white southern economist, published a rare study, *The Southern Urban Negro as Consumer*. In the 1934 study, Edwards observed, "more people read newspapers and magazines than circulation figures indicate." A practice of "occasional borrowing" among African American consumers derived from the expense of "subscription rates of 5 cents to 10 cents per copy." Edwards also found that "many white homes" passed on older magazines (undoubtedly, white publications) to "Negro servants."[4] While Chicago's midwestern urban locale did not necessarily preclude these interracial reading and borrowing trends, it underscores the magazine and newspaper as movable objects that potentially could travel without being officially tracked, as well as reinforces the vital role of magazines and newspapers among urban African Americans. Williams's complaint confirms a disjuncture between subscription figures and readership. Whether her appeal worked or not, the magazine survived and thrived. Published between 1916 and 1925, *Half-Century* achieved a longevity that matched and even surpassed some of the better-known periodicals of the New Negro era.[5]

Williams's reference to the magazine cover's "brown-skin color" hints at the magazine's work to depict the darker complexions associated with African American people; it also reveals her popular association of that color with brown. Catering to an aspiring, urban, middle-class, woman-focused readership, *Half-Century* regularly featured photographic images of ordinary looking, dark-complexioned women dressed in the latest fashions which set a good example for middle-class and aspiring urbanized women who constituted the magazine's main demographic. Similar to other publications of the era, *Half-Century* relied on advertising, attributing one-third of its space to publicize products deemed suitable for urban, middle-class New Negro consumers.[6]

Finances matter in any publishing enterprise. One newspaper, the *Nashville Globe*, was cofounded and financed in 1905 by Reverend R. H. Boyd, a former slave, prominent Baptist minister, and wealthy entrepreneur. In 1896, Boyd founded the National Baptist Publishing Board, which grew into "the largest and most successful African American publishing company in the world."[7] In 1905, in response to a streetcar boycott, the *Nashville Globe* emerged with the intent to "provide boycotters with a forum for protest" in the southern city.[8] The two-year-long boycott failed to quell widening Jim Crow practices on city transportation, but coverage in the *Nashville Globe* provided ongoing endorsement of accommodative resistance as a primary strategy to attain civil rights.[9] The *Globe*, Nashville's first secular African American newspaper, was also relatively free from external financial demands; furthermore, it widely touted support of African American–owned businesses and in doing so upheld Washingtonian principles of self-help and middle-class class ideals of respectability as cornerstone values for Nashville's growing African American middle class.[10] R. H. Boyd, a prominent local businessman, Baptist minister, and secretary of the National Baptist Publishing Board, financed the newspaper while his son, Henry A. Boyd, oversaw the newspaper's editorial tone and content.

One editorial defined Nashville as a vibrant urban center and reflected on the growing numbers of race-proud aspiring New Negroes whose need for guidance on matters of business, consumption, and racial progress the *Globe* aimed to fulfill. It noted, "the people of Nashville are ever on the alert for live and interesting items. Unlike most cities there seems to be a greater development of race pride, thrift, and energy shown in every way of life."[11] Whether these tenets were particularly unique to Nashville is difficult to say, given the parameters of this book, but it is clear that Nashville was among the South's fastest-growing urban centers; between 1880 and 1910, the city's African American population increased by 49 percent.[12] Although the *Globe* never attained nationwide circulation like the *Chicago Defender* or the *Pittsburgh Courier*, between 1910 and 1930 it was the largest-circulating African American newspaper in Tennessee.[13] By 1929, 20.5 percent of African American families in Nashville subscribed to the *Nashville Globe*.[14] Jessie Carney Smith describes the paper during these peak years as "community's griot [and] chronicler of events."[15] It ceased publishing in 1960 following the death of Henry A. Boyd and the changing political sentiment and action around civil rights.[16]

In Harlem, another publication emerged during the first decade of the twentieth century to espouse a message of the New Negro, but its strategy, voice, and vision were decidedly different from the Nashville newspaper. Originally intended "first and foremost" to take the form of a newspaper,[17] the *Crisis* appeared in 1910 as the official organ of the NAACP and maintained a clear civil rights agenda under its founding editor, W. E. B. Du Bois. The prominent intellectual directed the magazine's internationalist vision and integrationist agenda as it not only celebrated the New Negro in the modern world but also provided "A Record of the Darker Races." The popularity of the *Crisis* grew rapidly—an inaugural print run of a thousand doubled by its second issue; a decade later, circulation climbed to an impressive one hundred thousand copies—doubling its count from 1917. Although he was not the sole advocate of education, respectability, and race responsibility as vital markers of New Negro womanhood, Du Bois was certainly among the most influential; as it grew in popularity and reach, the *Crisis* provided one crucial venue for disseminating these prescriptions.

Scholarly attention to the *Crisis* during the years of Du Bois's tenure (1910– 34) largely focuses on literature, art, and politics, but advertising also played an integral part in the magazine's overall tone and vision. From the outset, the magazine embraced upwardly mobile advertising as a crucial arm of its political agenda. While attracting an interracial and international audience, the *Crisis* most directly addressed upwardly mobile and middle-class aspiring African Americans who were reconstituted within the magazine as educated, urban, middle-class New Negroes. The *Crisis* was clearly directed at those who were expected to fulfill the modern dictates on race womanhood. Displays in the *Crisis Advertiser* complemented the essays, editorials, poems, short fictions, and photographs that advanced the magazine's broader claim to prideful racial identity and rightful place of New Negroes in U.S. society. One of the first sightings of brown-skin beauty as a consumer-driven ideal appeared in advertisements geared toward young children. These advertisements were also directed to adults who, as readers of these publications and as parents, guardians, teachers, and owners of small retail businesses were the ones most likely to purchase these products for young New Negroes.

From "Negro" to "Real Brown Doll"

By the early twentieth century, the "Negro" or "Colored" doll accumulated significant meaning for the race-proud socialization of New Negro children. Specifically seen as capable of promoting race pride among girls, the brown-skin doll offered girls one material means to make connections between the race body, physical complexion, and gendered identity. Religious and moral reformers and other race leaders espoused the value of the toy as a socialization tool for children to learn prescribed gender roles, norms, practices, and behaviors. In 1908, the Negro doll gained new importance when prominent southern businessman and Baptist minister Richard Henry Boyd founded the National Negro Doll Company (NNDC) in Nashville, Tennessee.[18] The NNDC planned for an on-site factory to manufacture these toys and won the favor of the (Colored) National Baptist Convention in Lexington, Kentucky, when it took a "decided stand in favour of Negro dolls for Negro children."[19] Some convention members were critical; they argued that as a private enterprise the NNDC should be administered as such rather than under the remit of the National Baptist Publishing Board, overseen by Boyd.[20] Still, the National Baptist Convention gave "hearty approval of the Negro doll factory," passing a resolution that encouraged the embrace of Negro dolls by "people of our churches" and "the race at large."[21] "For half a century," the convention reasoned, African Americans "spent thousands of dollars on white dolls for Christmas," doing so because of the "uncomely and deformed features of Negro dolls."[22]

Numerous distorted representations of African Americans circulated broadly during the first decades of the twentieth century. The NNDC reported that countless "hideous objects," "caricatures," and "scarecrows" were marketed and sold as Negro dolls.[23] One mainstream southern daily newspaper, the *Atlanta Constitution*, reported on the resolution of the National Baptist Convention, approving of the convention's "profound conclusion" as one "well reached." Drawing on the rationale of the convention, the article surmised, "the negro baby must have a doll at Christmas that looks like itself and must not be deformed until it looks like something else."[24] The author seemed approving of the clear division of race by visual ideas of difference.

The NNDC promised to supply "a beautiful Negro Doll" to "anyone who wants one or knows of any friend who wants [one]."[25] One year later, the company directly linked the 1908 resolution to the sale of three thousand dolls that ranged in price from fifty cents to $8.50.[26] That same year, the Illinois Federation of Women's Clubs held the first "Negro Doll Fair" in the United States, intending to "introduce[e] into the homes of Negroes dolls that will not be a reflection upon the moral standing of the race and the infusing of race pride in children."[27] In 1911, the *New York Age* reported on Boyd's tour of nine states to promote the dolls as an overwhelming success, celebrating "Negro dolls for Negro children" as the "right thing." As it reported on the "Progressive Company in Nashville," the *Age* claimed the availability of thousands of Negro dolls, informing readers that "hundreds of churches [were also] contemplating doll bazaars."[28] In like spirit of racial uplift, Baptist women also organized doll clubs and hosted doll bazaars that were especially popular during the Christmas season.[29]

Women were targeted as being responsible for the purchase of appropriate dolls for their children. Among the many childcare duties and obligations facing early-twentieth-century mothers, tutelage in Christian morality, gender propriety, and race pride appeared topmost. Extolling the virtue of the Negro doll as a tool for the development of race pride among children, the *Nashville Globe* insisted that the "real development of the Negro race in America must come from an inborn and innate self" rather than solely from "external agencies," namely church, school, and colleges. Reaffirming much of the Progressive era's conservative sentiment toward the maternal role of women, the *Globe* writer declared, "We must begin at the cradle.... The mother must begin with the little infant.... It must be taught by both precept and example that the race of which it is identified is capable of becoming a model in beauty, virtue and in moral development as any other race."[30]

Mothers were cautioned against committing the grave "mistake" of presenting their children with "a flaxen-haired, blue-eyed, rosy-cheeked waxen figure of the pure Anglo-Saxon race"; doing so was "almost a crime." Play with white dolls potentially harmed African American children because they emphasized white aesthetic standards of beauty and in doing so supported cultural beliefs in racial difference and inferiority. The *Globe* warned that this "early impression" threatened to "linger in [the] breast" of the adult woman, thereby enticing "further mixing and mingling of the races."[31] This trope on the Negro doll contributed to the debate on race suicide among intellectuals that, throughout the first decades of the twentieth century, particularly targeted elite and middle-class African American women.[32] This public discussion on women's reproductive rights and responsibilities as one consequence of migration will be fully developed in the following chapter, but here it is important to note how, in the spirit of racial uplift, Boyd employed the eugenicist discourse of race suicide to reinforce the key expectation of motherhood among young girls.

Letters from African American children published in the *Nashville Globe* showed the desire among children and adults for Negro dolls; at the same time, these letters highlight the gendered expectations exemplified by the doll and the cultivation of the child's desire for the toy. No doubt assisted by their parents or other adults, children ranging from one to twelve years old penned letters to Santa Claus with their specific requests for toys. Most frequently, girls asked for a "Negro doll"; at times, they specified further by describing the doll's physical features that included the capacity to "open and shut its eyes." Children also itemized a list of domesticizing accessories needed for doll play; for example, Irene Belephant of Columbia, Tennessee, wanted "a doll buggy, a set of doll dishes, a table . . . four chairs . . . and a doll stove," while twelve-year-old Zenobie Walker of Centreville, Tennessee, requested "a little set of doll dishes, a doll and a little doll bed for my doll to sleep in." Three-year-old Lucile Mai Nicholson of Columbia, Tennessee, was particular in her request for the doll, a buggy, and a cooking stove. "I want to learn my doll to cook," she explained. "You brought me a piano last year and I will give my doll music lessons too."[33] A perusal of letters from the *Nashville Globe* shows that during the early 1910s, children characterized doll play as largely oriented around domesticity. Beauty had not yet emerged as the doll's key characteristic, nor was it seen as a driving desire among these children for the Negro doll.

Letters from children also underscore the desire of children and adults for dolls as friendly playthings. Until the first decade of the twentieth century, dolls, figurines, and other doll-like figures reflected denigrating and distorted views of African American people that enshrined their enslaved past as justifiable racial domination; these stereotypical images were so pervasive that few twenty-first-century readers require explication. Racist views of African American people showcased them as rooted in a primitive, oversexualized, and/or desexualized, "happy-darky" past. The *Nashville Globe* condemned these "hideous objects" as "black, blared-eyed, flat nose, red lips, with great tusks, with woolly, knotty or kinky hair, all out of proportion to any human being, and modelled after the lowest form of the monkey, orang-outang, or gorilla," concluding that these dolls "serve for nothing but to create a stigma and thought of inferiority."[34] The writer reported that the NNDC's efforts to make more realistic and pleasant-looking dolls in its Nashville factory met with a "vexatious problem" in shaping this representation. It explained that after two-and-a-half centuries of enslavement, African Americans in the United States had become "so intermixed with other nationalities that there is no feature or color nor one characteristic by which he can be traced." The writer acknowledged a great variance among people, and that a wide diversity of features and complexions characterized modern African American people. Despite framing this difference in a positive comparative—complexions are presented as "colors as numerous as the rainbow"—the writer maintained an elitist, sexist, and colorist bias in determining the look of the Negro doll. He vehemently rejected representations that featured darker-complexioned bodies and unprocessed hair, arguing that "it is a fact that a real black Negro of today is an exception rather than the rule: and a kinky, wooly-haired Negro woman is only found in the insane asylum."[35] Certainly, "a real black Negro" can be understood in various ways but the writer's signaling of natural hair and dark skin color showcases the destructive social commentaries on womanhood that featured in the process of modernization. Dark-complexioned women were viewed as anomalous, ungroomed, and mentally ill.

The design, manufacture, and sale of Negro dolls also relied on technological advances in the American doll-making industry to shape the doll's new image. No doubt the material mattered in modern manufacturing, but material also long shaped the preference of girls for their dolls. During the late nineteenth century, dolls made from cloth and fabric—rather than from tough materials like wood, or more fragile ones like china—were popular playthings of young, white middle-class girls: "black" rag dolls ranked as their most beloved toys. Made by white middle-class mothers, these dolls were rendered as "mammy" figures. Dressed in servant's clothing, Mammy dolls seemingly paralleled the role played by countless African American women between the antebellum period and the era of Jim Crow, but the historical meanings of attempts to represent that role through the doll figure are more nebulous.[36] As historian Kimberly Wallace-Sanders explains, these Mammy dolls "appear, disappear, and reappear in the American marketplace." By the 1920s, these dolls appeared on trend. In 1926, the "Beloved Belindy" rag doll debuted as a "mammy" to two red-haired, red-cheeked characters known as Raggedy Ann and Raggedy Andy.[37]

Dolls also symbolized the social and sexual order of race in the antebellum South. One such plaything, the Topsy-Turvy doll—a two-sided rag doll that appeared white on one side and black on the other—complicates further the histories behind dolls about the girls who played with them and the women who made them for their children. Wallace-Saunders questions the political meanings and use of Topsy-Turvy dolls during the antebellum era and rallies against dated views that African American–enslaved girls longed for white dolls as their playthings due to underpinning psychological desires to be white.[38] Rather, in considering the reasons enslaved women made these dolls for their own children, Wallace-Saunders views the Topsy-Turvy doll as representative of the period's "reality of racial interconnections" through its "subversive act of binding together black and white bodies."[39] Karen Sanchez-Eppler finds that the Topsy-Turvy doll mirrored the "logical dualism of segregation" that was reproduced in the doll's body to support a "binary structure of difference" by the stable racial division between black and white. Sexualized views of racial difference were also endorsed since "lifting the [doll's] skirts" revealed its other side. For Sanchez-Eppler, "the Topsy-turvy transformation lies in their ability to mask and deny a national history of miscegenation."[40]

By 1900, technological transformations had made possible "real" "Colored" dolls whose lifelike faces and movable joints assured more interactive doll-play, but the small number of African Americans who could afford such a purchase was forced to rely on imports from Europe. Production of "Colored" dolls began during the late 1880s when German technology invented bisque. A corruption of the word biscuit, bisque originally referred to the undecorated "pure white ware" that emerged from the kiln. As Genevieve Angione explains the changing meanings of bisque, showing how bisque developed "to mean an entire doll, a doll head . . . or doll limbs which are tinted to some semblance of skin tone."[41] This bisque-making process facilitated the modern finish of dolls in "an array of brown tints" to color the face and bodies of "Negro" dolls.[42] Tinting the bisque bodies of dolls was a painstaking process that depended on the labor of multiple workers, and helps explain why "pastel" rather than "intense color" dominated the look of late-nineteenth- and early-twentieth-century dolls. "Built up of thin painted layers," manufacturing dark-skinned dolls appeared costly and labor intensive; as Angione explains, the "beautiful satin-black complexion coat known generally as 'Nubian' may have taken up to five or six trips to the kiln."[43]

Between 1902 and 1914, U.S. doll manufacturers, working to squeeze out their German competitors, "continued to bumble through production successes and failures" but were unable to reproduce German-made bisque that made doll heads 'light, durable and realistically colored.'"[44] While the majority of "American products were heavy, coarse, breakable, and far too pink," two U.S. companies were successful in producing an "acceptable bisque." As historian Miriam Formanek-Brunell explains, the marketing of products using "buzz words" such as "'bisquette,' 'bisque-finish' and 'Newbisc'" hints at the continuing dominance of European doll aesthetics.[45] This marketing language foreshadowed the coming of the brown-skin doll.

The outbreak of World War I in Europe limited the ready trade of dolls, doll parts, and doll accessories, and some U.S. manufacturers exploited this insecurity by "running their factories around the clock"; by 1916, toy manufacturing was perceived as an enterprise holding vast and lucrative potential. By 1920, *Scientific American* reported on the growth of the U.S. doll manufacturing industry to a record 125 new factories appearing in Manhattan alone.[46] Less capital intensive than other manufacturing enterprises, doll manufacturing proved a relatively easier business for African American entrepreneurs to start up. But, as historian Juliet K. Walker explains, racist attitudes also strengthened African American enterprises through a relative lack of competition in the Negro doll business that also lured white consumers.[47] Among the most successful were Berry and Ross Doll Manufacturing, the first African-American woman-owned doll manufacturing enterprise in the nation. The company sold their dolls to customers—African Americans and others—doing so in large department stores on the East Coast as well as in the South.[48]

Less than a decade earlier, the success of the Negro or "Colored" doll was not easily assured. Competition remained fierce among U.S. doll manufacturers who were still trying to gain a foothold in the competitive transatlantic market. Negro dolls attracted hostile attention in Tennessee as vicious journalism attempted to derail the efforts of the Nashville-based National Negro Doll Company. In December 1908, R. H. Boyd, founder of the NNDC responded to a news report in the *Nashville Banner* that dismissed his vision for a Negro doll factory as a "dim, distant future" as the writer, Dan W. Baird, speculated on the look of Negro dolls. An elderly white Southerner, Baird recounted a distorted history of African-descended people's subjugation, savagery, and enslavement in the United States. "Invariably," Baird argued, dolls could only take on the look of a "prisoner of war or slave." Posing as an ally to African Americans, Baird condemned Negro dolls modeled on what he perceived as the totality of African American experience, concluding that this imaging was distasteful to "respectable Negro mothers . . . [who] will not buy colored dolls, and the other sort can't."[49] Playing on ideas of maternalism, claims to respectability, and insecure class status, Baird framed women as potential villains for purchasing the Negro doll.

As Baird gave alleged voice to a respectable African American mother who rejected a foreign-made colored doll, he used a distorted dialect to do so. The anonymous woman was reported as stating, "G'way fum here wid your old Dutch nigger doll. My chilluns' jest as good as anybody's and they are goin' to have just as purty dolls and playthings as anybody's." Clearly angered by the writer's racist assumptions on the look of dolls produced by the NNDC, Boyd upheld the doll's beauty. He explained how "Negro Baptists . . . had taken a long step in the right direction to develop the real, characteristic beauty and lovableness of Negro features and virtues for themselves as the Anglo-Saxon race has done for themselves." Equally exasperated by Baird's use of "Negro dialect" when "quoting the words of a respectable Negro," Boyd further defended the respectability of African American women, arguing that "the characteristic features of the refined gentlewoman of the race" provided the bases for modeling the Negro or colored doll. Roundly rejecting any claim made by the seventy-year-old white Southerner, the *Nashville Globe* lionized the NNDC with headlines that announced: "Dolls Being Shipped All Over the United States—Demand Great—Prospects for a Doll Factory Bright."[50]

Attacks like Baird's continued. The following year, the *Globe* condemned another news article as a "Damaging False Report" intent on "destroying the Negro doll industry." Within the *Banner* report, the *Globe* writer found "the most unkind cut . . . ever given to a Negro enterprise," which claimed that African Americans were rejecting the purchase of Negro dolls. The report alleged, "Negro mothers have set their foot on the Negro Doll Movement in Nashville, and no matter what church, conference, or religious and educational associations advise Negro dolls for Negro children, they will not be able to make it work." The news report professed that one woman rejected a sales pitch by one of Boyd's "clever salesgirls." Like the article that appeared one year earlier, the news item invoked a contorted dialect to give voice to the African American consumer. This time, the mother spurned the doll, exclaiming, "Git out! My baby shan't play wid any ob dem baboons. Dey's just as good as anybody's chilluns, and is gwine to hab pretty white dolls to play wid."[51]

In its defense of Negro dolls, the *Globe* article cited "Dr." Boyd's overview of the market as it connected the popularity of Negro dolls to the flailing sales of white dolls during the previous Christmas season. The writer surmised that "thousands of dollars' worth of white dolls left on hand from last season" fueled the current fears among white southern merchants who worried about a repeated poor performance. As well, the *Nashville Globe* writer challenged the item's source of information and showed the weak base for its declarations.

Finally, the writer confirmed the popularity and beauty of Negro dolls as produced by the NNDC. The news article concluded, "these Negro dolls are not uncomely, but are the nearest approach to the refined and cultured Negroes of today that the artist could possibly produce."[52]

The Negro doll might have fared better in northern and midwestern urban centers, but evidence shows that real advances in the production and sale of the Negro doll following the Great War. By 1920, advances in U.S. technologies in doll-making and the growth of U.S. doll manufacturing intersected with the rising tide of New Negro sentiment, expression, and enhanced political outlook. At the same time, the growth of mass consumerism, increase in leisure time, and relative rise in wages for African Americans in urban, industrialized centers translated into the increased buying and selling of consumer goods. By the 1920s, advocates of the Negro or "Colored" doll included clubwomen, middle-class reformers, Garveyites, journalists, and magazine editors who all espoused the value of dolls in the socialization of girls alongside the demands of middle-class respectability. As historian Michele Mitchell explains, "Material culture and race consciousness converged with a reformist preoccupation over sexuality to make the colored doll an exemplary racial tool."[53] The black press helped to circulate modern messages that Negro dolls facilitated a child's development by imparting values of respectable sexual conduct, moral maternalism, and domesticity as cornerstone values of the New Negro woman.[54]

By the second decade of the twentieth century, larger numbers of African Americans, if they so desired, could afford to purchase more realistic looking and pliable dolls that continued to be marketed as "Colored" or Negro. However, this did not mean that dolls caricaturing African-descended bodies disappeared. For example, as late as May 1927 the *Crisis* editorial "Postscript" published but offered no comment on a photographic image of "a Josephine Baker doll as sold in Paris" (fig. 2.2). Trading in a series of primitivist embodiments of the African American entertainer, the doll's fabric-clad body encased its depiction of Baker in a shape and color that seemed entirely unrepresentative of the entertainer, who was all the rage in 1920s Paris and who, in the same issue of the *Crisis*, was described as a "slim autumn brown girl."[55]

Language arose as powerful marker to annotate these dolls as "Negro." Descriptors of brown skin seeped into advertising text, but they did not fully displace older terms including "Colored" and "Negro" that continued to describe dolls. This interchangeability of language reveals much about the fluid and changing meanings of racial identifiers in the era of the New Negro. The early efforts of the National Negro Doll Company to recast the view of Negro dolls as beautiful took up the issue of nomenclature in an editorial; the essay de-

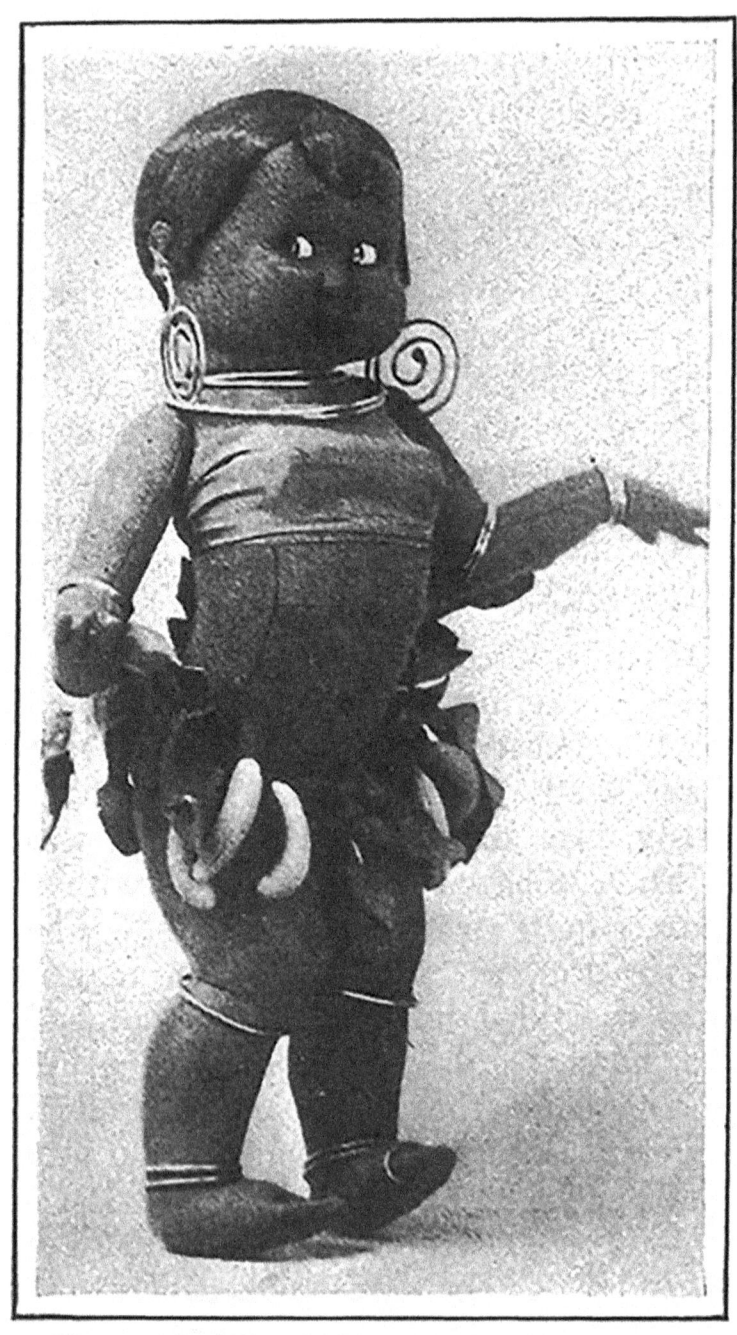

A Josephine Baker doll as sold in Paris

Figure 2.2. Image of a Josephine Baker doll, 1927 (*Crisis*).

duced, "The word Negro almost throughout the civilized world means black. In the United States, however, it has a very different meaning." Setting the United States against the "civilized" world, the article hinted at the promise of "black" as an inclusive identifier of Africans in the diaspora; at the same time, it drew out the problematic of "black Africans and their descendants" in the eyes of the white southern legal system. It critiqued the so-called "one drop rule" that condemned interracial heterosexual couplings by denying whiteness as an identity for offspring produced from those unions with as little as "one-eighth or one-sixteenth of Negro blood." While the author engages no more particular effort to devise a better name for people of mixed ancestry, it appears he found the designation of "black African" a poor fit to describe these folk, as might be explained in the continuing media discussions and advertising for the "Negro or Colored Doll."[56]

As marketing language, "brown" and "brown skin" first developed in advertising for the NNDC. The company largely advertised in various outlets including the *New York Age* and the *Crisis*. More regularly, it relied on the *Nashville Globe*, where it occupied significant space in half-page advertisements featuring a range of proclamations on the virtue of their dolls, which were clearly advertised as "Negro Dolls." Finally, the company boasted of selling "Great Big Beautiful Dolls" that were singled out as "the most beautiful of all toys on the market"[57] Indeed, beauty arose as an important selling point that linked the doll's beauty to the emotional health of girls. The advertisement claimed: "No girl is happier than when she has a beautiful doll."[58] Advertisements displayed curly-haired dolls of dark complexions and text captioning these images described the item with promises that "the features, the hair and the appearance of the toy endear them to the children."[59] Among the earliest of its advertisements, the NNDC cited *Collier's Weekly*'s positive reflection on "encouraging little Negro girls to clasp in their arms pretty copies of themselves."[60] In this decade, beauty, though celebrated, did not dislodge Christian morality and race pride as major factors in the doll's appeal. From all accounts, the NNDC was a self-sustaining enterprise; over the course of its twenty-year lifespan, it showed a steady though not entirely profitable trade in Negro dolls.[61] To market its product, the company engaged multiple methods including the appropriation of color descriptors to describe the Negro doll.

By 1913, the NNDC's marketing campaign showcased the sale of "High Brown" Negro dolls. Photographs of the dolls show ones that appear no different than others sold by the company and captions continued to rely on "Negro" to describe both dolls and children. Two advertisements suggest that the NNDC hoped to boost their sales by invoking this language of color. In

October 1913, the NNDC headlined their advertisement, "Great Big Beautiful Dolls / These 'High Brown' Negro Dolls Given Away." Two images accompanied the text: one portrayed a "Negro girl and Negro doll," the other a well-dressed thirty-six-inch Negro doll. One week later, another advertisement touting the Beautiful High Brown Negro Doll read, "Other Girls Have Gone to work to Secure One of these Dolls / Why Not You?"[62] The employment of "high brown" as a modifier appears to function by generating interest, desire, and a sense of girlhood responsibility for acquisition of the doll. To heighten desire for the doll, the NNDC relied on the connotations of beauty embedded into the term rather than on the real or perceived class status of lighter-skinned or "high brown" women.

At the same time, the doll company foregrounded the doll's accessibility to many. In 1911, as it advertised the "opening of the Negro Doll season," the NNDC assured consumers that "anyone who wants one or knows someone . . . can be supplied." Stoking enticement among *Globe* readers to see the doll, the NNDC underlined its slogan "No Trouble to Show the Goods" as it provided details on viewings.[63] By 1913, the NNDC introduced a new plan to facilitate the purchase of dolls by young people. Offering girls "the chance to get a Negro doll free," the company provided a detailed plan of the work needed to secure a doll that "depend[ed] on how much you talk." The newspaper explained how their work at securing yearly subscriptions would yield a free Negro doll that ranged in size from twelve to thirty-six inches. As the number of subscribers increased, so too did the size of the doll available to the child.[64] The *Globe's* clear interest in gaining new subscribers suggests that the use of "high brown" was meant to enhance the appeal of the dolls. In this case, "high brown" was used to modify "Negro"—it did not substitute or eradicate racial terminology. By the following decade, a significant shift occurred with the broader manufacturing, sale, and distribution of Negro and Colored dolls. As modern media advertising for the Negro doll intersected with and expanded upon these earlier efforts of religious leaders and moral reformers, beauty moved more to the center in marketing the Negro doll; modifiers of "brown" and "brown skin" came to supply a new understanding of the virtues of the Negro doll.

The doll business continued to grow. In 1920, as the *New York Age* reported on "New Departures in Harlem Business," it found "Colored Men Breaking Away from Traditional Enterprises," doing so with "Capital and Courage." Among the "most unique Negro businesses in Harlem" appeared to be "the manufacture of brown-skinned dolls—something practically unthought of, or at least not attempted before in Harlem." The article described the Berry and Ross Manufacturing Company as a Harlem-based factory "equipped with thirty electric power machines and . . . employ[ing] fifty colored girls." Selling to "jobbers and department stores," Berry and Ross also had a storefront at 135th Street to "retail its clothing and dusky dolls to Harlem people."[65] Incorporated in 1918, Berry and Ross represented the first large-scale manufacture of Negro dolls by an African American company.[66]

Victoria Berry and Victoria Ross, founders of the Harlem-based company, evoked brownness to affect the sale of dolls that they also marketed as "Colored Dolls." One advertisement appearing in the *New York Age* announced the sale of "Berry's Famous Brown Skin Dolls." It included descriptions of five different models of dolls that emphasized their different attributes. Still, "light or dark brown skin," "long flowing curls," and "shape and features" appear as key selling points of these dolls. Accompanying the text, a photographic image of a doll with a headband, long hair, and somewhat rustic-looking dress complicates the view of these Famous Brown Skin Dolls as colored or Negro dolls.[67]

Dolls were not always pictured in advertising. For example, in January 1920, Berry and Ross advertised in the *Crisis* and, like many other smaller businesses, relied on text rather than image to advertise its product. The large font advertising "Colored Dolls" announced: "Berry's Famous Unbreakable Brown Skin Dolls," and while disclosing no price it asked readers to "Send for catalog."[68] In 1922, the Harlem-based company was acquired by Garvey's Universal Negro Improvement Association, and as Mitchell explains, "whether UNIA dolls were identical to those produced by Berry & Ross is open to question," although the historian confirms that "dolls produced by the UNIA's own Negro Factories Corporation had 'brown skin.'"[69]

Both African American and white-owned companies appealed to consumers by employing a marketing language of beauty and brown skin; in addition, the doll's other attributes and accoutrements of style further enhanced social prescriptions on femininity, dress, and gendered composure, and in doing so underscored them as appropriate markers of New Negro girlhood. For example, in December 1923, with no particular appeal to the Christmas holiday or to present-giving, the *Crisis* ran two advertisements for dolls whose lifelike qualities drove their marketing; the first of these, the previously discussed O.K. Colored Doll with "beautiful brown-skin" (fig. 2.1) was followed, three pages later, by announcement of "Brown Skin Dolls: Beautiful Unbreakable Walking and Talking Dolls with Real Black Hair and Beautifully Dressed." Sized at eighteen inches, Department C of Bell Manufacturing Company, based from a mailbox in Jamaica, New York, sold "Brown skin" and "also other dolls of different prices and styles," although these varieties were not described or depicted (fig. 2.3). The Brown Skin Doll sold for $2.98 each or

$24 for a dozen, and appeared somewhat less "white" than the O. K. Colored Doll; the photographic image (presumably of the real doll), appearing under the capitalized, bold-font "BROWN," complimented the doll's long dark hair that might well have "passed" for not-white.[70]

Other manufacturers marketed their dolls as being of mixed ancestry, relying on both brownness and reference to "real hair," "dark hair," and "long curls" in their appeal to the New Negro consumer. One of the longest-running advertisers in the *Crisis*, the Bethel Manufacturing of Jamaica, New York, promoted "Colored Dolls and Novelties," privileging in its 1927 text "Pretty, Light-Brown, and Mulatto Dolls with Real Human Hair Curls"[71] (fig. 2.4). Three years earlier, this same company's nearly consistently run advertisement for dolls omitted any racial categorization of "mulatto," relying entirely on color, beauty, dress, and the doll's modern capacity of movement to announce the sale of "Light-brown dolls with Long Curls, Unbreakable, Walking and Talking Dolls with Beautiful dresses, shoes, and stockings."[72] Little is known about the Bethel Manufacturing Company of Jamaica, New York, that between 1924 and 1929 advertised the sale of dolls in almost every issue of the *Crisis*. More research into the doll-making industry and into marketing trends directed toward African American consumers is needed to determine if changes to the advertising text, though not the image, addressed any larger specific agenda in doll purchases or demographics. Whether this company aimed to attract a more specialized market of African American consumers as mixed-race people, or if it simply found light-skinned dolls with black long curls easier to pass off as "Colored" dolls remains speculation only.

What is clear in this perusal of advertisements for Negro or Colored dolls is the increasing use and reliance on the verbal language of brown as a racial marker in advertising text. By the 1920s, the mass manufacture and sale of dolls relied upon verbally defined brown complexions to bolster race pride among a younger generation of New Negroes as lifelike race images interacted with modern consumer products. Materializing as "real" through the brown-skin doll were gendered values, norms, and practices that signaled to young girls a conservative set of values that situated physical looks and adornment of the brown-skin doll's body as a key display of girlhood and womanhood. A tool of socialization, the brown-skin doll presented to girls a material association of race with brownness, brownness with beauty, and beauty with the accoutrements of style that for girls and women included hairstyle, color and texture, clothing, stockings, and shoes. When taken together, these material markers announced their importance in making beautiful the New Negro girl and woman. Certainly the most direct marketing of goods to New Negro women appeared in advertisements geared toward the

BROWN Skin Dolls

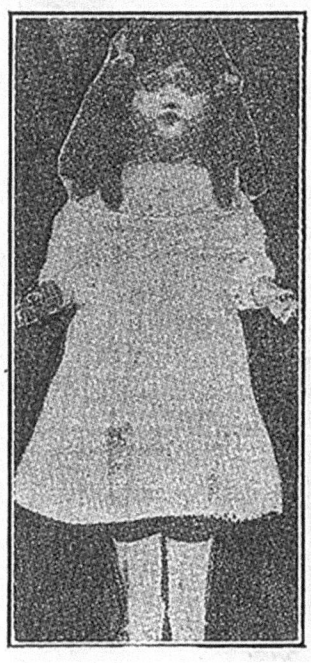

Beautiful Unbreakable Walking and Talking Dolls with real Black Hair and Beautifully Dressed.

Size 18 in.

$2.98 each; $24.00 Doz.

We also have other Dolls of Different Prices and Styles. Write for Free Catalog. Agents and Dealers Wanted. Photo Medallions, Photo Jewelry, Negro Post Cards, Pictures, Enlarged Portraits and lots of other novelties.

We copy from any photo you send us and return your photo with your order. Prompt shipments.

BELL MFG. CO.,
Dept. C
Box 103, Jamaica, N. Y.

Figure 2.3. Bell Manufacturing advertisement for Brown Skin Dolls, 1923 (*Crisis*).

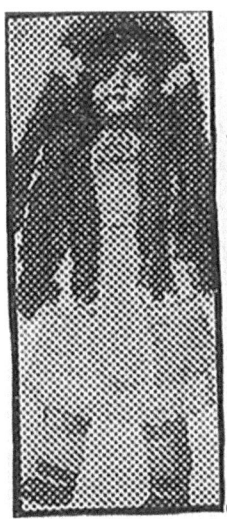

COLORED DOLLS AND NOVELTIES

Pretty, Light-Brown and Mulatto Dolls with Real Human Hair Curls. They Sleep, Walk, Talk and Cry. Sizes 14 to 30 inches. 15 different styles. 100 other novelties. Free Catalog.

AGENTS WANTED

BETHEL MFG. CO.
Dept. C, 97 South St.
Jamaica, N. Y.

Figure 2.4. Bethel Manufacturing advertisement for Colored Dolls and Novelties, 1927 (*Crisis*).

cultivation of feminized beauty through the use of cosmetics. Throughout the 1920s, advertisements in popular weeklies and literary monthly magazines celebrated women's outward show of made-up beauty as a key marker of New Negro women's middle-class modernity.

The Duty of Brown Beauty: Cultivating with Cosmetics

"From the beginning," Du Bois wrote in the *Crisis* in 1930, "[the magazine] has had the right to be proud of its advertising pages." Within the pages of the official journal of the NAACP, Du Bois assured readers that there they would find "no puffs or unwarranted facts" to undermine the magazine's commitment to advance "legitimate enterprise and the employment of Negroes at profitable work." Reflecting on the magazine's "recent efforts" to impart "the necessity of advertising" to social uplift organizations, the *Crisis* editor applauded the Walker Manufacturing Company as a chief innovator among other "purveyors of recreation and luxury." In particular, Du Bois applauded the beauty and cosmetic company for employing a host of modern marketing methods that included radio broadcasting, print media advertising, and a "moving picture film." The journal's editor praised the company's illustrious founder, C. J. Walker, for this creative harnessing of media to disseminate the message of racial uplift through consumption of beauty products and services.[73]

Du Bois's laudatory praise of the Walker Manufacturing Company was hard-won. Walker may readily be recognized by contemporary readers as one of the most successful African American beauty culturists whose line of hair and skin-care products made her the first African American woman millionaire. When she died in 1919, Walker's daughter, A'Lelia Walker Bundles, inherited her mother's fortune and assumed directorship of the company. Her daughter's notorious rise to fame as a Harlem socialite intersected with the dynamic growth of mass consumerism, the rise of modern sex standards, shifting gender roles, and celebration of alternative sexualities amid the vibrant cultural celebration of the Harlem Renaissance; at the same time, the Walker Manufacturing Company continued to flourish throughout the decade.[74] Du Bois's praise for the company's innovative advertising methods followed the death of C. J. Walker. Indeed, Walker was prominent among those African American women who, by working in beauty industries in the first decade of the twentieth century, faced accusations of subverting racial uplift and race politics by mimicking white aesthetic standards. The company's profitable line of products fostered this dubious reception. Featured regularly in the African American press, advertisements for "complexion soap," "Tan-

Off," and the "Wonderful Hair Grower," also secured the back cover of each monthly issue of the *Crisis* between 1924 and 1929.

Hair-straightening products; creams that promised to whiten, brighten, and lighten; and cosmetics appropriating ideals associated with white women's beauty presented a startling paradox to the race-proud messages circulating in the *Crisis*. Indeed, moralizing debates over skin lighteners and hair straighteners continued throughout the age of the New Negro at the same time that advertisements for these very products circulated widely in a broad range of African American publications. Influential weeklies, including the *Chicago Defender* and the *Pittsburgh Courier* often carried the same, but certainly not all, advertisements for consumer products as those that appeared in specialized and literary-oriented magazines like the *Crisis*, the *Messenger*, *Opportunity*, and *Negro World*. In 1925, Guy B. Johnson explained, "larger papers emphasize the advertisements that have national appeal at the expense of the local type of advertising." Johnson, a white southern social scientist, based his findings on a study of advertisements found in a representative sample of African American newspapers. These included two "large metropolitan newspapers," namely the *Chicago Defender* and *Negro World*, and three smaller weeklies—the *Norfolk Journal and Guide*, the *Atlanta Independent*, and the *Houston Independent*; "more or less," Johnson concluded, these publications commanded "local influence in their respective section of the South."[75] Johnson defined three main groupings of products and services advertised for sale and found the most ample grouping held "a prestige out of proportion to their actual worth." Within this grouping, beauty preparations "easily held first place."[76] Still, Johnson cautioned against assigning too firm a link between the dominance of beauty related advertisements and the meanings they held for consumers based on quantitative findings alone.[77] "Beauty preparations" included a broad range of skin care, hair products, and cosmetics for applying makeup. While the manufacture and sale of these products elicited debate among reformers, feminists, journalists, and race leaders, beauty itself was not the centrally contested claim. By 1920, important media venues regularly avowed the moral and physical beauty of African American women and girls doing so in the name of race pride. Kathy Peiss shows how claiming "women's beauty as a sign of racial pride" was a bold assertion that African Americans "had the same 'natural' right as all women to be beautiful."[78] This rights-based discourse on beauty intersected with the rhetoric of New Negro womanhood. The public celebration of women's pleasing physical attributes materialized in the press through numerous commentaries and photographic displays.

Beginning in 1891, the African American press played a pivotal role in celebrating the beauty of women. In that year, the *Chicago Appeal* questioned,

"Who is the Most Beautiful Afro-American Woman?" The newspaper supplied ballots for voting and prompted its readers to weigh in on the key concern.[79] In 1914, the race-proud paper *New York Age* set out to find the "Fifteen Most Beautiful Negro Women in the U.S.," soliciting photographs from readers to help overturn degrading "caricatures and exaggerations" of African American women.[80] As readers responded with interest, one letter writer, Demond Lewis, signaled the potential of the contest to define the "Ideal Type of American Negro Beauty."[81] As it reprinted the letter, the *Age* highlighted the concerns of "students of ethnology" like Lewis who charged the contest with finding "a typical representation of the cosmopolite beauty of the Negro women of the United States."[82]

The newspaper qualified the issue of "representing different types of women of the race showing various strains which have amalgamated into the race body through assimilation," and publicized Lewis's suggested method for finding the "composite" "ideal type." As he hailed an "Egyptian Type" as the basic model to form this composite, Lewis enumerated five groupings by "scientific order," ranking them as "The True Negro Type; The Mulatto Type; The Quadroon Type; The Octoroon-Type and the Near-White Type." He proposed a complicated arrangement of portraits according to these groupings to help "indicate the salient characteristics of the ideal composite type."[83] As promised to readers in its initial call, the *Age* published photographs submitted by contestants on a weekly basis and attempted to show "different types of women of the race showing various strains which have amalgamated into the race body through assimilation."[84] When the militant race paper published photographs of beauty-queen hopefuls on its front pages, it presented a range of looks; still, the winners of the competition were all light toned in complexion, suggesting a continuing colorist bias against darker skin tones. As previously discussed, the address of "type" was a scientific and social concept that gained currency and found broader application during by the second decade of the twentieth century. The popular discussions of beauty as racial type underscores the broad reach of intellectualizing about race that helped legitimize public discussions of women's bodies by race identity.[85]

By the mid-1920s, this concern over racial type as an amorphous amalgamation of racialized characteristics seemed to give way to a somewhat more inclusive though equally ambiguous celebration of brown skin as a dominant type of beauty. For example, in 1925, the first national beauty contest for African American women appropriated the language of brown as a marketing tactic and an appeal to communities of New Negroes. The Miss Golden Brown Contest was brokered by Mamie Hightower, a fictitious "beauty culturist of international repute" who fronted the all-male, white-owned company that manufactured Golden Brown beauty products.⁸⁶ Hightower touted race pride and race progress as the main agenda of the Miss Golden Brown Contest. The *Pittsburgh Courier* lauded her "inestimable service to our Group as a beauty culturist and benefactress" as it reported on the appointment of Hightower's longtime "admirer" and friend, Hallie Q. Brown, a renowned African American lecturer, as the judge of the contest.⁸⁷

Based on "preaching the gospel of complexion for ten years," Hightower claimed to find "our type of beauty rivals that of all other people" and urged the "develop[ment] in every member of our group that quality known as pride." Advertising for the contest included Hightower's appeal to race pride to urge on participation: "It is not enough that some scientists are admitting that the glorious Cleopatra was of our race—let us prove it once and for all that we have here in America some of the most beautiful women of the world."⁸⁸ Attracting more than 1,400 applicants, the Miss Golden Brown Contest was widely publicized in the African American press. Full-page advertisements declared the winner, Broadway performer Josephine Leggett, as a longtime user of Golden Brown's line of cosmetics.⁸⁹ The crowning of the light-skinned Leggett in Atlantic City in October 1925 disrupted little of the white aesthetic of beauty. The company encouraged women to follow the beauty queen's lead by using their products. "You, too," it counseled, "can have the light bright complexion that is the heritage of our race. You, too, can have soft, wavy hair that can be dressed in any style."⁹⁰

Important scholarship on beauty pageants shows their significance in contesting beauty as the domain of white womanhood and, in doing so, helped to shape and define a modern ideal of African American womanhood.⁹¹ The color used to indicate racialized beauty is particularly striking when understanding how some, like Lewis, impressed the importance of these contests in identifying a modern racial ideal that accounted for the diverse complexions and looks of New Negroes. By 1925, the Miss Golden Brown Contest underscored this view by appropriating color in the nationwide beauty competition. As Maxine Leeds Craig explains, while national beauty contests were not seen again for decades, beauty pageants did not disappear; local communities, institutions, and organizations continued to celebrate and define women's beauty through smaller-scale pageants.⁹² Close study of these pageants no doubt yields even more diverse representations of beauty according to community desires and standards. And, as much as "brown" proliferated as a key descriptor to define the beauty of African American women, other color-inflected descriptors also circulated during the 1920s. For example, Kathy Peiss reports that, beginning in 1927, a national Miss Bronze America pageant arose to directly redress the white-only Miss America pageant that originated six years earlier.⁹³

Certainly these broad and popular claims to beauty attested to its modern concern. Still, commentators, educators, writers, and journalists embroiled in the debates on race responsibility and the role of the New Negro woman assessed the importance of beauty by expanding upon an older politics of middle-class respectability that connected cosmetics to wanton sexuality. Some elite and middle-class clubwomen continued to espouse traditional values when defining the parameters of modern womanhood. Between 1924 and 1928, these views appeared in the *Messenger*'s monthly symposium entitled, "Negro Womanhood's Greatest Needs." "Leading Negro clubwomen" characterized the New Negro woman as a cheerful homemaker, a socially committed race woman, and a patient, genteel wife who "never forgets her tender womanly and great motherly heritage."[94] At the same time, clubwomen endorsed advancements of the age, including women's formal political inclusion with the franchise to vote, continuing entry in higher education, and expanded economic opportunities in various professional roles.

Still, morality persisted as a gendered responsibility that rested solely on women. Mrs. Bonnie Bogle of Portland, Oregon, emphasized the need of New Negro women "to build strong character by embracing all that is good and noble."[95] Other clubwomen, including Claudine Johnson Bass of Little Rock, Arkansas, found modern women faring poorly against "the noise and speed and disgust" of the Jazz Age. Johnson Bass judged women were "less discreet and less cautious" than "sisters in the years gone by." The loss of "timidity and modesty peculiar to pure women of yesterday" was particularly upsetting to this clubwoman, who called for the "restoration of decency."[96] Indeed, for some clubwomen and other middle-class moral reformers, little about the modern condition garnered full respect for women. The emphasis on women's moral character appeared to supersede all. Among these middle-class reformers, beauty was construed in moral terms.

Others jeered at physical beauty as a trade-off for women's other redemptive qualities. In July 1925, the *Messenger*'s editorial, "Beautiful but Dumb," claimed beauty as the domain of less intelligent women, arguing that "nature ... doesn't give women everything in one package." Characterizing smart, successful women as either "homely, little, dried-up looking soul[s]" or "huge elephantine Amazon[s]," the male author endorsed modern beauty culture as a salve to women's physical failings, arguing, "if she is ugly she needs everything to make up for the absence of pulchritude." Beautiful women were also trivialized. The *Messenger* editorial droned, "if she is beautiful, normally she doesn't make any sense." The likely provision made for "beautiful but dumb" women was security through marriage or a man's economic support in exchange for a "pretty woman to look at."[97]

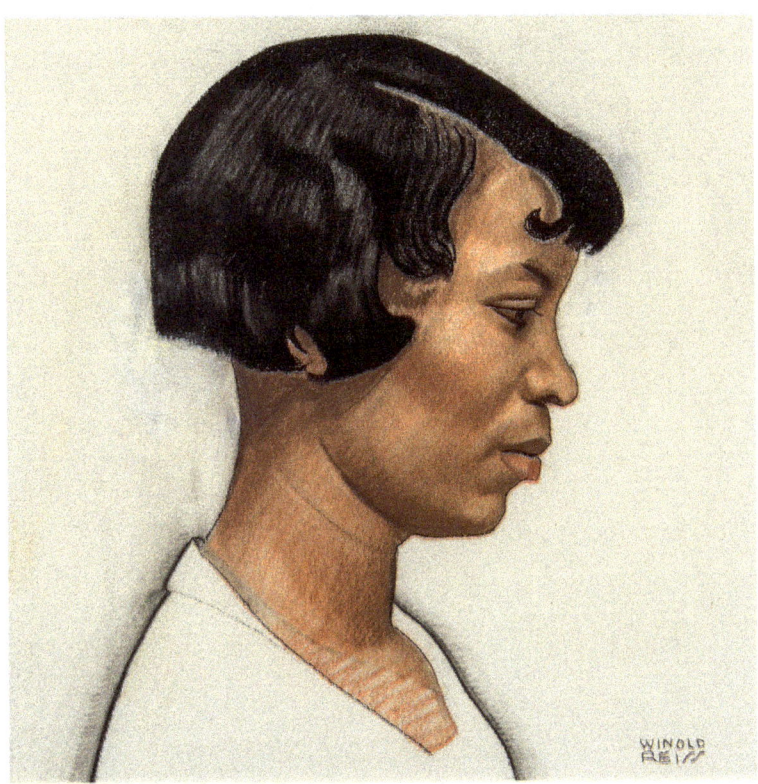

Plate I.1 Winold Reiss, *Miss Hurston* (Zora Neale Hurston), c. 1925, pastel on Whatman board. Gift of the artist. Image courtesy of Fisk University Galleries, Nashville, Tennessee. Photo by Jerry Atnip.

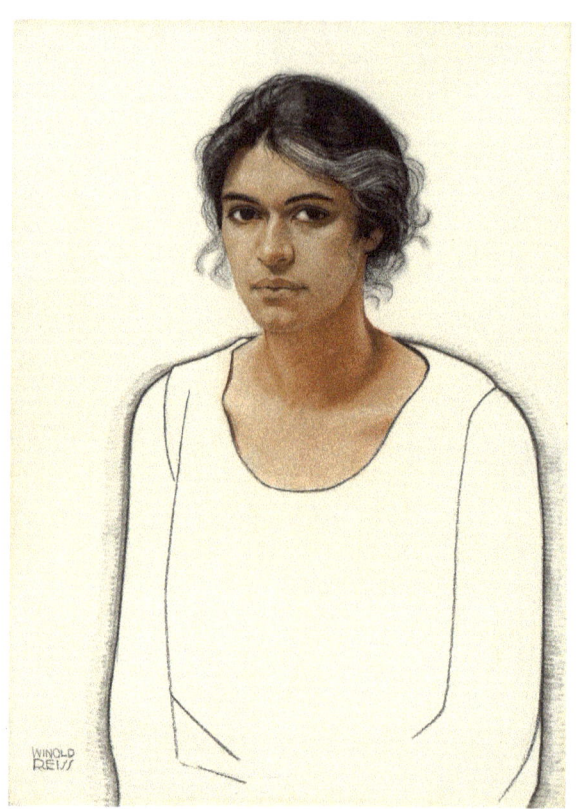

Plate I.2. Elise J. McDougald, 1924. Artist, Winold Reiss. Pastel on board. Image courtesy of National Portrait Gallery, Smithsonian Institution; gift of Lawrence A. Fleischman and Howard Garfinkle with a matching grant from the National Endowment for the Arts.

Plate I.3. Harlem Girl 1, 1925. Artist, Winold Reiss. Image courtesy of the Museum of Art and Archaeology, University of Missouri-Columbia.

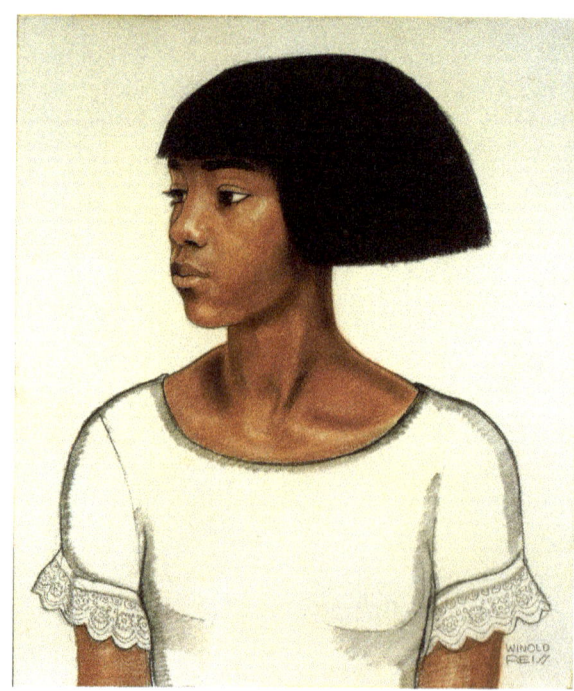

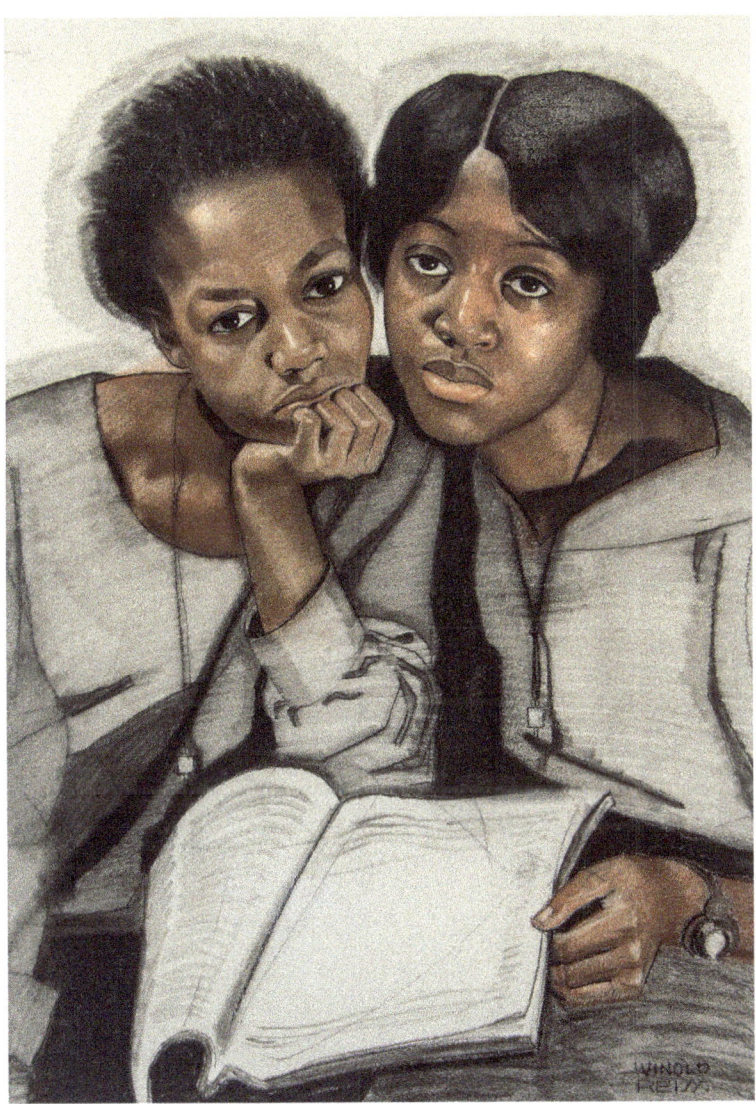

Plate I.4. Winold Reiss, *Type Study, II* (Two Public School Teachers), c. 1925, pastel on Whatman board. Gift of the artist. Image courtesy of Fisk University Galleries, Nashville, Tennessee.

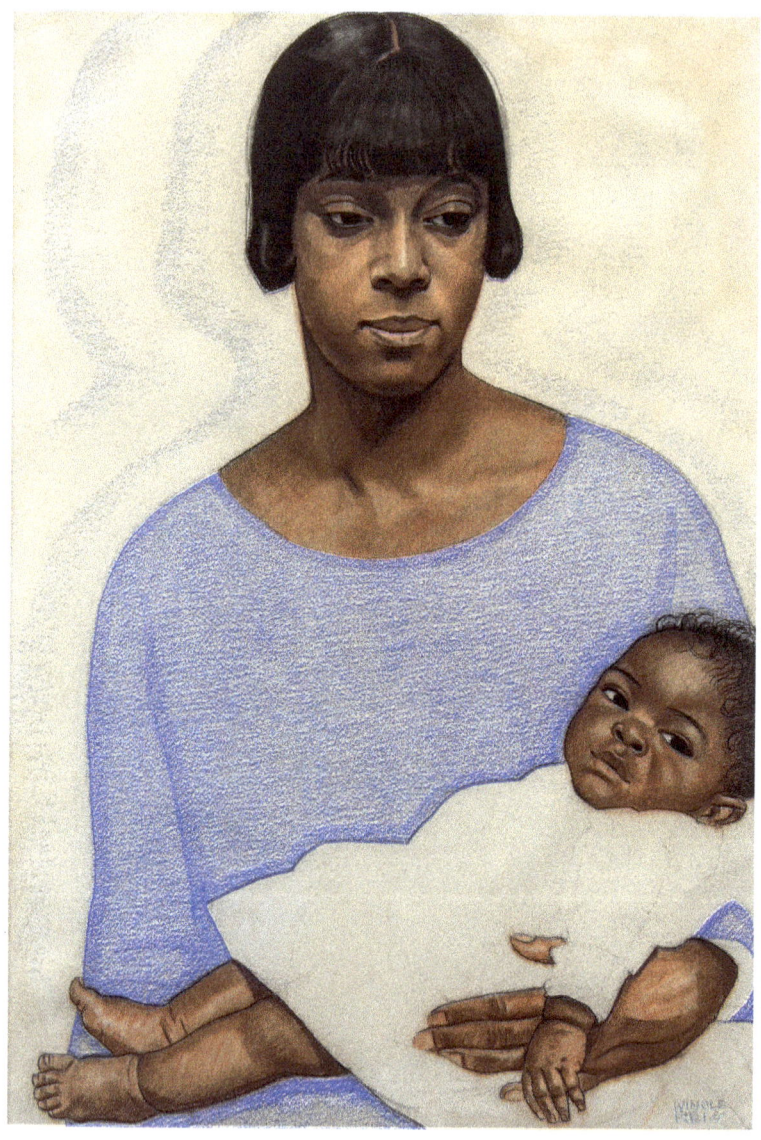

Plate I.5. Winold Reiss, *Brown Madonna*, circa 1925. Image courtesy of Fisk University Galleries, Nashville, Tennessee.

Others vocalized support for cosmetic use in more positive terms. Louis W. George, advertising manager for the *Messenger*, noted the broader cultural idealization of beauty among white people through the concerted efforts and expenditure of "those not beautiful ... to become beautiful or as near so as possible." He reasoned that "the colored girl today would greatly limit her opportunities did she not make use of hair dressing, manicuring and facial massaging" to advance her place in society. While endorsing modern beautifying practices, George also touted the "sound hygiene and sanitary advantages" derived from cosmetic use, and in doing so sanctioned moralizing tenets of good grooming on the path to racial uplift.[98] Still, George urged the embrace of beautifying products geared toward women, and championed cosmetic use as a broader cultural trend and modernizing apparatus. George was certainly not alone in this foregrounding of women's self-help beauty activism, which developed into a powerful discourse to ground respectable beauty as a cornerstone value of middle-class New Negro womanhood.

The dominance of white aesthetics persisted and proved critical to debates on beauty. Political commentators such as George Schuyler, a regular columnist for the *Messenger*, voiced firm concern over the expenditure on skin-lightening products and the racial self-hatred they seemingly underscored.[99] Others, such as Guy B. Johnson, found that "practically all the beauty preparation advertisements now make their appeal to the desire for straight hair and a light complexion." Hinting at fierce competition in the beauty and cosmetic industry, the white Southerner noted that "few ... can afford any longer to advertise their products in a conservative way." As he speculated on the pressures facing cosmetic companies, Johnson considered that "perhaps a few unscrupulous companies" forced others to follow suit, but without evidence he pushed no further. He provided his readers with excerpts from a representative sample of newspapers advertisements that clearly showed the consistent celebrations of a white aesthetic standard of beauty—indeed, the first skin-lightening product listed promised "White Skin Beauty Overnight."[100] Journal editor Charles S. Johnson critiqued the findings of the white Southerner, claiming their potential to "draw hot protests from many Negroes and gleeful snickers from many whites." The *Opportunity* editor reasoned through the findings as he questioned the role of the "most race conscious papers" in endorsing "the mechanism for obliterating racial characteristics." Crucially, Johnson noted the lack of autonomy among New Negroes to create their own "modes and fashion." "There are no special Negro styles," Johnson noted as he observed the "penalty of nonconformity" engendered "bitter ridicule." With this view, the journal editor reasoned that when enacted by African Americans and other marginalized people, cosmetic use and ascriptions to dominant standards of beauty formed "an unconscious protest against an inferior status."[101]

Others condemned the desire for "white skin beauty" as a "fake concern." *Half-Century* magazine blasted "some . . . Colored editors" for "accepting ads from white concerns knowing full well that the concerns are selling our people fake preparations." The author chastised "Betrayers of the Race" who sold "fake white concerns" to their readers and admonished newspaper editors for "cheating the Colored people out of what they are paying for." The author also considered how African American women were not immune to the demands of beauty that were shaped by white standards. Rather than condemning African American women who attempted to bleach their skin, the writer reasoned fashion's cause. "They, like all other daughters of Eve, want to do the thing that is most fashionable." Like most white women, the writer continued, "darker sisters" would "rather be dead than out of style." In making this case for the fashion sensibilities of African American women as both modern and natural, the *Half-Century* writer underscored the responsibility of newspaper editors to reject advertisements for products that promised "white skin beauty."[102]

Distinctions between white and African American–owned cosmetic companies underscored the ethics of cosmetic sale and consumption. Rapid changes in science and technology buoyed significant advances in the cosmetic industry and augmented competition in the consumer marketplace. In addition, during the first three decades of the twentieth century, white companies "increasingly impinged upon the black cosmetic market." Historian Blain Roberts explains how more expansive budgets and wider distribution links to drugstores and national chains provided an advantage to white-owned cosmetic companies.[103] Some consumers openly criticized the manufacturing of cosmetics by whites; they underscored matters of health and safety, believing that white-owned companies cared little for their welfare. In a letter to *Half-Century*, Mrs. Mary Vaughan recounted her visit to a white-owned manufacturing plant where she learned how the company's face powder was made. Her guide readily disclosed that rice powder was one main ingredient but was secretive about other components. When asked about her own cosmetic use, Vaughan expressed satisfaction with her regular brand of face powder because "it matched [her] complexion perfectly and always looked smooth."[104]

Apparently she was wrong. Her guide criticized Vaughan's face powder, finding it was "not very good, your face is shining now." Not surprisingly, Vaughan was coaxed into using a "sample box of light brown powder." Happy with the product, she purchased more later, only to suffer distasteful results.

"Within a week," she wrote to the magazine, "my face became sore and in two weeks' time it was covered with unsightly pimples and blackheads." When the white-owned company advised that the breakout was merely a transition process between the products, Vaughan was placated, investing further in the company's "products, soap and cleansing cream." The results were horrific. Vaughan reported, "my skin seemed to have been poisoned in some way." Suffering from "neuralgia and sick headaches," Vaughan fell under her physician's care. When the offending product was examined, Vaughan's doctor found "deadly drugs and deadly minerals, mixed into the very small percentage of rice powder." The ordeal confirmed Vaughan's commitment to "us[e] powder made by members of my own race." She resolved, "If I live a hundred years I will never put any powder on my face that is made by white people. I feel confident knowing that no colored person would knowingly make a preparation that would injure our women's skin." Certainly, Vaughan's letter appealed to the responsibility of manufacturers to produce safe, quality products and declared belief in African American enterprises as businesses that cared for the welfare of its people.[105] By design or fortune, Vaughan's letter appeared next to an advertisement for High Brown Soap, a product made by the African American–owned Overton-Hygienic Manufacturing Company of Chicago. The advertisement proclaimed the safety of its product and boasted attainment of an "acme of perfection in scientific soap-making." The company's founder, Anthony Overton, was also underwriter for *Half-Century* magazine; the clever placement of the letter next to the advertisement could not hurt his business.[106]

Though not immune from criticism, African American–owned companies, along with "manufacturers, newspapers, tastemakers, and consumers," played important roles in casting "hair and skin preparations" in race-positive terms.[107] One of the most successful, the Walker Manufacturing Company, worked to offset criticism through advertising that reinforced the promise of beauty products that are meant to temper social and economic exclusions based on race. The company's advertising refuted accusations of white mimicry and racial self-hatred by marketing these products as treatments for the growth of hair and repair of damaged hair and ailing scalps. Products like the Wonderful Hair Grower promised success as it had for its founder, a washerwoman turned millionaire. Walker's washerwoman-to-millionaire story formed an integral role in the company's marketing approach and open endorsement of capitalist enterprise as a key strategy for social mobility.

Frequently, African American–owned beauty enterprises were also the same ones to filter money back into their communities through the employment of women, civic donations, and fundraising efforts.[108] As historian Tiffany Gill shows, Walker triumphed over her critics through engagement in a "combination of economic opportunity, philanthropy, and institution building," and contributed generously to various African American institutions; nevertheless, her efforts met cool reception from many, and outright contempt by some.[109] Still, by the 1920s, the rhetoric of economic nationalism provided the most tangible justification for beauty culture entrepreneurs.

In Harlem, the business of beauty emerged as an important and visible venture that was scrutinized by white observers. Nancy Cunard, an elite British writer, noted the "innumerable 'skin-whitening' and 'anti-kink' parlors" in the "Negro capital."[110] Another white writer, H. A. Haring, expanded this voyeuristic lens as he described Harlem beyond the well-known vibrant scene of nightlife and cabarets. In 1928, his contribution to the trade journal *Advertising and Selling* provided "first-hand daytime information" on the "buying ground for about 125,000 people" who constituted "the most populous group of Negroes anywhere in the world outside of Africa." Beauty appeared to be big business in Harlem. Within "even half a day," Haring reported his encounter with many window displays for "drug lines" that promised "Brownlight Beauty Powder—lightens the skin."[111] Haring also claimed that beauty parlors were "three times as numerous, in ratio to population, than anywhere else in New York." These parlors beckoned and welcomed patrons with windows that advertised hair straightening and skin whitening through a language of color that privileged brown. Salons advertised the services of "specialist[s] in brown skin" while others welcomed patrons to "come in and become a brownskin tulip."[112]

No doubt Harlem's beauty culture presence exposed the blatant contradictory forces that shaped women's beautifying in the modern consumerist trend. Many profited from marketing their goods and services in a rhetoric of self-improvement that highlighted collective "race progress." At the same time, these very businesses appeared to cultivate white aesthetic standards of beauty, offering services and products for hair straightening and skin bleaching.[113]

Harlem beauty shops ranged from home-based small enterprises to swanky salons and African American–owned beauty shops that were both small and booming. Beauty parlors also represented an important work and social space for women. In 1939, writing for the Federal Writers' Project, Vivian Morris described beauty culture as a profession. Morris reported that the industry "takes care of over fifty percent of Negro professional women" and "suppl[ies] jobs for a goodly portion of the male populace in the role of salesman, advertisers and . . . male beauticians." As she ranked beauty shops into "Average Harlemite," "Theatrical," "Elite," and "Hometown," Morris explained that beauty work was "no bed of roses." Morris reported the view of one "tall operator" who explained her pursuit of training in beauty culture was aimed "to get away from sweating and scrubbing other people's floors." Another beauty operator agreed, "You sweat just as much or a damn sight more." Still, this "short woman" deemed laboring in the field of beauty as "a little better than housework—it's cleaner and you don't have no white folks goin' around behind you trying to find a spec [sic] of dirt." Certainly, the absence of white bosses buoyed a greater sense of independence for these beauty workers, but the constancy of white dominance in the lives of working-class urban women was difficult to avoid. The frustrations recounted in Morris's report highlighted the importance of the salon as a vital haven for working women on both sides of the beauty operator's chair. For example, one beauty worker complained about her clients, finding that not only were "most of 'em in a hurry," but they also seemed unable to enjoy the beauty services she provided without talking about their own work and the white women for whom they labored. Such talk bothered the beauty operator, who complained, "you'd think on their day off they'd forget their madams."[114]

Women were not the only patrons of beauty shops. On her visit to beauty shops in the "Theatrical" area on Seventh Avenue, Morris found one male operator "washing a person's hair whom you assume to be a woman in slacks," and the customer turned out to be a man. Without further critique, she confirmed for the reader, "Yes, the theatrical men and a few non-theatrical men get their hair straightened and waved." Even so, "theatrical men" appeared less commonly than did the female customer, who remained the mainstay of this era's beauty industry. As Morris explained to her reader, the "desire [for] beautiful hair and soft attractive skin" resulted in a number of beauty "systems . . . used by the several hundred beauty shops . . . sprinkled through Harlem."[115]

This responsibility to race also appeared in a long-running advertisement for the East India Hair Grower that in April 1930 proclaimed, "It is the Duty of Human Beings to be attractive" (fig. 2.5). An image of a somewhat plump-faced, middle-aged woman appears in the center; readers of the *Crisis* learned through the photo illustration's caption that pictured here was Mme. S. D. Lyons, representative from the Oklahoma City–based business. Although the company's appropriation of "Madame" was not unique to the era, it did invoke the view of a maternal, married woman, thereby rendering traditional respectability to this beauty. Between the early 1920s and early to mid-1930s, S. D. Lyons consistently advertised its beauty hair-care products in the *Crisis*.[116] For over one decade, the company marketed the jar of hair grower as salve to a host of hair problems that included "falling hair, dandruff, itching scalp or any hair troubles." Marketed as the "best known remedy for Heavy and Beautiful Black Eye Brows," the India Hair Grower also worked to "restore Gray Hair to its Natural Colour." S. D. Lyons appealed to women's sense of "duty" in their efforts to cultivate well-groomed, youthful beauty by taming this host of unseemly hair problems. Indeed, when the April 1930 advertisement appeared to appeal to the "duty" of New Negro women, the advertisement was positioned to follow Du Bois's postscript that espoused the "very definite social value" of modern advertising.[117]

Youthful standards of beauty further defined the parameters of these displays of commodified beauty. Markers of youth, namely bobbed hair and cosmetic use, dominated, but they were also matched by efforts to hide signs of maturity. Gray hair was advertised as a "worry" that should no longer plague women and men who could rely on Eau Denna hair dye; formerly advertised to "anyone" could use the product to affect a "natural" look that would not interfere with other modern processes such as "permanent waving."[118] Another solution for hair problems was advertised through wigs that included the Adeline Wig. For $13.50, the Alex Marks Company of New York City advertised the sale of the handmade "youthful looking wig" that not only affected the short bobbed modern style, but could be also be parted on either the right or left side, thereby suiting individual taste and changing fancy.[119] Certainly African American women were not the only women to face these enticements and pressures. The wide availability of cosmetics and products in broader U.S. culture promised youthful beauty with its practiced cultivation to help characterize the dominant ideal of feminized beauty as it emerged during the early 1920s.[120]

At the same time, brownness was becoming a fashionable trend. As early as the 1890s, the New Woman's burgeoning interest in athletics curried some favor for a healthy, darker complexion.[121] Still, when contrasted with the class-based exultation of "lily-white" skin, the tanned tone was not readily acceptable as stylish, especially in hot and dry climates, as well as in regions of the U.S. South where associations of darker complexions with servile slave status endured.[122] But, by the mid-1920s, after its earlier raging success in France, the "Brown-Skin Fad" grew in such popularity across the Atlantic that "suntanning had turned into a craze" through mass marketing of consumer cosmetic products.[123] Suntanning's faddish growth in the United States was partly in response to tabloid images of French fashion designer Coco Chanel leisurely tanning on the Riviera. A fevered response to dancer Josephine Baker in Paris can also explain the rising appeal of brown skin, although that connection is replete with irony. In 1921, Baker auditioned for Eubie Blake and Noble Sissle's Broadway musical *Shuffle Along* and was measured as too dark

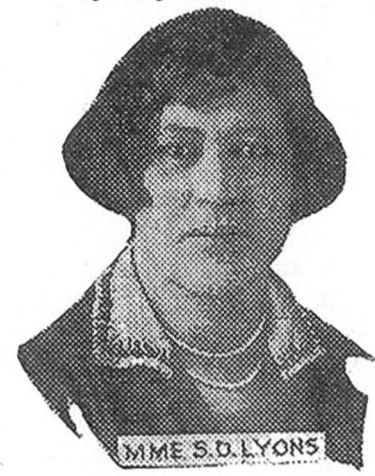

Figure 2.5. S. D. Lyons advertisement for India Hair Grower, 1930 (*Crisis*).

to join the lighter-complexioned chorus line who sang and danced in support of the "Brown-skin" Florence Mills. According to Baker's own account, her dark brown complexion was viewed as a potential upset to the visual impact of a chorus line of "high yella girls."[124]

Indeed, in his review of *Shuffle Along*, Jamaican-born Harlem writer Claude McKay applauded the comedic burlesque show but found "the ensemble a little disappointing and lacking in harmony." In particular, McKay lamented the show's lost opportunity "to accentuate the diversity of shades among 'Afro Americans' and let the white audience in on the secret color nomenclature of the Negro world." While calling attention to "colorphobia" and rumored elitist practices of intraracial color snobbery, McKay was more concerned with presentations of African American life to the white world. Despite deflecting intraracial color discrimination as a declining practice and viewing the "diversity of shades" of African American people as mostly incidental, McKay advocated for more diverse representation in the chorus line: "For, as the whites have their blonde and brunette, so do the blacks have their chocolate, chocolate-to-the-bone, brown, low-brown, teasing-brown, high-brown, yellow, high-yellow and so on. The difference on our side is much more interesting and funny."[125]

Nothing was funny about colorist practices in hiring that were not unfamiliar to those seeking employment in the 1920s entertainment industry. The Cotton Club was among the most notorious. The elite Harlem cabaret catered to white audiences by supplying a steady stream of African American talent, including chorus lines of women who were described as "tall, tan and terrific."[126] Still, this colorism is qualified by cultural critic Jayna Brown, who explains, "the preferential hiring of light-skinned women, was true to an extent, but only to an extent; the women of the chorus line came in all shades of brown."[127] One of those fabled "lucky breaks" brought Baker to the Broadway stage, and to the director's surprise she was a smash.[128]

The tanned brown complexion was a slow-growing trend. At first, the U.S. cosmetic industry was slow to respond, but when it did it acted with a vengeance. The industry flooded the U.S. market with tanning lotions and darker face powders advertised with images of (made-up) brown-skinned Nubian princesses and Indian maidens at once supplying mythologies of the regal, remote, and colonized. Never once was the suntanned complexion marketed in the United States as an emulation of the lowly and local: the African American complexion. Indeed, the racial politics of brownness appeared an ongoing debate. As Peiss notes, "it took the African American press to expose the easy co-existence of the tanning aesthetic with white supremacy."[129] African American *Plain Talk* writer Eugene Gordon poked fun at these advertising ploys, describing these products as "science's latest aid to niggerizing the Nordics." Gordon praised the natural brownness of African American women to highlight the seemingly absurd practice of skin whitening through products such as Madame Walker's Tan-Off, which promised to lighten skin discolorations.[130] Amused at the efforts of white women to "brown themselves" in the name of style, Gordon underscored the temporary nature of these "white brownskins." With some disdain, he noted, "a brownskin is now a badge of distinction, like the bizarre tags that amateur travelers paste on their luggage." Gordon concluded that for some women the trendy embrace of the suntanned complexion existed merely as "a matter of fashion."[131]

Brown complexions became a special feature through the mass marketing of cosmetic products. In her consideration of 1920s cosmetic consumer and business culture, Peiss concludes, "the ideal of brown-skinned beauty was vigorously promoted by the African-American beauty trade."[132] The expansion of African American–owned businesses during the interwar era translated into efforts to attract an African American clientele through storefront service or print advertising; beauty products enticed modern New Negro consumers through the language of brown. High Brown Face Powder, a popular cosmetic produced by the Overton Hygienic Manufacturing Company of Chicago was never marketed as a skin-lightening product and packaging for the product remained free of imaging—no face depicted the color of High Brown. As Blain Roberts notes, Overton himself joked that this absence of image "allow[ed] his consumers to envision themselves as that woman, regardless of skin tone." Despite this democratizing view, the names of the shades of powder told a different story. By the 1930s, women could choose from "brunette, high-brown, pink, flesh-pink, and white," suggesting that the powders were also used for lightening effects.[133] White-owned companies also utilized color-inflected language not merely to lure the consumer but also to present themselves as African American enterprises concerned with racial uplift. The Golden Brown Company used "brown" in the company's title and marketed its cosmetic line in race-positive terms. Advertisements explained that Golden Brown cosmetics would not "whiten your skin—as that can't be done" but would help produce a more even and "bright" complexion.[134]

A different view of this appropriation of the language of brownness explicates its far-reaching appeal. The Kashmir Chemical Company incorporated in Chicago in 1918 employed a "positive approach." Its sophisticated advertising methods referenced color as an important marker of modern beauty. One of the company's five male investors, Claude Barnett, fostered much of the company's "rapid success." Barnett, a migrant from Florida and a Tuskegee graduate, helped found the first press service for African American newspapers in 1916. The Associated Negro Press provided an extensive network for Kashmir. The company's access to influential publications, including the *Chicago Defender*, *Messenger*, and the *Crisis*, facilitated the broad advertising of Kashmir's products.[135]

The Kashmir Chemical Company referenced the distant disputed region of India in its company name while advertisements relied on color descriptors to enumerate complexions, beauty products, and public identities. Complexion dominated as a key concern for the company. Kashmir preparations included a Cream Brown Face Powder that topped its list and was advertised as helping "complexions tak[e] on the charm of color and youth." During the war, the cosmetic company endorsed traditional gender roles for women as advertisements conjured and conjoined beauty with patriotism, depicting women as mothers, nurses, and smiling, caring beauties.[136] Postwar advertising addressed beauty as a practical issue. One advertising brochure questioned "Why Women Want Beauty" and asserted the importance of beauty to a woman's power, explaining, "A woman's appearance has more influence upon her career than any other thing." The "Kashmir Way" promised to teach women to "live in the fullest measure . . . by mak[ing] the most of [their] opportunities to look well."[137]

The natural beauty of African American women was celebrated by Kashmir. One advertising brochure asserted, "There is just as much real beauty in the colored race as in any people of the world if it is properly developed." Kashmir compared the beauty of African American women to their white counterparts, arguing, "Only by the most careful make-up can the Caucasian equal the creamy yellow, the matchless browns, and the satiny, glossy dark skin of the Colored Woman." The company noted that North American climates—so far removed from the "mild, balmy atmosphere of India, Africa, southern Italy, France and Morocco"—were less forgiving to African American hair and complexion and offered various salves as treatment.[138] From this broad vision of people of color, Kashmir asserted that African Americans could achieve beauty with knowledge and proper care. The possibility of "pretty skin and hair" appeared within reach of readers who were assured that Kashmir products were not only "wonderful" and "startling in [their] effect," but also "harmless."[139] Subsequent advertisements dropped references to the safety of their products and assured women of the item's transforming effects, promising, "You won't know yourself in a few days!"[140]

The company forged an internationalist outlook in its very name. When forced to settle a battle over its trademark, "Kashmir," it opted for another reference to "exotic" and distant beauty. Renamed "Nile Queen," the company drew reference to the famous Egyptian Cleopatra, marketing its namesake as "Kleopatra, Queen of the Nile, The World's Famous Brown Beauty."[141] Exoticizing Cleopatra as a "dusky beauty" and a "beautiful creature of African birth," Nile Queen claimed "brown beauty" as the heritage of African-descended women. Kashmir further exploited this internationalist view. In the company's advertising for beauty training and an announcement of a correspondence beauty college, the company boasted of being the "best equipped" in the world.[142] Still, despite listing offices in Paris, Tokyo, and Calcutta, the Chicago-based company had no such foreign offices.[143]

The internationalist vision of women of color also appeared in advertising that appeared before its name change. For example, in November 1916, the "Kashmir Girl" appears in what appears to represent traditional Japanese style (fig. 2.6). Dressed in a kimono, she poses with an Asian-inspired fan; the image of the raced model sits in between two captions that announce, "Skin Beautiful" and "Hair Beautiful." In no way could one confuse the model depicted for a Japanese woman; despite her straightened hair, her complexion, features, and look announce her as a woman of color but perhaps one of indeterminate race background. Kashmir's connection of Asian womanhood to products intended for African American women relied on descriptors of brown skin tones to identify products related to boosting complexions as both youthful, charming, and beautiful.[144]

Another long-running advertisement in the *Crisis* marketed the East India Hair Grower. Appearing on an almost regular monthly basis between 1924 and 1928, an image of the "East India Girl" testified to the abilities of the hair preparation (fig. 2.7). A young African American woman looks out in a three-quarter profile gaze, her features and complexion announcing her racial identity as African American, but her long hair—plaited and falling in one solid braid toward the reader—celebrates darker-complexioned beauty as "Indian" in look and fashion.[145] The very origin of this Indian-inspired beauty was found in the United States rather than on the South Asian continent as the descriptor "East" would imply. The product's creator, Sidney Daniel Lyons, was born in 1861 in the "old Choctaw nation" that would later be reorganized as Perry Cliff, Arkansas. Born to a "full blood Choctaw Indian" woman and a man of "Africa[n] extraction," Lyons concocted his hair grower as the "Texas Wonder." When he moved from Texas to Oklahoma in 1889, Lyons renamed the product East India Hair Grower.[146] For over two decades, Lyons amassed his wealth by peddling the hair grower "over the countryside" in his horse and buggy.[147] At the time of his death in 1942, Lyons had amassed such wealth that news announcing his death at the age of eighty-one described a "valiant, resourceful man" whose "active mind and will to improve his finan-

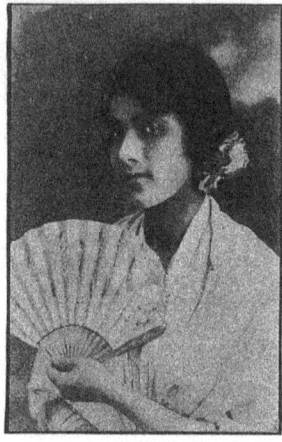

Figure 2.6. Kashmir advertisement, 1916 (*Crisis*).

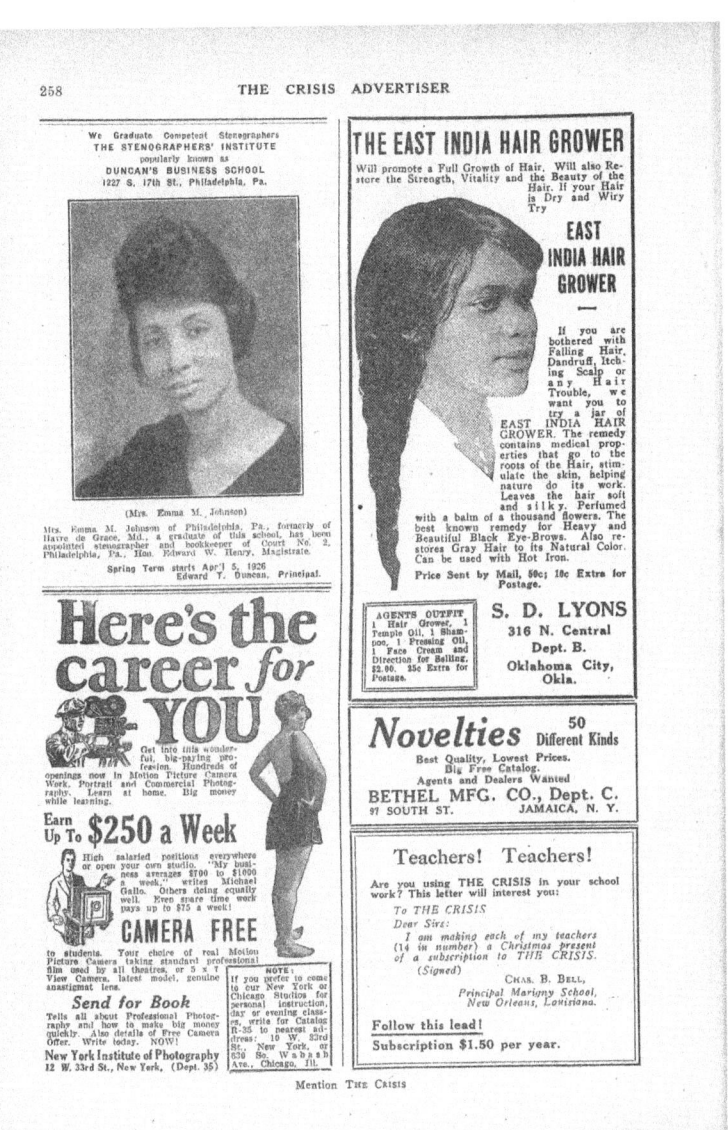

Figure 2.7. S. D. Lyons advertisement for East India Hair Grower, circa 1926 (*Crisis*) and Duncan's Business School advertisement, 1926 (*Crisis*).

cial condition, and those of his race," accorded him the status of "one of the wealthiest toilet goods manufacturers among Negroes of the nation."[148] As the Oklahoma City newspaper the *Black Dispatch* recalled Lyons's great rise from "Texas farm boy," it underscored the importance of the East India Hair Grower to his great achievement. The company's success allowed him to open a grocery store, and later to become "owner of considerable oil holdings" and property in Oklahoma City. Production of the East India Hair Grower was discontinued in 1935 when Lyons turned his attention and profits reaped over the years to focus on investments in oil.

Despite the broad internationalist vision and incorporation of "other" raced women to emphasize modern beauty, the brown-skin beauty ideal remained limited and limiting. Images accompanying the text of these advertisements also challenged the ability of New Negro women to embrace fully—if they so chose—stylized markers of modern womanhood. For example, when imaged throughout the 1920s, consumer-based representations of women's beauty frequently rejected the modern style of bobbed hair, illustrating models with long, wavy hair or the "Indian mane."[149] In this case, long hair did not appear as an emulation of white women's beauty. Rather, it reinforced the connection of long hair with femininity, doing so through the localized and exotic performance of physical characteristics associated with American Indian women.

An advertisement for the East India Hair Grower further challenged readers to consider beauty as individual potential in need of cultivation. Between the late 1920s and 1935, advertising for the product expanded the very definition of beauty. In November 1931, the advertisement read, "Beauty? No, we cannot all be beautiful but we can be neat and attractive. Let Mrs. Lyons show you how."[150] The image representative of Marie Anthony Lyons underscored the connections between good grooming, successful enterprise, racial uplift, and marital status. Certainly advertisements in the *Crisis* that featured images of women expose some of the broader rationale used to present women's applying makeup as both "duty" and strategy for personal advancement. Of course, beauty's tenets buoyed celebration of women's heterosexual appeal, but even more consistently, women's beautifying appeared as testament to preparedness to assume respectable work.

Beauty culture emerged not merely as an expense but also as an avenue for a potential career, a fallback in times of emergency, an avenue for steady income, and freedom from drudged labor; furthermore, training in beauty work offered the advantage of less time-intensive training for women.[151] Indeed, when the back cover of the June 1928 issue of the *Crisis* featured the monthly advertisement for the Walker Company, it proclaimed training in a "few short weeks" at one of the seven branches of Madame C. J. Walker Schools of Beauty Culture; the full-page advertisement offered comparative rates of instruction time and earning prospects in six respectable occupations opened to African American women. The potential income for beauty agents of the Walker system to earn fifty dollars weekly appeared to be double the wages of "stenographers, expert file clerks, and pharmacists." Based on figures supposedly obtained from the U.S. Government Census, the Walker Company determined that their agent generated higher wages than trained nurses who earned an average thirty-five dollars weekly, while "grade school teaching" amassed the lowest regular pay packet of twenty dollars.[152]

Advertisements featuring photographic images of attractive, well-groomed women underscored the value of cultivating a modern look in other types of work. In particular, clerical work dominated as one continuously advertised labor role where images of individual, ordinary women testified to their successful training in this field. Throughout the 1920s, "The Stenographers' Institute, popularly known as Duncan's Business School" boasted of such success through its consistent advertising in the *Crisis*. By August 1928, reporting on "Social Progress," the *Crisis* noted how the resources of the Philadelphia-based institute included "$21,000 worth of real estate," "$6,000 worth of equipment," and a "large library."[153] On a handful of occasions, Duncan's Business School used the image of individuals to tout the success of training at the institute that in 1928 offered "dormitory accommodation for girls." The school extended a broad welcome to all, explaining, "We help anybody—clerical, domestic, or otherwise"; in a sizably bigger font, the advertisement highlighted that its principal, Edward T. Duncan, was now Reverend Duncan.[154]

In March 1926, Duncan's Business School featured a photographic portrait of former Marylander, Mrs. Emma M. Johnson, whose image and story acted as testimony to the success of their graduates (fig. 2.7). Johnson now resided in Philadelphia where her appointment as "stenographer and bookkeeper of Court No. 2," presided over by the "Hon. Edward W. Henry, Magistrate," proved her success not merely in attaining white-collar employment, but doing so in the civil service. The image depicts a somewhat fine-featured, simply styled woman whose upswept hair and unadorned neckline announce a professional look. The following month, Duncan's featured Miss Roberta Carr as another success story by headlining, "They came from the South." Due to her lack of bouffant hair and modern neckline, Miss Roberta Carr appears somewhat less glamorous than Johnson; her simple dress and her everyday hairstyle highlighted a practical, modern look. Her promotion from stenographer to cashier at the Mutual Life Insurance Company of Durham, North

Carolina, appeared to suggest that even in the Jim Crow South, training from Duncan's Business School, coupled with respectable self-presentation, was a winning combination.

Men were also featured as success stories from the Duncan's Business School. In December 1926, an advertisement in the *Crisis* explained the illustrious rise of Herbert C. Nelson, Esq., from stenographer in the U.S. government service to prosperous real estate business owner. Underscoring the opportunities for employment in "government service and business offices," Duncan's Business School framed stenographer training as work suitable for both women and men. Still, the image of a bespectacled Nelson in suit and tie used to accompany the narrative of his ascent to business owner bore little resemblance to the three other advertisements that featured the profiles of women; these women were appointed to civil service positions, but gained no independence as business owners.

Steady, respectable employment certainly endured as one mainstay in the brown-skin discourse on New Negro beauty. Beauty, respectable comportment, and modern dress along with middle-class standards arose to counter to discriminatory hiring practices. In November 1928, a report on "The NAACP Battlefront" that headlined "Color Discrimination in Government Service," featured photographic images of six winners of the California NAACP Popularity Contest, which no doubt acted as a euphemism for a subscription drive. The six diversely complexioned New Negro women smiled out at readers as the value of their monetary prize formed the caption to their image. The article referenced the contentious demand on candidates to furnish a photograph with their applications as the photo discourse of young, smiling, modern New Negro women challenged the embedded assumption that raced bodies were different, unattractive, and distinctly unsuited for integrated work in the modern environment.

Conclusion

By the 1920s, brown-skin beauty developed as a marketing device and consumerist discourse directed at diverse constituencies of urban African Americans. Appropriations of brown beauty featured in newspaper and magazine advertising for dolls and cosmetics, sending crucial cues to girls and women on the significance of beauty, youth, and respectability in defining the gendered identities of New Negro girls and women. Rising in tandem with the broader racialized collectivizing around the modern identity of the New Negro identity, the advertising discourse of brown-skin beauty adhered to, reflected on, and expanded broader cultural, consumer, and fashion trends.

At the same time, brown skin developed into an important gendered synonym for African American women's modern beauty.

Important shifts demonstrate the growing currency of brown skin. It appeared as central to definitions of modern beauty that were rooted in race pride and values that upheld social and economic progress as vital to the advance of the New Negro. First, the marketing of dolls progressed from an emphasis on maternalism and domesticity in the socialization of girls to the celebration of beauty as the doll's chief attribute. Secondly, public debates on beauty presented conflicting viewpoints on cosmetic use despite the clear consensus that African American women were beautiful, too. Efforts to define a beauty ideal erupted through the display of women's self-submitted photographs in newspapers and magazines as they facilitated and reported on national and local beauty contests. Technological constraints notwithstanding, the privileging of light complexions in the physical look of dolls, beauty contest winners, advertising language, and imagery contradicted views of brown skin as a clear departure from whiteness; at the same time, advertisements appeared in major African American newspapers and magazines, making evident the racial identity of women judged as brown-skinned. In sum, the consumerist discourse helped shift the parameters of womanhood from respectable "race woman" committed to the service of home, family, and community to feminized beauty, successful worker, and modern New Negro.

The public imaging of women's brown beauty erupted beyond the back pages of the *Crisis* or amid the pages of mass-circulating newspapers and journals. It formed a central thread in the literary and artistic output of the Harlem Renaissance movement to mark a unique expression forged in the literary arts–based movement. A close examination of representations found in Harlem's literary print culture exposes some of the contradictions, tensions, and critiques embedded in these depictions. It shows how women's bodies were centrally figured as the constant gaze on New Negro women showcased their modern status during a period of mass migration, ongoing racial discrimination, and shifting norms and values around sex and gender. The chapter that follows considers how the visual and textual discourse on beauty and brownness reinforced interpretations of women's beauty along a dominant feminine ideal; at the same time, representations of brown beauty presented potent challenges to racist stereotyping, underemployment, and the political and social exclusions endured by New Negro women.

3

"Of the Brown-Skin Type"

Madonnas, Mulattas, and Modern Women in Literary Print Culture

The heroine should always be beautiful and desirable, sincere, and virtuous. The hero should be the he-man type, but not stiff, stereotyped, or vulgar. . . . Above all, however, these characters must live and breathe, and be just ordinary folks such as the reader has met. The heroine should be of the Brown-skin type.
—George S. Schuyler, "Instructions for Contributors"

In 1928, in a set of "Instructions for Contributors," African American editor, journalist, and social commentator George S. Schuyler advised aspiring writers on what he perceived to be the key formula for those seeking entry into the literary marketplace of Harlem Renaissance fiction.[1] As he advised the author-aspirant, Schuyler warned against the use of colloquial language and "over-artistic" expression, urging the cultivation of an "intimate manner" with one's audience. "Gloomy" subject matter, Schuyler warned, held little appeal for "people [who] have enough trouble without reading about more." He also cautioned against a critique of the white world, reasoning it was better to stick "exclusively" to representations of "Negro life" and African Americans as "ordinary folks," or people with whom they would likely be acquainted. Writers seeking to market their work as New Negro during the late 1920s when interest in this fiction was its height were counseled to veer away from the "erotic" and maintain "clean and wholesome" representations of African Americans in depictions that avoided open engagement with "contemporary moral or sex standards."[2] The brown-skin type appeared the best representative to absorb and reflect the values characteristic of the New Negro heroine. In these editorial guidelines, the brown-skin type was predicated on her object position as both desirable beauty and reliable mate to the fiction's sophisticated "he-man."

Schuyler's "Instructions" described the brown-skin type as a gendered counterpart to the New Negro man rather than a subject unto herself. Her figure embodies a series of characteristics that illuminates a contradictory race politics in relation to African American women's modern and urbanized condition. Schuyler endorsed an older, middle-class politics of respectability for this "heroine," whose "sincerity" and "virtu[e]" offered a "defense" against sexual debasement; at the same time, Schuyler's insistence that the heroine "always be beautiful and desirable" championed a resolutely modern ideal of feminized beauty as gendered quality hosted in the physical appeal of the brown-skin body. In Schuyler's expert editorial and journalistic opinion, the successful enterprise of representing the New Negro woman relied on a modern beauty aesthetic that asserted brown skin as indexical to women's normative heterosexuality; at the same time, the heightened appeal of the brown-skin type forged a buffer against sexual debasement.

Schuyler's "Instructions" were first printed in the "Illustrated Feature Section," a magazine insert that was distributed in forty African American newspapers with an aim to "secure the patronage of nationally advertised merchandise for Negro Newspapers." Published between September 1928 and January 1929 by the white-owned William B. Ziff Company of Chicago, the "Illustrated Feature Section" appears to be one of the earliest print media strategies used by some white-owned businesses and national corporations to appeal to African Americans as modern consumers. Historian Robert Weems Jr. explains how the Ziff Company worked as a "white intermediary" to help white-owned businesses reach the "Negro market" through the "Negro press" when the same efforts by African American newspapers were "ignored and rebuffed."[3] Vishnu Oak's 1948 study of "Negro" newspapers notes how the Ziff Company "partly offset" the "lack of recognition of the Negro Press . . . as an advertising medium," doing so with some success until the late 1930s.[4] As Jeffrey B. Ferguson reports, the magazine's "sensationalistic" content and blatant agenda to lure African American consumers resulted in Schuyler's resignation as editor of the magazine he later characterized as "moron fodder."[5] Still, in 1928, Schuyler found the "Illustrated Feature Section" to be a useful platform to address African Americans as producers of Harlem Renaissance literature rather than as mere consumers of "Camel cigarettes, White Owl Cigars, Lifebuoy soap, Chevrolet automobiles, and Bond bread"—the few major national brand-name products marketed to African Americans.[6]

Schuyler's "Instructions" championed the interest of Manhattan's new publishing houses in Harlem literature. While viewing the literary marketplace as one avenue to socioeconomic progress, Schuyler underscored the still-limited opportunities for African American authors. As George Hutchinson explains, "contrary to the exaggerated accounts of the 'vogue' of the Negro, the overwhelming majority of publishers showed absolutely no interest in publishing the work of black authors." Hutchinson points to an "amazingly small, though historically significant, group of interconnected firms" as responsible for Harlem Renaissance book publishing. These mostly Jewish publishers were relative outsiders to New York City's publishing world; Hutchinson explains their dual interest in promoting works of cultural pluralism and their desire to "disaffiliate 'American' from 'Anglo-Saxon' literature."[7] With this view, Schuyler's advice on crafting the gendered brown-skin type appears as much a strategic brokerage between aspiring African American authors and white publishers of Harlem Renaissance fiction, as it does a mediation on race relations, a term that historian Ariela Gross explains was newly made in the 1920s.[8] Likely finding a broad but disparate audience as it circulated within the pages of forty African American weeklies, "Instructions to Contributors" found second life one year later in an essay that appeared in the *Saturday Evening Quill*. The small-scale publication was financed solely with resources contributed by members of the Boston Saturday Evening Quill Club. This self-described group of mainly "unprofessional" writers included poet Helene Johnson, novelist Dorothy West, and Eugene Gordon, a journalist and writer of fiction. With an annual print run of 250 copies, the journal was not made available for sale until its final issue in 1930.[9] Despite its particular address to a small group of presumably African American Bostonians, the magazine very likely circulated among literati in other urban centers that were engaged in the cultural Renaissance of the New Negro. The *Quill*'s reprint of "Instructions" affirmed Schuyler's counsel.

Penned by Eugene Gordon, "Negro Fictionist in America" assessed the modern literary marketplace that catered to a new white readership. Gordon noted that "until recently . . . Negro fictionists" felt compelled to depict "the hero [a]s bronze or black" with "godly virtue ooz[ing] from his manly pores." "Black," Gordon argued, "was always right. But now the situation is different." Gordon explained how this different situation compelled a reorientation of representation: he mandated a widening embrace of more complex literary characters and greater nuance when depicting interracial interactions between African Americans and whites. Gordon offered no explicit reason why "black" was no longer "always right": there was no open rejection of black as a descriptor of color and character; rather, Gordon hinted at the shift to an alternative set of racialized characteristics as a strategy to access the modern literary marketplace. To these ends, a new directive on color was confirmed by Schuyler's bolstering of the brown-skin type in Harlem Renaissance fiction. As Harlem Renaissance scholar Henry Louis Gates Jr. notes, Schuyler's "Instructions" were "widely circulated among black writers," and within one year this guidance was "ironclad."[10]

The representation of brown-skin types erupted into a dynamic repertoire in Harlem Renaissance print culture, both in text and imagery. This chapter traces that development by studying the gendered tropes that prefigured the emergence of "brown" or "brown skin" in this era's print renditions of modern African American womanhood. First, the image of the "Brown Madonna" materializes as one key representation at odds with the changing status of New Negro women in the modern, urban environment. The chapter then turns to study the trope of the "brown-skin mulatta" as a popular device that projected a series of anxious distortions onto the mixed-race gendered body, doing so during a period of heightened antimiscegenation rhetoric. Finally, the chapter reflects on the more nuanced and diverse imaging of modern brown-skin womanhood and studies brownness as an uneven marker of class, race, and nation that was used to identify African-descended women and "other" non–U.S.-born women of color in Harlem Renaissance print culture.

These tropes are deciphered as separate and distinctly powerful manifestations of New Negro womanhood; they highlight the differently sexed, classed, and gendered meanings accorded to brown complexions in the modern environment. At times, celebrations of these brown-skin types seemingly reinforced old notions of middle-class respectability that revered motherhood, service to race, demure self-conduct and self-presentation as key dimensions of urbanizing "race womanhood." On other occasions, brown-skin types emerged to challenge ongoing racist attitudes that were reinforced by antimiscegenation laws and the racist science of eugenics that defined raced bodies as degraded in their difference. By the late 1920s, Harlem Renaissance literary print culture increasingly featured brown-skin types as mothers, mulattas, and modern women. This embodiment of New Negro women formed a counternarrative to virulent racist stereotyping that justified the continued socioeconomic and political exclusion of African Americans in modern America.

Focusing on the representation of the brown-skin type in Harlem Renaissance print culture, this chapter examines the gendered depiction as it appeared in a range of novels, anthologies, plays, short fiction, and poetry. It also draws on Harlem Renaissance magazines as important places to feature the work of New Negro writers, artists, and commentators. With particular focus on those publications geared toward the urban, educated middle classes, this chapter examines a range of representations produced in the *Crisis* and *Opportunity*, magazines organized by influential organizations, the National Association for the Advancement of Colored People (NAACP), and the National Urban League, respectively. It also studies the *Messenger*, the magazine of Schuyler's association, which reflected the somewhat more militant views of its socialist publishers, A. Philip Randolph and Chandler Owen. In addition to the iconography crafted in these magazines, other critical reflections on New Negro womanhood appeared in specialized journals including *Survey Graphic* and the *Birth Control Review*. Circulating among educated, liberal, reform-minded, radical, socialist, and feminist white and African American women and men, these Manhattan-based magazines offer variegated views of classed, gendered, and raced values, contested and celebrated throughout the decade noted for the rise of the New Negro and the modern New Woman. This chapter explores the artwork, photography, and textual representations of New Negro women as cultural products that, for the vast part, were produced by African American women and men. It studies how writers, poets, and artists utilized the language of color in general and brown in particular to enunciate the modern conflict around class, color, race, and gender. Amid the variety of brown-skin types to emerge, the maternal model set one key coordinate in the middle-class discourse on New Negro womanhood.

Brown Madonna

The original frontispiece to the 1925 critically hailed anthology of the Harlem Renaissance, *The New Negro, Brown Madonna* (plate I.5), in color, vividly depicted the brown complexion of its subject. Edited by Howard University philosophy professor Alain Locke, the collection introduced readers to the New Negro through the visual of a brown-skinned mother and child, heralding the birth of a new era using conventional forms in unconventional ways. This depiction relied on the classical iconographic imaging of the Madonna holding her infant child to signify raced, gendered, and sexed identities as emblematic of the New Negroes' modern condition. In Winold Reiss's full-color portrait—the only one of the two portraits in the anthology to exhibit the color of the subject's apparel—the Madonna is dressed in celestial blue, a color historically associated with the Virgin Mary and with the broader realm of the saintly and the spiritual.[11] While ambiguously gendered and appearing in a soft and clean pinkish-white gown, one may assume the infant child is male as would be consistent with representations of this embodiment of the Madonna (with child); he too is brown in complexion and appears both relaxed and alert as his eyes fix on an object in the distant foreground. The Brown Madonna's dark brown eyes are also averted. Her lowered gaze remains close to the body, asserting distance between the viewer and the New Negro woman who appears as the revered universalized Mother. While nothing of the Brown Madonna's face, body, or hands appears markedly those of a "young" woman, her bobbed hair, which is obviously black as it frames the

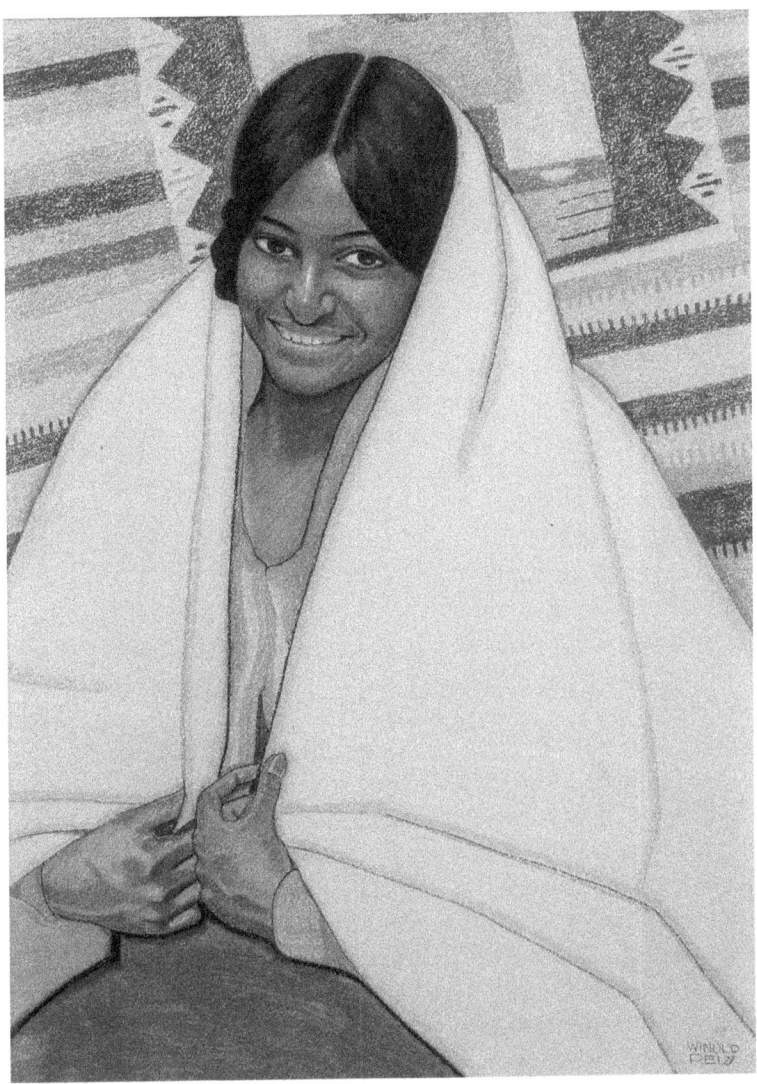

Figure 3.1. Winold Reiss, *Type Study, I* (Ancestral), c. 1924, pastel on Whatman board. Gift of the artist. Image courtesy of Fisk University Galleries, Nashville, Tennessee.

face of a body that is captioned as "brown," declares the modernity of the figure, who remains forthright in commitment to her womanly status as mother.

The name of the Harlem woman and the child she holds who was not her own is unknown to scholars. The portrait was chosen and captioned by Locke, who selected the image from among the thirty-seven portraits produced by Reiss to appear as the frontispiece of the anthology.[12] The portrait of the Brown Madonna mirrored an older tradition found in slave narratives that displayed informative illustrations of the author at the novel's outset. Unlike slave narratives, the portrait of the Brown Madonna carries no name. It was one of the few images of unnamed, non-elite African Americans to appear in Locke's anthology. The depiction celebrated the New Negro woman's primary role as mother; in body and spirit, the *Brown Madonna* appears to represent the racial collective. Capturing and captioning the New Negro woman in ways that positioned women as spiritual mothers rather than smiling mammies, the frontispiece of *The New Negro* celebrated the view of a brown woman holding a brown baby as central to the politics of modern African American womanhood.

Reiss's use of brown as bodily complexion of both Madonna and child and Locke's captioning of the image announce with certainty that this is the color of the New Negro. Brown's emergence as a crucial visual language in an era when the mass communication of ideas and images relied largely on black-and-white print culture highlights the role of artists and editors in helping to configure alternative visions of African Americans. Appearing in 1925 as the first representative image to officially encode the New Negro in figurative form, this portrait powerfully depicted the brown complexion of modern, urban, and race-proud African Americans. Crucially, Reiss's full color portrait and the captioning of the Brown Madonna as "brown" helped make brown distinguishable to the lexicon of the modern eye.

While the Brown Madonna may have helped readers orient themselves to new visuals of African Americans, the ideological construction of New Negro motherhood engaged biological deterministic views of African American women as gendered bodies whose reproductive capacities promised a literal rebirthing of African American culture. This focus on maternity as destiny reflected an older view of reproduction that was premised on the middle-class Victorian valuation of "true womanhood." Motherhood was situated along judgments of women's purity, piety, submissiveness, and domesticity, as womanhood's central defining characteristics.[13] These Victorian values appear to resonate with modern notes. As Anne Stavney demonstrates in her study of "the politics of maternal representation," the era's masculinist impetus sought to "reclaim and desexualize the black female body while also rebutting the corresponding racist iconography of the sexless, nurturing black mother, the black mammy."[14] Locke's celebration of the New Negro presented a rebuttal against these negative aspersions of the black mother by recasting—in language and visual—the black mother as the Brown Madonna.

As revered as she appeared, the *Brown Madonna* illuminated few of the decade's protracted concerns over falling birth rates or the reproductive politics of birth control and abortion. Between 1890 and 1930, birth rates declined among white and African Americans. Whereas white women birthed an average of five children during the 1860s, that number, by 1920, fell to three; among African American women, birth rates dropped from seven children during the 1870s to an average of three or four by the 1910s. Although variations across class, region, and occupation influenced the number of live births among African American women, birth rates remained lowest among urban dwellers and college-educated women.[15] Particularly after World War I, with the growing flow of native-born migrants to urban centers, reactionary concerns over "race suicide" emerged among both African Americans and whites, doing so with very different rationales.[16]

As Linda Gordon explains, the panic over race suicide developed as a backlash against changes in the lives and choices of women that began with the social purity campaign for "voluntary motherhood" during the 1870s. Although voluntary motherhood did not disassociate maternity from marriage, it did specify the socioeconomic and physical conditions for successful mothering.[17] By the first decades of the twentieth century, declining birth rates among white Americans sharpened fears of "race suicide" that were fueled by anti-immigrant sentiment; women's modern status as political subjects; and women's relative growing access to education, public forums, and medical interventions such as birth control and abortion.[18] White Americans who scrutinized declining birth rates among African Americans reinforced racist views of racial inferiority as they indicated untamed sexual desire and poor health and hygiene as the main causative factors. Historian Jessie M. Rodrique challenges this stultifying view of African Americans showing how "ideological bias and research design have tended to foreclose the possibility of Afro-American agency, and thus the conscious use of contraception."[19] As Darlene Clarke Hine argues, as a modernizing force, the Great Migration enhanced women's deliberate and active choices to limit fertility and reproduction.[20] As it facilitated greater access to birth control for broadening groups of women, urbanization played a crucial role in the modernizing trend of lower birth rates among women.

No doubt, women practiced birth control for a range of reasons, but aspirations for greater freedom clearly impinged on the choices made by migrating and urbanized women. Some elite women, such as Alice Dunbar-Nelson, expressed narrower views, denouncing the use of birth control as a means to "preserve . . . economic independence." Dunbar-Nelson indicted "the more cultured and more leisurely classes" for the "sharpest decline of the peak" in falling birth rates among African Americans and held younger women as particularly responsible. While she applauded their interest in "the new Negro" and recognized the capacity of younger people to "do big things," Dunbar-Nelson cast a dim view of these "race-loving slips of girls and ardent youths" who advanced distorted views of "freedom of the individual and the rights of the Negro." To emphasize her point that youth held a skewed commitment to progress, she railed, "No race can be said to be a growing race, whose birth rate is declining."[21] The Bureau of the Census reported on a shrinking African American population, noting changes from 14.1 percent in 1860 to 9.9 percent in 1920. Dunbar-Nelson was not alone in articulating a view of race suicide.[22]

Race suicide reflected eugenic concerns over the breeding of better or superior human beings. Among whites, the precipitous decline in reproduction heightened nativist worries about being overrun by immigrants, African Americans, and "mixed-race" others; after 1921 and 1924, with the closing of doors to America's "new" immigrants, this concern turned more sharply to African-descended people and the so-called "mongrel" groups that increasingly populated urban landscapes.[23] While not departing entirely from concerns over "better" bodies, African American elites, race leaders, intellectuals, churches, and secular organizations engaged more directly with ideas of racial progress under the rubric of race suicide. Frequently emerging as the central focus of these debates were urban middle-class, educated, and professional women; protests against race suicide either rarefied or vilified New Negro women as potential mothers of the race.

In 1925, the same year that Locke's *New Negro* appeared in print, another Howard University academic vocalized concerns over the changing status of women, underscoring the threat of race suicide. Biological deterministic views of women's bodies and sexist interpretations of their duty to the race collective emerged in the views of some elite African American men. Writing in the *Messenger*, Harlem writer J. A. Rogers evaluated the comments of Howard University's Dean Kelly Miller, critiquing his view that "the liberalization of women must always be kept within the boundary fixed by race." The Jamaican-born Rogers applauded women's growing independence: "I give the Negro woman credit if she endeavors to be something other than a mere breeding machine. Having children is by no means the sole reason for being."[24]

Like much else in the 1920s, men dominated the public discourse on women's reproductive rights. As Jamie Hart shows in his examination of the writings of African American intellectuals between 1920 and 1939, issues of demography, eugenics, public health, and theology were critical to debates on either side.[25] In particular, African American intellectuals emphasized women's responsibilities to the racial collective as they underscored the avenues to fulfillment that matched little with women's growing independence, freedom of movement, and increasing access to birth control and abortion in the urban environment. This is not to say that women were silent on the subject, but questions about freedom of expression linger. For example, Alice Dunbar-Nelson's denouncement of young, urban, educated women as responsible for falling birth rates is complicated given her own status as a thrice-married, childfree, professional woman and her personal writings that reflect the "deference and dissemblance uplift ideology imposed upon black women." Kevin Gaines's sensitive analysis of the "everyday struggles and contradictions of uplift ideology in the life and writings of Alice Dunbar Nelson" cautions against accepting too readily her political commitment to this stance on reproduction. Gaines argues that "within uplift, black women cannot exist for themselves, but only insofar as they serve the utilitarian project of race building." Gaines complicates linear readings of Dunbar-Nelson's view on women's reproduction by underscoring the "status benefits of voicing... outmoded, if not oppressive, ideas" that equated "the patriarchal family with respectability and bourgeois stability."[26] As we shall see in the chapter that follows, Dunbar-Nelson was not unlike other women who wrote creatively during Harlem's Renaissance. The vital characteristics of age, occupation, marital status, and sexuality at once limited and expanded opportunities for acceptance into respectable circles of the literati as premised by women's performance and articulation of middle-class tenets of New Negro womanhood.

In other places, elite and upper-middle-class African American women also reinforced women's maternal role. Between 1924 and 1928, the *Messenger* ran a monthly series dedicated to "Negro Womanhood's Greatest Needs." The series took the form of a symposium "conducted by the leading Negro clubwomen of the United States," offering elite and middle-class reformers a new space for racial uplift efforts that were now honed and presented within the journal as modern self-help strategies. Contributors including Mrs. Bonnie Bogle of Portland, Oregon, reinforced the bourgeois characterization of the modern African American woman as a cheerful homemaker, socially committed race woman, and patient, gentle wife. As Bogle reminded readers of the *Messenger* forum, this New Negro woman "never forgets her tender womanly and great motherly heritage."[27]

Race leaders of this era also espoused motherhood as an important marker of womanhood, but when "envision[ing] a 'future' woman," prominent race leader W. E. B. Du Bois pictured one who "could enjoy unrestricted access to education, financial independence, and motherhood at her own discretion."[28] Despite this feminist reasoning, Du Bois's advocacy for birth control, like for some other members of the African American middle class, was tied to elitist ideals of race progress rather than the eugenic embrace of "race suicide."[29] Others, including Blanche Schrack, the white associate editor of the New York–based *Birth Control Review*, defined the aim of the journal's September 1919 issue as educating "colored mothers [who] are no more able to help themselves than are white women under similar circumstances."[30] While Schrack appealed to white middle-class women's "obligation to aid them to make their lives decent and livable,"[31] African American writers, social commentators, and creative writers also emphasized moralizing, classist judgments against working-class and working-poor urban and rural African American women and men.

Unable to produce an article for the special issue on birth control, Du Bois wrote to acting editor Mary Knoblauch reaffirming his "very firm" belief in "birth control." In lieu of a longer essay, Du Bois provided a short verse that highlighted the moral dimensions of race progress: it began, "Save us, World Spirit, from our lesser selves!"[32] This moral vision of birth control was also reflected in the *Crisis*. One 1931 advertisement in the journal showcased a handbook and directory for birth control clinics, thereby offering readers a chance to locate those of "professional standing . . . in th[is] work." Positioned below advertising for "Modern Sunday Schools," the advertisement for the birth control handbook seemingly adhered to core principles of Christian spirituality and self-help education that, under Du Bois's founding editorial leadership, the *Crisis* regularly espoused as markers of modern womanhood.[33]

Modernization of the African American condition was a central concern for the socialist-leaning *Messenger*, whose editor, Chandler Owen, also advocated for birth control through the rhetoric of race progress. In his interview with white birth control advocate Margaret Sanger and editor of the *Birth Control Review*, Owen reinforced elitist attitudes and moralizing judgments on modernity's influence on African American women. His perspective on "Women and Children of the South" justified "limiting the number of children born to Negro mothers" to "afford opportunities for education and more time and money for a general improvement in conditions." Owen emphasized "material" gain as not only better access to food, housing, education, and clothing, but also as means for southern cultural development. He continued, "When people have more money and fewer children, they read, go to theatres, take small vacations, travel a little, and—of great importance—they engage in athletics."[34] Owen found urban, educated, and presumably middle-class women less inclined to view "gratification of desire" as the mainstay of their interactions with the other sex. By reference, Owen applauded "Negroes in cities today." In Boston, Philadelphia, New York, Washington, and Baltimore, Owen claimed: "it is difficult to find the more intelligent Negro woman who have any children at all." In contrast, the backwardness of southern women surfaced with their narrow ambitions that foregrounded "marriage the sole aim of existence" and the "fear of becoming an old maid" appeared as "a serious problem" to this cohort of women. Despite his touting of material gain and access to leisure and consumer culture as an index of modern race identity, Owen castigated this gendered anxiety as "a capitalistic institution, having its roots in the desire to be 'respectable,' to leave legitimate children who can inherit property."[35]

In this same issue, women's creative writing highlighted the material, physical, and psychological effects of motherhood. Among the nonfiction commentaries, short fiction also addressed the birth control cause. Angelina Weld Grimké, whose poetic expressions of sexuality, brownness, and womanhood feature in the next chapter, contributed a short story entitled "The Closing Door." Written especially for the *Birth Control Review*, the short story appeared in two parts beginning with the September 1919 special issue.[36] Narrated by a self-described "yellow scrawny, unbeautiful girl" named Lucy, the story follows her friendship with Jim, "a brown, good-natured giant with a slow, most attractive smile and gleaming teeth" and his wife Agnes Milton, who is not described by color but by "the wonderful quality of her soul." The twenty-five-year-old Agnes is supported by her husband's "easy money," but as Lucy notes, "Oh! [Agnes] didn't love the money for itself but him for trusting it." The distinctly modern note of companionate marriage appears most celebrated, but despite this happy, modern partnership, unwrought by economic deprivation, squalid living conditions, or immoral sexual behaviors—the typical concerns of elite and middle-class reformers in their efforts of "racial uplift"—the reader is warned, early in the story, that the couple's "happiness will not last."[37] Agnes's pregnancy, while first a blessing, coincides with the horror of lynching. Upon learning of her brother's brutal murder in Mississippi, Agnes withdraws from the world around her and descends into darkness. The story ends tragically as Agnes sees herself as a "cursed" "instrument of reproduction!—another of the many!—a colored woman—doomed!—cursed!—put here! willing or unwilling! For what? to bring children here—men children—for the sport—the lust of ... mobs."[38] The door closes unhappily with infanticide at Agnes's hand, her subsequent mental breakdown, and death.

"The Closing Door" portrayed the harsh realities of lynching as physical and psychological violence against African American bodies transcendent of gender, place, or social status. The story also highlights how male-oriented crises helped situate the concerns of the race in the first decades of the modern era. African American women's activism against lynching, especially as terrorism rooted in antimiscegenation hysteria and efforts to protect "white womanhood," melded further with efforts for re-emasculation of the New Negro in the post–World War I era. As historian Nikki Brown shows, these concerns resulted in "black women's activism" shifting more "tightly [to the] prescribed roles in the era of the New Negro."[39] Furthermore, as historian Clare Corbould explains, "women, mostly writers, . . . saw how the ideology that linked mother and home made it impossible to speak truthfully about the conditions in which black American women lived, trying to hold together families in mostly adverse circumstances."[40] Indeed, Grimké's short story, which foregrounded women's reproductive politics, appeared against the backdrop of continuing agitation for passage of the NAACP-sponsored Dyer Anti-Lynching Bill.[41] In "The Closing Door," Grimké highlighted the modern era's link to an enslaved past as Agnes's desperation and mental instability leads her to infanticide in an effort to break the violent cycle of domination, ownership, and control.

Maternal status also found little celebration in women's creative writings. As feminist scholars Hazel V. Carby, Thadious Davis, Cheryl Wall, and Ann du Cille demonstrate, African American women shaped their own expressions of womanhood that considered the complex intertwining of sex, race, class, and gender and often reached different conclusions on motherhood.[42] Women novelists of the Harlem Renaissance demonstrated little interest in motherhood. In the novels written by Nella Larsen, Jessie Fauset, and Zora Neale Hurston, independent women are largely childfree and unconcerned with maternity as they search for (predominantly heterosexual) sexual pleasure, intimate love, and sexual subjectivity. When children are produced, as in Larsen's *Quicksand* (1928), they weaken the biracial brown body of the protagonist, Helga Crane, who verges close to death. And, as Angela Davis notes, other powerful voices of the period, namely those of blues women, also eschewed the reproductive trope.[43] Certainly blues women and women writers addressed different class- and race-based audiences, but it is notable that when representing womanhood during the 1920s, both groups of cultural producers failed to celebrate motherhood or to position maternity as central to women's sexual and social identities. Further removed from hagiographic depictions of women as Brown Madonnas, women's poetry reflected a broader range of emotive, intellectual, and individual responses to the classed, racial collectivizing effort that positioned women as guardians and mothers of the next generation. In a diverse set of cultural expressions, color materialized as a metaphor to facilitate divergent positions on maternal matters. During the Harlem Renaissance, poetry emerged as one important expressive means to do so.

"'Tis a noble gift to be brown, all brown," declared the opening line of "The Bronze Legacy," which appeared as one of two poems positioning motherhood as subject in the "Child's Number" of the *Crisis* in 1922. The poet Effie Lee Newsome (1885–1979) celebrated the racial legacy of youth through positive associations with color.[44] Bracketed with a dedication "To a Brown Boy," "The Bronze Legacy" advised,

> 'Tis a noble gift to be brown, all brown,
> Like the strongest things that make up this earth,
> Like the mountains grave and grand,
> Even like the trunks of trees—
> Even oaks, to be like these!
>
> To be brown like thrush and lark!
> Like the subtle wren so dark!
> Nay, the king of beasts wears brown;
> Eagles are of this same hue.
> I thank God, then, I am brown.
> Brown has mighty things to do.[45]

Triumphant, resolute, and proud, the poem invokes qualities engendered traditionally as male as it pronounces the "mighty things" awaiting brown skin's doing. Like the "king of beasts" and the "trunks of trees," impending brown manhood, or boyhood allusion to manhood, appears as mighty, powerful, and inordinately tasked to function in meaningful ways. The speaker of the poem also claims brownness for themself. If read as a woman's voice addressing a "brown boy," Newsome's lines, "to be brown like thrush and lark! / like the subtle wren so dark!" perhaps most clearly appear as imagery gendered as feminine. The poet then offsets the warmth and independence of the bird-like with robust, masculine imagery: "Nay, the kings of beasts wears brown / Eagles are of this same hue." In this reading, the speaker of the poem's happy claim to brown relies on less subtle displays of brownness as she reasons and rejoices, "Thank God, then, I am brown."[46]

"Bronze" appears in the title of Newsome's poem where the color brown performs the central task of identifying racial identity. As seen in the previous chapter, this conflation of bronze and brown was not uncommon to the era. In literary works of the period, bronze was frequently employed as a linguistic derivative of brown to describe glimmering and majestic bodies, sometimes emphasizing mixed-raced people as African American under the broad umbrella of colors perceived as lighter than "black." In Newsome's poem, the use of bronze as "legacy" hints at more precise meanings of this color descriptor. Here, it suggests the winnowing of mixed ancestry to more fulsome visions of the darker-complexioned brown body as modern representative of the New Negro.

Another poem on motherhood was published in the "Child's Number" in April 1922. Georgia Douglas Johnson's "Motherhood" appeared alongside aside Newsome's "Brown Has Mighty Things to Do." This poem struck a vastly different tone and position on "race motherhood" and gendered guardianship. Douglas Johnson, a conservative and respected "woman's poet," employed the formulaic representation of New Negro woman as a potential mother to reject the role; the speaker warns, "Don't knock at my door, little child / I cannot let you in." The poet soothes the unborn child in her reinforcement that it is not a lack of desire for birth and life that motivates the speaker from barring its entry to a "world . . . of cruelty and sin," but rather the speaker's interest in protecting "my precious child" from "monster men / inhabiting the earth."[47]

A wife and mother, Douglas Johnson was possibly the poet who most clearly adhered to the identity of New Negro womanhood in her public embrace of the role as literary hostess, and as "lady poet" of the era.[48] Douglas Johnson, one of the few women poets who was both married and a mother, captures the overall place of motherhood in women's creative writings. Women's reproductive politics appear to be framed entirely within the era's racial ideology, and the poet endorses a conservative stance that positions the imagined welfare of the unborn child over women's independent choice to become, or not become, mothers. During an era of increasing popularization of birth control, declining birth rates, and feminist politics buoying modern notions of America's "New Woman," the poem "Motherhood" hints at a rejection of women's maternal role, pointing to an important shift in African American women's reproductive politics.

Black rather than brown appears to be the color descriptor of choice in a poem that embraces motherhood while acknowledging harsh constraints on maternal status. Anita Scott Coleman's "Black Baby," published in *Opportunity* in February 1929, invokes blackness in the poet's pragmatic, yet romanticized imaging of motherhood. The poet's voice reveals,

> The baby I hold in my arms is a black baby
> I toil, and I cannot always cuddle him
> I place him at the ground at my feet

> He presses the warm earth with his hands...
> I watch to discern which are his hands
> Which is the sand
> Lo... the rich foam is black like his hands.

Here, blackness finds connection to the "earth" and "sand," which in their natural brown tones are framed as black displayed at the hands of the child. The speaker of the poem is pragmatic about her inability to comfort her child due to back-breaking labor that appears reminiscent of slavery.

Yet, told in the modern voice, the speaker reinforces her commitment to the black baby, who, though mired with his mother's toil and economic struggle, looks at her with promise. The poem ends: "My black baby looks at me / His eyes are like coals / They shine diamonds." Juxtaposing the blackness of coal as "costly fuel" derived from men's sweated labor, and commodity paid for by her own, with the glimmering hope of "diamonds" the black baby's mother finds her ultimate worth in the gaze of the black boy. Her willingness to venture forth into motherhood, despite hostile conditions, redeems her as a New Negro woman.[49] Herself a married mother of four and one of the few women of the era to publish their own collections of poetry, Coleman championed the black baby.[50] Still, brown bodies, rather than black, found broader celebration as New Negroes in their distancing from the drudged and impoverished conditions so frequently connected to the representative Old Negro, materializing most powerfully in the literary and visual trope of the brown-skin mulatta as a bridge to this divide.

Brown-Skin Mulatta

Readers may hardly recognize Winold Reiss's portrait of Elise Johnson McDougald (plate I.2) as the mulatta figure who seems to dominate the visual and literary landscape of Harlem Renaissance cultural production. McDougald's brown-skin color, unfashionable hairstyle touched with grey, and shapeless body garment, out-of-step with the narrow lines of modern clothing, underscores her distance from figurations of the modern mulatta whose youth and sexualized beauty permeates most representations. Displays of mulatta womanhood rarely engaged with these complex personal histories that situated race, class, and gender conflicts as unduly burdensome not only for New Negro women of mixed ancestry, but also for white working-class women who entered into partnerships with African American men. Certainly, Reiss's portrait of the educator could not possibly convey this complicated past, but the image of McDougald transcends reductionist views of the mulatta even as the portrait appears in *The New Negro* as the only representation of a woman of mixed ancestral heritage. Yet, the brown-skin mulatta figure dominated the period's representations of New Negro women in the decade when the very classification of "mulatto" ceased to exist. Developed from an older antebellum literary convention, the mulatta was a readily recognizable literary character who frequented the pages of 1920s Harlem Renaissance fiction, poetry, and plays. As the boundaries that officially measured white and African American mixed-ancestry status eroded by 1920, the mulatta figure endured as a key gendered trope in Harlem Renaissance representations.

A testament to the era's heightened political debates, shifting definitions of race, and interracialism of Harlem's movement of arts and letters, the mulatta figure also reinforced the binary of racial difference established by the past generation. The mulatta thereby served two important purposes in crafting this era's representative ideal of womanhood. As Hazel V. Carby explains in her groundbreaking work, *Reconstructing Womanhood*, the mulatta figure operated in an intermediary capacity; her ability to move between the races, in a period when such movements were increasingly proscribed, provided writers with creative latitude. Carby explains the role as "a vehicle for an exploration of the relationship between the races and, at the same time, an expression of the relationship between the races."[51] By employing the mulatta convention, authors enabled white readers to envision the workings of their own privilege, and the distinct lack of opportunity among African Americans. Furthermore, the mulatta figure's movement between the two worlds, and her struggle within those realms, permitted the African American literati to reflect upon their own advantage as elite, middle-class, frequently lighter-skinned urbanites. This multivalent nature of the mulatta partially explains her literary popularity.[52]

African American women writers often employed the mulatta motif as a readily recognizable literary convention and least offensive literary image available to writers to depict African American womanhood in the era of the New Negro. Other accessible literary models involved "Topsy," the impoverished, oppressed girl-child stereotype made famous in Harriet Beecher Stowe's 1852 abolitionist fiction, *Uncle Tom's Cabin*. As well, the desexualized mammy, whose image modern New Negroes rigorously worked to depose, first appeared between 1820 and 1852 "in southern plantation fiction, memoir and religious propaganda." By the 1890s, the mammy became increasingly distorted in terms of "complexion, dialect, and size" to reflect much of the heightening sentiment of Jim Crow in that era.[53] Finally, another nineteenth-century convention interpreted enslaved and African-descended womanhood through the stereotype of the oversexualized Jezebel whose circumspect class origins and insatiable sexual appetite were also frequently made apparent through her biracial, often light-complexioned body.[54]

By the Harlem Renaissance era, these older tropes dissipated neither in full nor in part. Still, an alternative figuration of New Negro womanhood endowed the modern mulatta figure with middle-class appeal. As Cherene Sherrard-Johnson astutely observes, "there was something feminine and flexible" about the mulatta that made her "irresistible to authors."[55] Writers including Jessie Fauset and Nella Larsen reworked the conventions to reflect their own creative visions and modern-day concerns. While they did so in different ways and with different emphases, both authors used the mulatta to indicate a dualism of mind and body, of societal expectations and sexual subjectivity. Both women were of mixed ancestry but occupied vastly different footholds within the community of Harlem's literati. Fauset, born to an elite Philadelphia family, and Larsen born to a Scandinavian mother and Afro-Caribbean father, both underscored the mulatta's modern tragedy as residing less in her warring physical body and more in the problematic of her outsider status in the various social worlds she inhabited.[56] For example, in *Passing*, a 1929 novel that won Nella Larsen wide acclaim, one central character, Clare Kendry, appears light enough to pass for white, although that "passing" is ultimately doomed.[57] Such representations remained close to an older, nineteenth-century convention. As Michelle Wallace explains, in literature of that era, characters that appeared almost white were the "only kind of mulattoes who seem to matter much."[58]

Still, modern representations of the mulatta relied only partly on descriptions of complexion in literary texts. People of mixed ancestry were also made visible by qualifiers of "dark" and "light" that proclaimed color as value rather than hue. For example, in 1922, poet Georgia Douglas Johnson, a child of two mixed-raced parents, described her poem "The Octoroon" in terms that seem to quantify rather than qualify color as complexion.[59] The poet writes, "One drop of midnight in the dawn of life's pulsating stream / Marks her an alien from her kind, a shade amidst its gleam." No doubt by referencing the "one drop rule" that by southern law and custom categorized race by "blood," this poem rejects the false construct by adopting a modern classification of race through color. In the last lines of the two-stanza verse we find a somewhat concrete reference to color as the poet defines the octoroon's plight for peaceful sanctuary: "For refuge, succor, peace, and rest, she seeks the humble fold / Whose every breath is kindness, whose hearts are purest gold." The poem evokes the idea of color in several ways without ever granting color a name; when it does so, it appears as gold—a glimmering, gleaming metal that is also associated with light rather than dark in its yellow base. Yet, the poet relies on "midnight" and "dawn" to imply that color is found in the "shade" or "gleam."[60]

When identifiable by skin color or complexion, the mulatta is frequently described as "light brown," "very light-skinned," or "creamy colored." At times, light-brown-skinned women also embodied the mulatta; Zora Neale Hurston's protagonist Janie Crawford in *Their Eyes Were Watching God* (1937) faces no emotional or physical struggle to choose between white and African American worlds despite her difference within the male-dominated space of Eatonville. Herself described as a "brown skinned.... striking woman," Hurston seemed less concerned with describing Janie's complexion than she did with attending to the crowning glory of her protagonist.[61] Hair, more so than complexion, appears to be the central feminized and sexualized characteristic that marks Janie as a New Negro woman and intimates further at the crucial variables of time, space, and place in determining the role of complexion in African American communities both real and fictional.

In other places, especially in stories of racial passing, brown complexions portend the inability of characters to pass for white. For example, in Jessie Fauset's *Comedy: American Style* (1933), Teresa, a light-brown-skinned girl relates to her mother the day's happenings at school; she tells how her friend Phebe, who all believe is white due to her fair complexion, confessed: "I belong to the black or Negro race."[62] Teresa's color-conscious mother, Olivia, who has championed her daughter's friendship with Phebe as the girl's "ethereal fairness" and "thick straight cap of pale gold hair" appeases Olivia's anxious and destructive colorism, is horrified by the "idea of a girl as white as [Phebe] saying that." Teresa explains, "Phebe showed [the teacher] a picture of her mother. She wears it in a locket around her throat all the time. And her mother is colored. Not black, you know Mamma, but real, real brown." Olivia understands "real real brown" perhaps *too* well; in the opening chapter of the novel, Olivia's friend urges her to leave the white world behind and join her in Boston. In this early scene, we learn of Olivia's disdain for any potential male Bostonian suitor. "All of them black or brown," she raged.[63] In this way, brownness signified the inability to pass for white even as it worked to denote biracial, triracial, and other mixed ancestral and ethnic immigrant identities. *Comedy*'s adult Teresa absorbs her mother's destructive colorism and pleads with her suitor Henry to "pass for a Mexican" in their new married life. Henry, a proud New Negro, is horrified at such suggestion, and *Comedy*'s omniscient narrator reports his bodily response: "Under his bronze skin he was ashen." Passing is unfathomable to Henry, and Teresa's willingness to do so renders the relationship unworkable; he leaves Teresa behind, heartbroken.[64]

Comedy: American Style shows how the insidious nature of colorism threatened the social and psychological well-being of the modern generation; here, too, Fauset signals the happy balance of brown. Indeed, while Olivia encourages her daughter's friendship with Phebe due to the girl's light complexion, she also censures Teresa's friendship with another girl, Marise, because she is brown-skinned. While Phebe must courageously announce her raced identity, and Teresa appears a character constantly anxious about her own light-brown complexion, Marise is described as a self-assured "nut-brown" girl who "can sing and play and dance. . . . and think up such smart things to say."[65] In *Comedy: American Style,* Fauset makes clear the gendered, generational, and classed issues shaping these concerns over color that first erupted during girlhood.

Whiteness was also used to describe the mulatta, but usually indicated when she was fair enough to pass with ease, although such passage was usually temporary and doomed. African American authors, and Harlem Renaissance authors, in particular, updated the convention, employing it differently from their white counterparts. In her address of fiction published between 1900 and 1930, Judith Berzon clarifies, "in the white version. . . . the mulatto usually dies; in the black version, he is summoned back to his people by the spirituals, or their full throated laughter, or their simple sweet ways."[66] By the early 1930s, writers empowered their light-skinned characters. This included poet Countee Cullen whose character Constancia Brown, an upper-class woman, resists "passing" for white—the crucial dilemma haunting the mulatta figure.[67] Indeed, as the official designation of "mulatto" disappeared from official terminology, the older, declining "mulatto elite" conceded authority to a new African American middle class. Many urban literati helped form this cohort of new authorities. Many had roots in the mulatto elite, but they openly rejected colorism as the New Negro movement embraced the diversity of shades seen to constitute African America.

However, as the literary role of color matured into a powerful visual language to announce an optics of inclusion when judging bodies of color as African-descended, other members of Harlem's literati sharply critiqued exclusions forged on judgments of color. Wallace Thurman, a young radical novelist, editor, and playwright who was also a bisexual man of dark skin tone, authored one of the rare novels where a dark-complexioned woman appears as the central figure. Published in 1929, Wallace's satirical novel, *The Blacker the Berry,* follows the tale of Emma Lou Morgan in her self-deprecating battle against intraracial color and sex discrimination. As Thurman moves his character from Boise, Idaho, to college in California, and to the pulsing streets of Harlem, New York, he portrays Emma Lou's dwindling self-esteem and internalization of inferiority as a response to intraracial color discrimination.

Among the range of judgments censuring Emma Lou's dark-brown body, beauty continually emerged as the most crucial dimension. Considering herself lucky to have been blessed with "a beautiful head of [straight] hair," Emma Lou pays singular attention to camouflaging her dark skin. While working as a teacher, Emma Lou quickly assesses the complexion of her colleagues to find that "the darkest was a pleasing brown." Determined not to be the darkest among them, Emma Lou relies heavily on cosmetics. She fails to see that her overuse of whitening cosmetics renders her a laughingstock at the school. Her oversensitivity to color and fragile self-esteem internalizes this mockery as an aspersion against her dark complexion. So dependent on cosmetics, Emma Lou cannot understand that "she was being discussed and pointed out, not because of her dark skin, but because of the obvious traces of an excess of rouge and powder which she insisted upon using." When she receives an anonymous letter suggesting "that she use fewer aids to the complexion," Emma Lou dismisses it as a joke: it "never occurred to her that the note told the truth and that she looked twice as bad with paint and powder as she would without it."[68]

Thurman critiqued the excess dependence on cosmetics and skin-lightening attempts by presenting Emma Lou masking her own image to the point where she cannot see her own reflection clearly. Unwilling and unable to find beauty in her skin color, Emma Lou strives to create an artificial complexion in closer approximation to the "pleasing brown" that appears throughout the period as an acceptable standard of aesthetic beauty. Descriptions of Emma Lou's preening and priming the skin for whitening effects border on the ridiculous. These scenes show Emma Lou eating arsenic wafers, using bleaching creams, and applying peroxide solutions, all in the hopes of lightening her skin. The process so blinds Emma Lou that she does not see her skin taking on an "ugly purple tinge"; rather, she believes these efforts "made her skin less dark."[69] These exertions to lighten her skin were all directed at appropriating an aesthetic of female beauty celebrated by some African Americans, like the light-skinned circle into which Emma Lou was born. These attempts to achieve an unattainable ideal of beauty distort her self-image, rendering her view of self as an unattractive, dark-skinned woman. While part of her effort at applying makeup was directed at attaining a more positive self-assessment, another obvious intent was to increase her sexual attractiveness.[70] In Thurman's fiction, Emma Lou struggles but finally approximates a degree of self-acceptance; with resigned pragmatism she understands, "she could strive for change of mental attitudes later. What she needed to do now was to accept her black skin as being real and unchangeable."[71]

Dark-skinned female characters were rare when compared to the modern mulatta who featured prominently in fiction, poetry, and imagery of the era. As Shane White and Graham White reflect, the political consciousness of the era "also entailed a deliberate and prideful display of black bodies, particularly those of women, in a manner that transcended white hoary stereotypes."[72] Cultivated in part by the rising militant consciousness and energies of the post–World War I period, the task of Harlem's literati task of representing New Negro womanhood was infused with a gendered urgency. As the imagery of New Negro womanhood acquired a more central position in the period's race politics, the public display of New Negro womanhood demanded greater responsibility.

The *Crisis, Messenger,* and somewhat less often, *Opportunity,* reflected the cultural nationalism dominant in the agenda of the Harlem Renaissance by regularly featuring portraits of women as gendered "race" ambassadors. In 1924, in the same year that the masthead of the *Messenger* shifted from its claim as "The Only Radical Negro Magazine in America" to "The World's Greatest Negro Monthly," the magazine promised its readers to "show in pictures as well as writing, Negro women who are unique, accomplished, beautiful, intelligent, industrious, talented and successful."[73] Throughout the 1920s, the display of genteel beauty, femininity, and accomplishment appeared central to respectable womanhood's visual trope. Harlem Renaissance literary journals pridefully featured on their covers illustrations and photographic images of women and frequently highlighted their genteel status when doing so. Within the magazine, editorials combined with images to report on women's beauty, education, service, and talent as proud attainments of New Negro women. As literary critic Nina Miller explains, captions and taglines touted women's individual accomplishment, "often reading like 'society' pages, publishing credentials and connections of the elect."[74] Still, complexion endured as a key motif in the representation of New Negro women.

Elite and upper-class women, many of whom were considered light-skinned, were utilized as icons of racial achievement because their very existence contradicted the beliefs of a prejudiced society; their realization of class and respectability—attained in spite of their race—triumphed over all possible odds. As literary critic Nina Miller explains, this imaging of light-skinned bourgeois women was a double-edged sword—the public nature of these representations "threatened to erode the very class-bound dignity it was intended to project."[75] The light-skin bourgeois symbol of the New

Negro Woman required a counterpart to absorb negative attention. Miller demonstrates that the representation of New Negro womanhood was "split to become two diametrically opposed figures: the 'exalted Negro woman,' icon of bourgeois gentility, and the primitive 'Brown Girl,' icon of racial authenticity."[76] Despite the oppositional construction of the "bourgeois woman" and the "brown girl," both images reinforced dominant views of modern African American womanhood. The first image—the exalted bourgeois woman—was the face of the race that adorned the covers of Harlem Renaissance journals. Respectable and responsible in her womanhood, this icon displayed a genteel, light-skinned, and feminized image of womanhood. The second image—the "brown girl"—offered a salve to this respectability and fulfilled popular perceptions of "primitive" female sexuality; her darker skin, youthful body, and lack of genteel status epitomized the primitive passion popular in imaginings of the authentic "Negro." According to Miller, the existence of the brown girl allowed the bourgeois woman to retain her social status, for the former "often absorbed the potentially degrading sexual implications which paradoxically emanated from the genteel woman's 'exalting' [public] performances."[77] These seemingly oppositional gendered figurations embodied traits favorable to the enterprise of re-presenting the modern public identities of New Negro women as respectable beauties.

Apparently, the photographic covers of lighter-skinned women did not always win open admiration. Arna Bontemps recalls the appearance of Regina Anderson on the cover of *Messenger* magazine in 1924 as a notable moment but discloses no particular fanfare around the imaging. Anderson, though still largely an unknown figure, contributed to the Renaissance movement in ways that Bontemps describes as significant.[78] She moved from Chicago to Harlem seeking "liberation . . . to discover her race womanhood," but as Nathan Huggins reveals, the "pert olive-skinned" girl seemed out of place, finding it "difficult to fit into the comfortable and complacent middle-class society that was expected of New Negro ladies."[79] Her roommate and friend, Ethel Ray Nance, who migrated from Duluth, Minnesota, to Harlem to work for Charles S. Johnson and *Opportunity* magazine, was also a fair-skinned woman whose beauty, Bontemps tell us, "was too fair to reveal her true identity in that black-is-beautiful environment."[80] Appropriating language that reflects black consciousness of the post-1965 era, Bontemps's recollection nonetheless invokes the spirit of the 1920s New Negro movement that embraced the dark complexions of African-descended people. By this Harlem-based standard and by his account, women like Anderson, or perhaps more so like Ray, did not appear as the best representatives of New Negro womanhood since their lighter complexions belied their status as African American. The discernibility of race by color appeared through the marrying of two different tropes.

The sentimental portrait of the light-skin mulatta and the eroticized display of the brown-girl provided a foundation for the fusion of these notional strands of racialized beauty in the literary imaging of African American women. By 1928, George Schuyler's "Instructions for Contributors" described the brown-skin type as the modern composite of an increasingly standardized representation of New Negro womanhood. As literary representations underscored the influence of complexion in shaping an ideal of modern womanhood, this imaging borrowed on and updated older gendered representations, doing so with intonations to the urbanizing circumstances and race collectivizing demands that confronted elite and middle-class New Negro women. The brown-skin type also transcended these modern tropes of motherhood and mulatta-hood and emerged most powerfully in visuals of the era. Certainly this imagery erupted in multiple spaces, but throughout the 1920s the enhanced prominence of brown-skin womanhood on the covers of *Crisis* magazine deserves special attention. This chapter's final section turns to study a diverse set of visuals that underscore the centrality of feminized brown-skin beauty. As a means to showcase the respectability of modern African American women, this imagery worked as a positive protest to advance the integrationist agenda of the *Crisis* under Du Bois's editorial leadership.

The Modern Brown Woman

Between January 1920 and December 1930, representations of women surpassed any other imaging of New Negroes on the *Crisis*'s monthly covers. Children were also commonly depicted on the magazine covers, but those displays were largely linked to the annual children's issue, and apart from that special issue, such imagery rarely depicted New Negro children and youth as independent subjects. In some instances, the Madonna figure reaffirmed the maternal body as necessary, and in doing so displayed the continuous gendering of girls and women from infancy to maturity. From its beginning and throughout the 1910s, the journal celebrated the accomplishments of New Negro men in its regular "Men of the Month" feature, but men were not commonly featured on its cover. By the era of the Great Depression, shifts in race collectivizing politics heightened even further the plight of men. At this point, women did not disappear from view, but the imagery of men increased in the print media's mass visual landscape. Other common variations away from the representation of women included the December issue, which regularly relied on illustrations to depict religious Christmas scenes; with these exceptions, covers of the *Crisis* were largely dominated by illustrations and photographs of New Negro women throughout the 1920s.

Between January 1920 and July 1924, *Crisis* cover art, though alternating between illustrations and photographic images, relied more heavily on hand-drawn images. Illustrations, like photographs, were solicited by the magazine and submitted by readers in response to the magazine's ongoing open call. Rejection letters to artists often included advice or explanation. For instance, Irene Baker of Dayton, Ohio, was advised to develop her talent as a painter by pursuing "an intensive course of study under an accomplished instructor."[81] Other responses to submissions underscored the practical limitations of reprinting artwork in the *Crisis*. In what appears to be a second rejection of her work, a letter authored by Du Bois explained to Martha Lucille Winston of Washington, D.C., that despite his great interest, "the expense of color reproduction is so costly just now that it will be some time before we would dare undertake it." Du Bois did not discourage the artist: "Some time in the future," he wrote, "when you have something that would make a good cover for the *Crisis* . . . send it . . . and let us see what we can do."[82] Unfortunately, Winston's subsequent submission failed to impress; a second letter (addressed by the *Crisis* rather than by Du Bois) rejected her artwork with the simple explanation that it was "not suitable for our purposes."[83]

Illustrations judged fitting for the covers of the magazine were produced by a number of professional artists, including Roscoe C. Wright, Laura Wheeler Waring, Aaron Douglas, Alan Freelorn, Bernie H. Robynson, Joyce S. Carrigan, D. Norman Tillman, and Vivian Schuyler.[84] The diverse styles of these artists produced a range of images for the magazine covers, although commissioned artists were also asked to edit their work according to the tastes of their editors. For example, in a 1919 letter to Laura Wheeler, Du Bois wrote to "retur[n] herewith one of the pictures which you made for Jessie Fauset's story." While "excellent," Du Bois noted that the magazine's new literary editor did "not like the young lady's face" and asked Wheeler to "fix [its] front line."[85] While it is difficult to know the precise problem of this "front line," the letter underscores a very literal dimension of the role of the magazine's editors in shaping the representation of New Negroes. Clearly, Wheeler heeded the editor's suggestions. For two decades, Wheeler was one of the magazine's most consistent illustrators.

Editors also solicited the work of artists. In December 1925, Du Bois wrote to Winold Reiss, noting the artist's "sale of reproductions of portraits of Negroes." The *Crisis* editor explained his intention to report on Reiss's work in a forthcoming issue and emphasized that such coverage "would help tremendously in the sale of these portraits." Du Bois was particularly interested in reproducing what he termed the "Madonna." He asked Reiss to "borrow the plate" to allow a reprint of the image for a future cover.[86] The image of the Brown Madonna never appeared in the *Crisis*, and no response to Du Bois's request has yet been found.

From July 1924 onward, a steadier stream of photographic images appeared on the magazine's covers. That year's annual education issue portrayed a woman graduate in cap and gown who, as the table of contents revealed, was "A Master of Arts" from the University of California. With a pleasant smile, the young woman, seated with diploma in hand, looks over her shoulder with quiet pride in this significant accomplishment (fig. 3.2). The image underscores some meaningful shifts in the magazine's modern imaging of women where ordinary-looking women of less ordinary accomplishment helped endow new meaning onto modern womanhood at the same moment that photographic renditions more consistently graced the magazine's monthly covers.

Photography itself was presented as an alternative modern employment and respectable profession for New Negro women and men. For at least two decades, Du Bois had personally espoused photography's potential in influencing and shaping new visions of African-descended Americans as U.S. citizens. At the Paris Exposition in 1900, Du Bois supplied 363 photographs for the American Negro Exhibit, the majority of which were uncaptioned images of unnamed people.[87] By October 1923, Du Bois encouraged the involvement of "young colored men and women" in this "fine and paying career." Du Bois underscored the unique strengths of New Negroes in this role, arguing, "The average white photographer does not know how to deal with colored skins and having neither sense of their delicate beauty of tone nor will to learn, . . . makes a horrible botch of them." The added incentives of "good incomes and excellent social service" elicited Du Bois's questioning, "why are there not more colored photographers?"[88]

Cover art for the *Crisis* offered a rare view of African American subjects as captured by what one might assume was a cadre of African American artists and photographers whose names were not always pronounced; frequently, the magazine's table of contents revealed only the name of the photographic subject. One early cover depicted a long-haired beauty in sensual dress and pose, and credited the image simply, "After a Photograph, posed by C. M. Battey."[89] The caption inferred a steamy dimension to the very work of being photographed, thereby hinting at the early problematic of the association of women's modeling with a compromised moral standard. The photograph sets

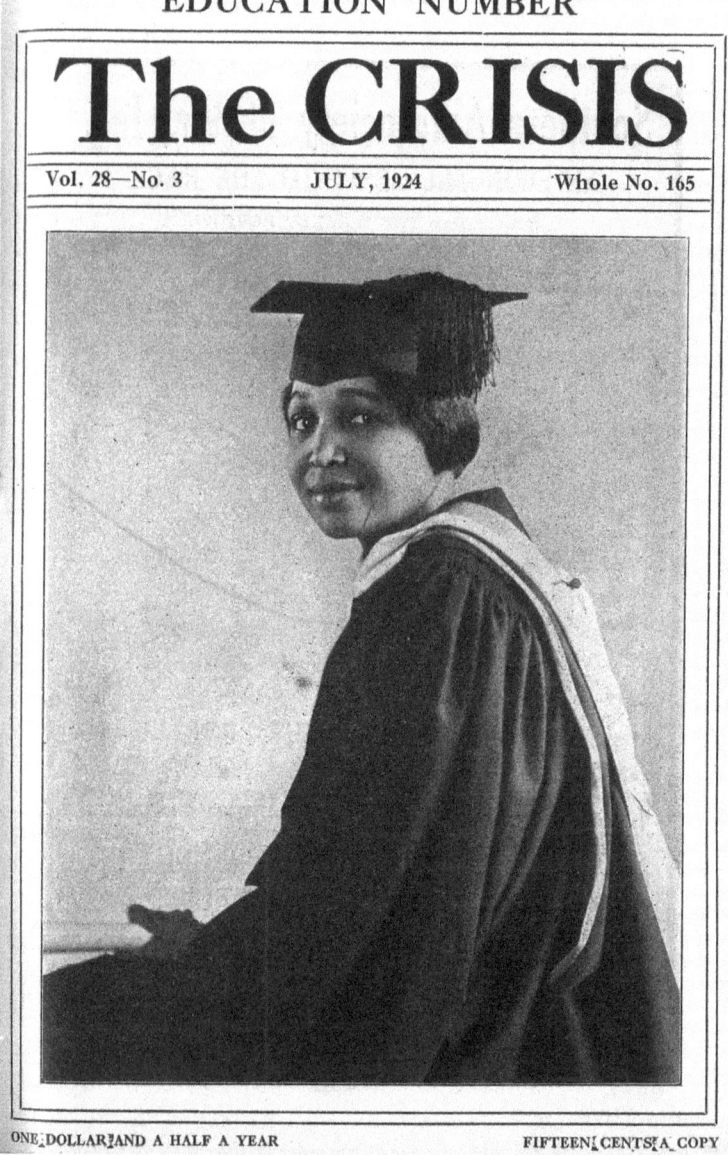

Figure 3.2. "A Master of Arts," *Crisis* cover, July 1924. Courtesy of the Crisis Publishing Co., Inc.

its subject in seemingly biblical or ancient times; a gourdlike object appears in the background, while an urn helps prop up the woman who, seated on the ground, looks into the distance and light. Sexual and sensual in her bare shoulders, beaded necklace, and draped clothing, the subject's religious posturing acquires redemption through this supplicant, sultry pose.

As well, beauty mattered. Cherene Sherrard-Johnson finds that, despite their lofty goals, Harlem Renaissance journals frequently relied on a "colorist conception of beauty and femininity" by prefiguring "mixed- and ambiguously raced women" on its covers and pages. According to these findings, the visual index of "light-skin" pronounced an elitist beauty ideal that discriminated against other African Americans based on classed associations with color.[90] No doubt lighter-skinned women attained a sizable share of this era's magazine coverage, but when searching through a decade of the *Crisis* cover art, a more complex view of New Negro womanhood challenges totalizing perceptions that women of light complexions dominated the era's representations in literary magazines. Despite their print image appearing in black and white, and the subjective nature of judging the "color" of complexion, women whose diverse complexions could well be categorized as "brown" were common in illustrations and photographic images. Modern women were imaged in numerous ways; three key groupings help organize the visual discourse of modern brown-skin womanhood as it began to emerge during the Harlem Renaissance era.

Youthful, feminized, and sexualized beauty characterized one significant series of representations of infants, girls, youth, and adult women. These depictions often relied on markers of hairstyle and texture, fashionable clothing and accessories, and skin tone. For example, in October 1922, the photographic image of a very light-complexioned girl child with wavy brown hair graced the cover of the annual children's issue. Perhaps the child, Valdora Turner, appeared white to many readers in 1922, as she might well seem to readers in the twenty-first century. Turner peered out at her audience, her head and shoulders bare except for swaddling cloth that modestly protected her chest, torso, and lower body from view. Adorned simply with a gold bangle and pendant crucifix, the photograph of young Turner professed degrees of modesty, religiosity, and material acquisition that also circulated as key tenets of African American identity during this era. Although Turner's ambiguously raced image graced the cover, the magazine pages revealed a compendium of values, norms, practices, and expectations. While the magazine never identified complexion or color as a prerequisite to respectable comportment, such imagery asserted a dutiful path to individual achievement in the name of race progress.

The children's issue ran almost continuously as a special edition of the NAACP magazine from October 1910 to 1934, the year of Du Bois's resignation. The issue interspersed a continuous display of African American babies, children, and youth from across the country with reflective and critical essays on a range of race issues. Historians Gregory Dorr and Angela Logan consider the special issue's heightened embrace of an "assimilationist eugenics." They demonstrate how the photographs of fit and healthy babies provided a "scientific counter narrative" to white eugenicist propaganda on the degenerate bodies of African American people.[91] As Daylanne K. English shows, Du Bois admitted that the photographs featured were secured through a selective process, but he softened these exclusions for the benefit of readers. In the 1914 children's issue, the *Crisis* editor explained how the photographic submissions provided a bounty of evidence of racial progress through the "larger and larger class of well-nourished, healthy, beautiful children among colored people."[92]

By the second decade of the twentieth century, the NAACP joined the popular trend of hosting baby contests that Daylanne English describes as the magazine's "most starkly eugenic feature."[93] These baby contests reflected the broader popularity of "Better Baby" and "Fitter Family For Future Fireside" contests that reached the height of popularity in white America by the late 1920s.[94] Historian Molly Ladd-Taylor explains, "Baby beauty pageants and parades were a popular form of working-class entertainment in the nineteenth century, but in the 1910s health reformers invested them with the higher moral and scientific purpose of combatting infant mortality."[95] Known as "The Tenth Crusade," the NAACP's baby contests ran between 1924 and 1934. They formed a central dimension of the NAACP's assimilationist agenda and played a vital role in fundraising to support the organization's antilynching campaign.[96] Much of the preliminary and ongoing work around the baby contest was orchestrated by Field Secretary William Pickens, who encouraged the activism of parents with reference to "brown babies." Official announcements and appeals to local branches for their participation rationalized the need for this ongoing fundraising, Pickens declared: "The Tenth Crusade is still on, and will be on as long as there are Brown Babies and Color Prejudice."[97]

Photographs of finalists were published in the children's issue as evidence of the fitness and health of the New Negro to form "a visual and literary blueprint for the ideal, modern black individual."[98] Parents, guardians, and other adults contributed photographs of children, very likely responding to monthly editorial selections, suggestions from professional photographers, and to their own modern sensibilities and preferences. Historians Shane White and Graham White describe a dizzying pictorial of "babies on the cover, pages with sixteen photographs of black babies, half-page shots of babies, babies in cute outfits, and even naked babies arrayed on rugs," and surmise how the magazine helped to "create a style in which young black children were henceforth often snapped."[99]

The *Crisis* regularly featured images submitted by New Negroes throughout the nation and readers responded enthusiastically to calls for photographs. So great was this response that the editor ruminated on the "heart-breaking work" of selecting for reproduction only half of the three hundred photographs submitted by "fond parents." Citing the limits of "space and . . . purse," Du Bois assured parents that images omitted were "just as striking and beautiful."[100] However, as the decade wore on, Du Bois sharply upbraided members of the community intent on self-aggrandizing publicity for their individual accomplishments. In February 1930, Du Bois scolded those who lamented "My Picture Did Not Appear." As he reminded readers that the magazine "exists to work for the uplift of twelve million American citizens," Du Bois begged sarcastic pardon from those whose "picture is omitted, or your effort forgotten or unknown" in "the storm and stress of this work."[101]

Beauty appeared as one dominant thread in the life cycle of New Negro women. The *Crisis* cover in October 1925 showed the second prizewinner of the NAACP's baby contest. Clad in white dress and bonnet, Ermine Casey Bush of St. Louis, Missouri, posed with a hand-held mirror as she looked to the foreground, likely meeting the eyes of the adult photographer and/or parents or guardians standing close at hand (fig. 3.3). Ordinary in her brown complexion, the child is posed to appear mindful of her own image: the immaculate dress confirms this effect demanded time and attention. Another cover appearing three years earlier featured the "Photograph of Misses Dents."[102] These two young girls, presumably sisters by their similar look and the comfortable closeness of their bodies, also appear as "ordinary" African Americans whose "real" complexions may very likely have been qualified as brown. Sober colors dress both bodies, but the hairstyles they don and the necklines of their clothing—though differently styled were both made of white lace—suggests age differences between the two that appear, at once, notional and significant. The apparently younger Miss Dent wears her hair in two rolls in a short style. She looks out with neither smile nor serious pose, but seems slightly forlorn; the older sister leans into her younger sibling, half-smiling at the viewer. The older, dimpled Miss Dent wears a more mature hairstyle, and her scoop-neck lace collar announces a womanly femininity. By contrast, her sister's girlishness is framed in a sailor-suit-type neckline that retains its gendered-as-female look through its white lace.

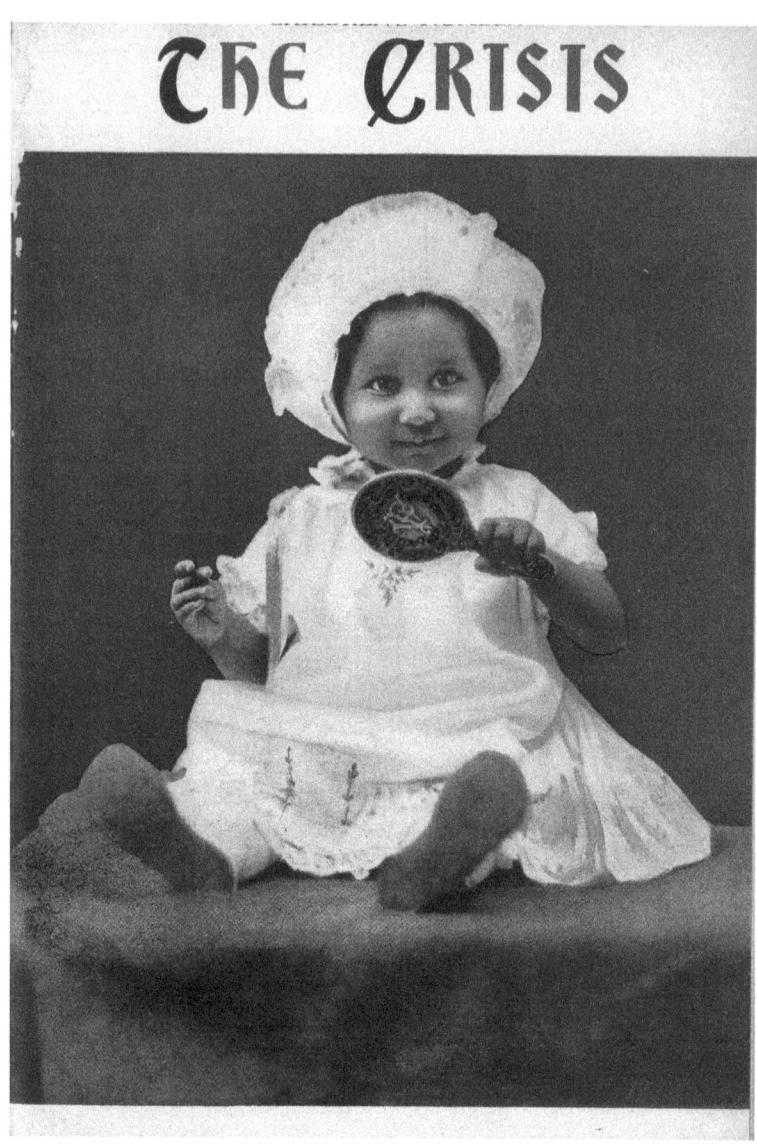

Figure 3.3. Ermine Casey Bush. *Crisis* cover, October 1925. Courtesy of the Crisis Publishing Co., Inc.

As it appeared in the *Crisis*, a photo discourse on the gendered life cycle of New Negro women affirmed an ascending hierarchy of color. Images of babies, youth, and women display somewhat greater acceptance for "average" or "ordinary" brown complexions in youthful years, but displays of womanly beauty show a chronologically associated celebration of women who, while increasingly of lighter complexions, nonetheless remain visibly racially "different," and in this sense, brown. Two covers, "Study of a Negro Girl" (fig. 3.4) and "Photograph from Life" (fig. 3.5), appearing respectively in July 1925 and November 1928, celebrated light-brown-skin beauty in its portraiture of unnamed women of apparent mixed ancestral heritage. Through the accoutrements of fashion and style, age is challenged and ordered in these depictions. No doubt the bobbed haircut, long stringed necklace, and dangling earrings help the "Negro girl" approximate the appearance of an adult woman; at the same time, her soft, sweet smile and interested though not bold look at the viewer mostly reveals her as a "girl." As well, November 1928's cover, simply titled a "Photograph from Life" offered a lively display of a young woman with neatly groomed short black hair and dressed in a fresh white bodice. Her smile is both suggestively knowing and strained as she looks askance into the foreground. Both images, while also relying on technical manipulation of lighting, capture youthful womanhood through the fashion and style as well as through their subjects' visibly not-white bodies.

Women's sensual beauty most boldly appeared in illustrations, but in November 1925, a "Photographic Study of the Head of a Negro Woman" powerfully captured the beauty of its subject through the display of her long hair (fig. 3.6). With her back to the viewer, the young woman appears in three-quarter profile as her averted eyes look slightly upward. Neither fair nor dark-skinned, this woman also appears to fit this era's visual imagining of "brown," but in this case, hair more than complexion emerges as the dominant marker of her status as New Negro woman: long hair that is beautifully textured falls down a seemingly bare back, doing so without apology or conceit. The captioning of this spectacular portrait appears to suggest an element of anthropological study and a positive learning outcome for any considered attempt to deny the beauty of African American women on the basis of hair. The unusual cover offers an oppositional view of African ancestry in photographic depictions of New Negro womanhood as they appeared in the *Crisis* during this era. One other image—an illustration rather than a photograph—complements this oppositional pose, while also presenting hair as a fundamental medium to display respectable feminized beauty. In July 1927, "Drawing from Life" (fig. 3.7) portrayed a young girl clearly marked as

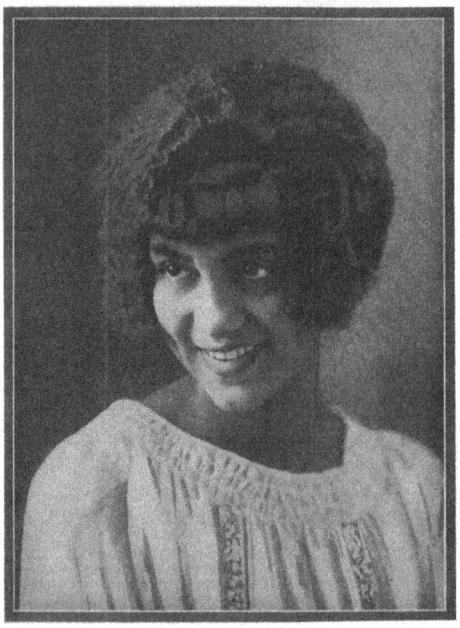

Figure 3.4. "Photograph from Life," *Crisis* cover, November 1928. Courtesy of the Crisis Publishing Co., Inc.

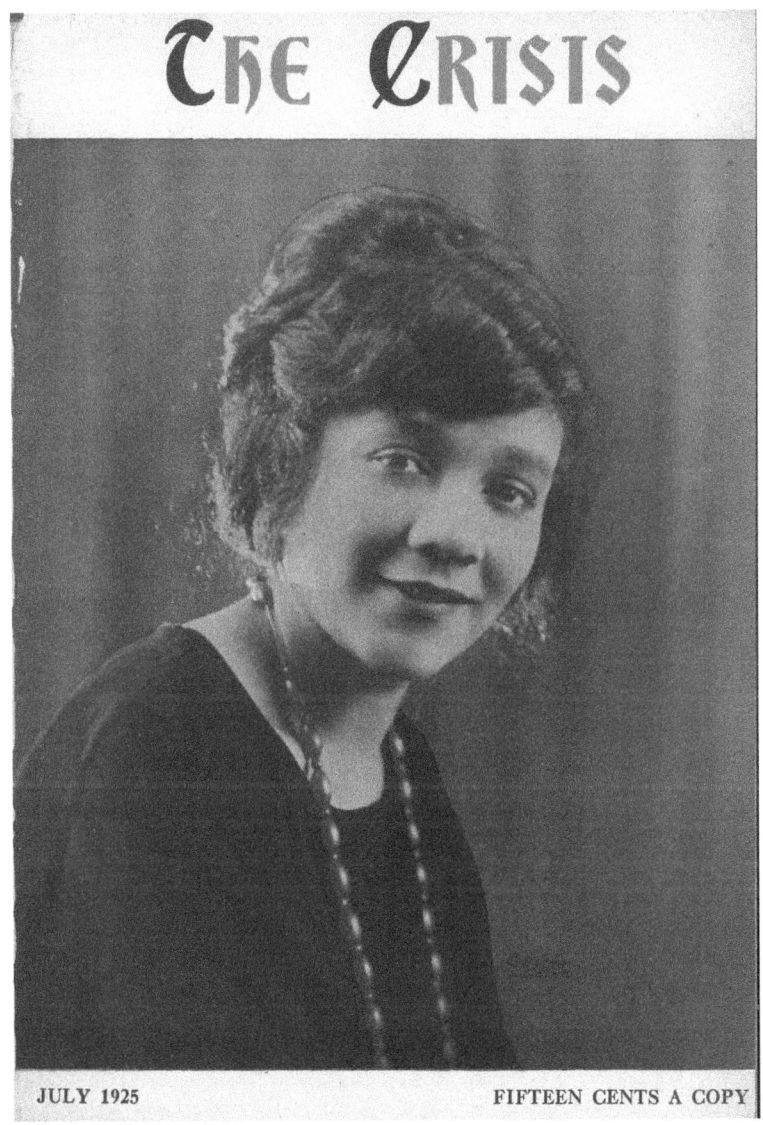

Figure 3.5. "Study of a Negro Girl," *Crisis* cover, July 1925. Courtesy of the Crisis Publishing Co., Inc.

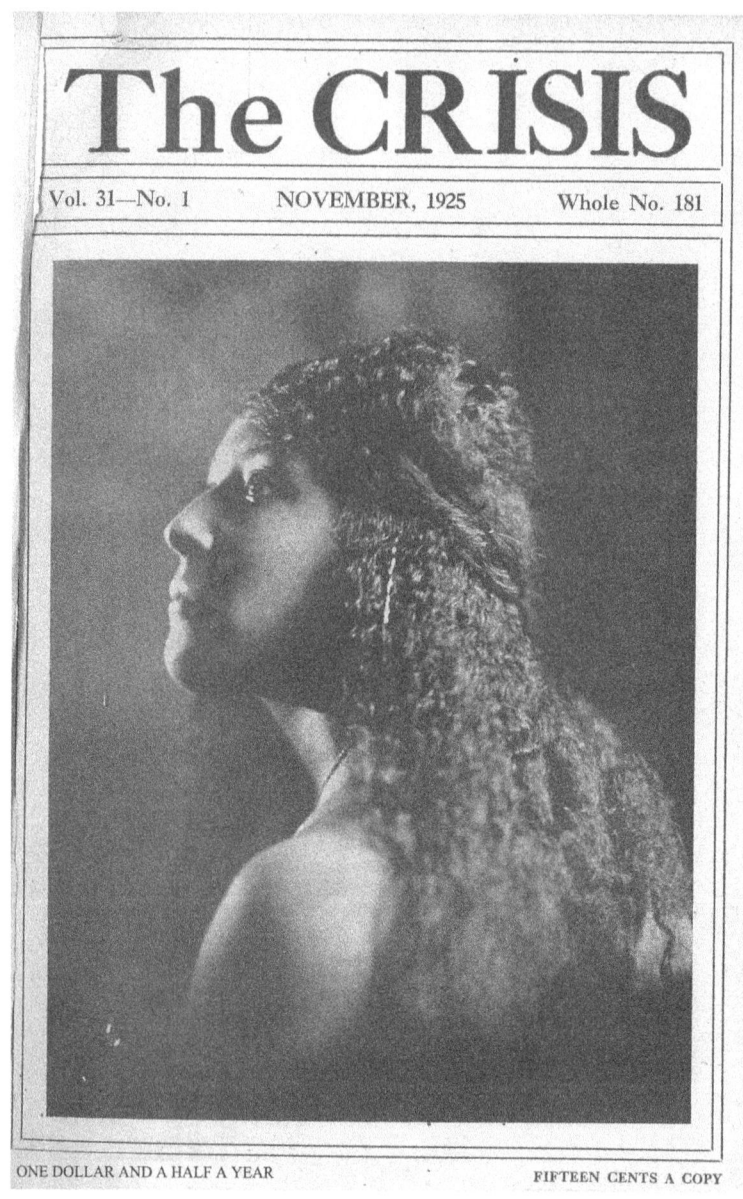

Figure 3.6. "Photographic Study of the Head of a Negro Woman," *Crisis* cover, November 1925. Courtesy of the Crisis Publishing Co., Inc.

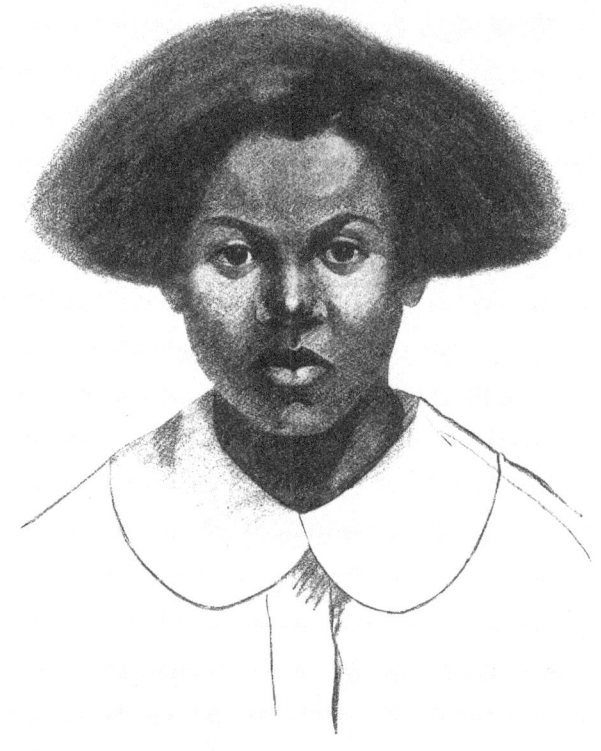

Figure 3.7. "Drawing from Life," *Crisis* cover, July 1927. Courtesy of the Crisis Publishing Co., Inc.

African American by her dark skin tone and hair that is styled in a modern symmetrical bob somewhat like Reiss's "Harlem Girl."[103] The artist D. Norman Tillman appears inspired by Reiss as he applies less focus on the subject's clothing. The pan collar of the white bodice adorns a dark girl whose eyes hold the gaze of her viewer.[104] The startlingly simple image of this New Negro girl avows an autonomous subject position.

"I am Black, but comely, O Ye Daughters of Jerusalem," announced the *Crisis* cover in February 1925. No photographic image of a beautiful woman accompanied the Old Testament avowal rendered in beautiful script. Framed by an intricate graphic, the pronouncement hints at foreign influences in its declaration of beauty, blackness, and womanhood, and in doing so captures a more expansive celebration of womanhood. Intermittently throughout the 1920s, images of non-U.S., African-descended, and "other" raced women graced the covers of the internationally circulating magazine. These covers also relied upon and relayed a growing racial imaginary of modern brownskin womanhood.

In January 1920, a dark-complexioned woman smiled at the camera as her patterned bodice and her unabashed headdress confirmed foreign status. The professional photography team of Brown and Dawson captured the Afro-Caribbean woman, who was captioned as "Woman of Santa Lucia." Other images of foreign women of color also relied on clothing to declare exoticized difference from the more regularly occurring New Negro woman. In 1925, a marked interest in North African and Arabic people was apparent. Photographic covers relied on depictions of beautiful women of color, while captions for the images asserted racial intimacy with a global community of people of color. These captions hailed, "Arabian Cousins of Ours" (January 1925), "A Moorish Maid" (May 1925), "A North African Cousin of Ours" (May 1926) (fig. 3.8), and "A North African Head" (January 1927). Each image depicted girls and women in boldly patterned, non-Western-style clothing or, as in the case of the "Arabian Cousin of Ours," traditional dress. As well, adornments of headdress, facial markings, and jewelry highlighted the foreignness of these light-brown-skin bodies that, in their difference from the white mainstream aesthetic ideal of beauty, were nonetheless "comely."

Filipina women also emerged as celebrated beauties. The presentation of these subjects as both foreign and familiar reflects the contradictory impulses that structured American imperialism through its colonization and Westernization of the formerly Spanish chain of South West Asian islands. Between the late nineteenth and early twentieth centuries, as western European nations "scrambled for Africa," the United States espoused a rhetoric of nation

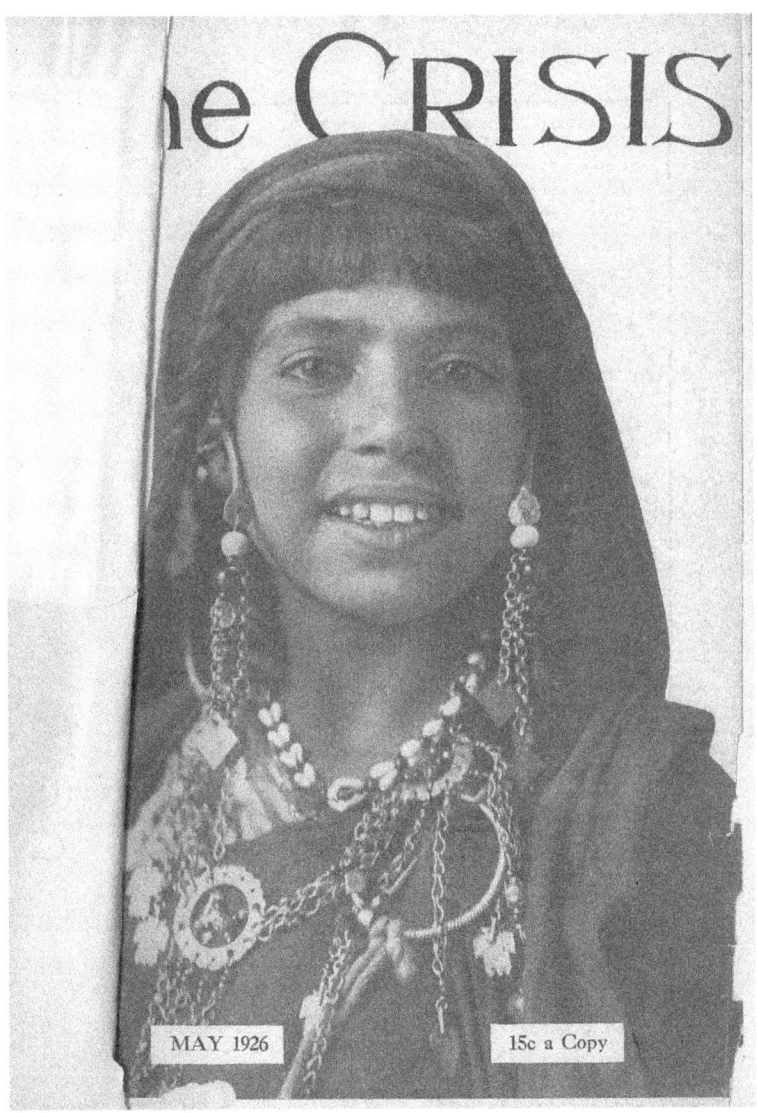

Figure 3.8. "A North African Cousin of Ours," *Crisis* cover, May 1926. Courtesy of the Crisis Publishing Co., Inc.

building on the islands; the interventions of white capitalist hegemonic powers on the global stage helped expand Du Bois's vision as he named the "color line" as the bane of the twentieth century. Writing at the time of the official end of the Filipino-American War (1899–1902), Du Bois highlighted "the relation of the darker to the lighter of the races of men in Asia and Africa, in American and the islands of the sea."[105] Despite this anti-imperialist stance and internationalist perspective, Du Bois's editorial view located, affirmed, and regulated conservative gendered norms as conducive to the assimilationist project of American colonialism.

For example, the magazine featured a cover image, Manila's "Queen of Carnival" in March 1925 (fig. 3.9). Beginning in 1908 and lasting until 1939, the Manila carnival was a two-week event that celebrated relations between the United States and the colonized territory. Among the carnival's many events, the selection of the queen quickly developed into an immensely popular cultural practice signifying the growing control of Filipinos over the carnival. Virginia Vidal Llamas, whose image appeared on the *Crisis* cover a few years after her coronation in 1922, garnered significant support of the recently established newspaper, the *Philippine Herald*, which buoyed her popularity. Similar to early African American beauty pageants, ordinary people voted for the queen of the carnival based on photographs of nominees that appeared in local newspapers. Between 1908 and 1925, beauty and social standing appeared to be the requisite criteria for selection, but an educational achievement was soon incorporated as an important category for judgment.[106] In March 1925, the display of feminized beauty by the Manila queen of the carnival announced modernity to its gendered colonized Asian subject who, decked out in a jeweled crown and dress, peers out with steady focus.[107] Indeed, Llamas appears far from brown in complexion, yet incorporation of her image into the magazine's long-running broader visual discourse of womanhood exposes the expansive boundaries of color, as well as the growing celebration of Afro-Asian connections.

Another cover image seemed to validate the fitness of colonized Filipinos as American citizens, doing so through an assimilationist embrace of education as an extension of U.S. liberal democracy. At first glance, the July 1926 portrait of a young girl in school dress might be interpreted as a very light-skinned or mixed-ancestry New Negro person, doing so not only because of the context in which it appeared but also because of the healthy wave of her bobbed hair. At closer glance, this child cannot pass; her features indicate Asian ancestry. Nonetheless, unlike the other images already described, she is clearly "modern," as told by her Western dress, hairstyle, and lack of jeweled adornment. The caption, "A Colored Graduate of the Philippine Normal

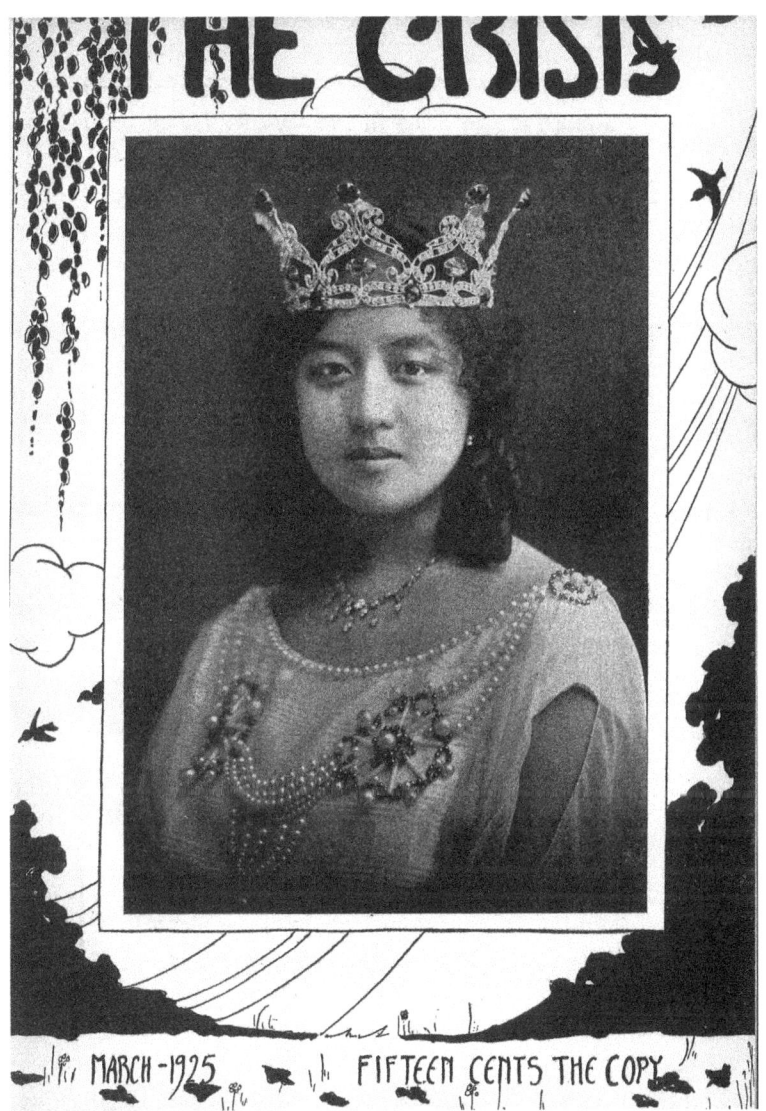

Figure 3.9. Manila's "Queen of Carnival." *Crisis* cover, March 1925. Courtesy of the Crisis Publishing Co., Inc.

School" (fig. 3.10), reasserts possibilities of a mixed ancestral heritage. More meaningfully, the photograph also poses a challenge to the boundaries defining "colored" people to include Southwest Asian girls and women whose "colored" identities relied less on dark complexions than on distance from other aspects associated with white looks. Furthermore, the girl's status as "graduate" of a "Normal School" intimates her identity as a modern educated woman; ultimately, this educated status emerged as the most powerful lens from which to view the shaping of brown-skin respectable beauty as a means to modern progress.

As Mina Roces demonstrates, during the American colonial regime in the Philippines, Western dress quickly grew to be associated with male political power. Many Filipino male nationalists embraced this "vestimentary code" as they ascended to political roles at the local and national level. At the same time, Filipino suffragists, many of whom were beauty queens and highly educated women, embraced customary dress also to declare their modernity, doing so in different fashion. Among these women, traditional clothing helped "make a statement that women were still 'traditional,' 'nationalistic' and 'Filipino.'"[108] Indeed, among the many markers that portray "A Colored Graduate of the Philippine Normal School" as modern the subject's wearing of a school uniform confirms this view. In 1917, women university students adopted uniforms, and this fashion quickly spread to announce "the impracticability of the Filipino dress for daily wear and an active life."[109]

Finally, educated beauty arose to powerfully assert the view of women's higher education as a socially responsible and sexually respectable gendered way forward. Usually in July, but sometimes also in August, and less often in September, the *Crisis* published its education issue. Each year, that issue surveyed and reported on movements toward integration at institutes, colleges, and universities as they happened, while also offering a yearly tally of numbers of African Americans enrolled in historically black colleges and universities and other educational institutions across the nation. As well, the pages of each issue were filled with images of graduating individuals and classes while the magazine's front pages maintained the regular task of providing advertising space for schools and colleges ranging from Knoxville College in Tennessee to Howard University in Washington, D.C. The former highlighted a spiritual and moral educational ethos and boasted of a "beautiful situation" and "healthful location," and among its other basic educational offerings, the college offered instruction in "Domestic Science, Nurse Training, and Music." The latter touted its prestigious claim as a "Great Institution" where a broad range of academic subjects was offered. Given the heightened attention to higher education as a foundational base for the magazine, it is not surprising

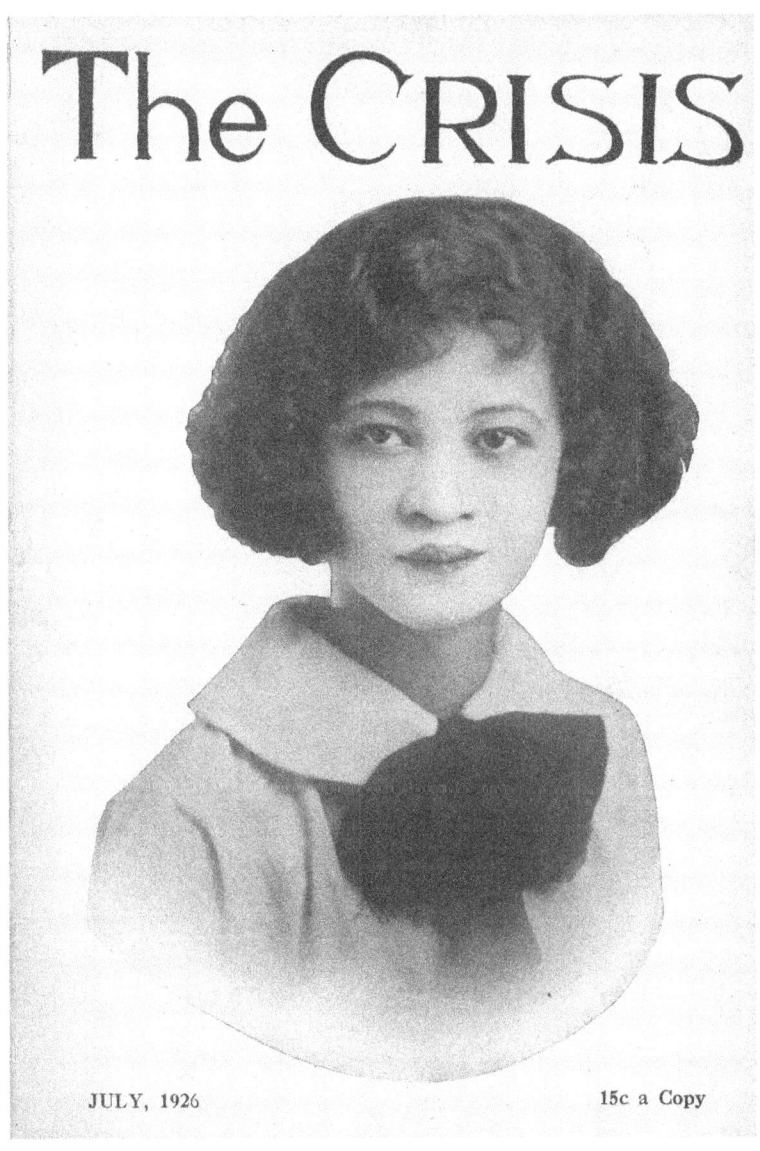

Figure 3.10. "A Colored Graduate of the Philippine Normal School," *Crisis* cover, July 1926. Courtesy of the Crisis Publishing Co., Inc.

to find the spotlight on educated women as photographic cover images on many of these education issues.

On such cover featured Clarissa Mae Scott, Phi Beta Kappa graduate of Wellesley College. The July 1923 issue featured Scott's genteel portrait, which hinted at possible mixed ancestral heritage (fig. 3.11). The *Crisis* named Scott as one of three Wellesley graduates that year as it tallied and enumerated graduates from around the country. Scott's father, Emmett J. Scott, was named as both former secretary to the late Booker T. Washington and current secretary of Howard University.[110] Scott's demure appearance revealed little of the poet who, as we shall see in the chapter that follows, penned powerful verses that centered on the plight of modern womanhood before her tragically youthful demise in 1927. In July 1924, the cover image for the annual education issue more formally announced its subject's membership in the educated ranks as a woman of ordinary brown skin tone appeared in cap and gown.

Conversely, when depicted as graduates, both lighter-skinned women and men appeared in less need of educational garb to assert their inclusion into the ranks of an educated, urban middle class. Two images published in August 1924 and August 1926 provide this contrasting view. The former (fig. 3.12) shows a "Bachelor of Philosophy" from the University of Chicago in profile, cameo-style, musing into the air, while the latter showcased "A Bachelor of Music from Oberlin" (fig. 3.13) as an equally fair-skinned woman whose fashionable hair, clothing, and long single strand of pearls accents her respectable beauty. Still, in this image, the graduate's slumped shoulders and rounded back suggest a quieter struggle than one might not expect for an Oberlin-trained musician of light-skinned privilege.

Finally, two images work to declare the triumph of ordinary brown-skinned women as ones most likely to succeed as the more difficult Depression years loomed. In August 1930, the magazine's education number showed an average-brown complexioned woman as "A Salutatorian" (fig. 3.14). By standard conventions, there is nothing particularly beautiful about the young woman, but her cap, gown, and dutiful smile help render her academic attainment even more noteworthy. The following month, another image appeared to seal the decade's celebration of educated women. "A Western School Teacher" looked out confidently (fig. 3.15). Professional in look and dress, she is not without adornment, but such detail appears well suited to her occupational status. A neat bob frames her face that is clearly African American in look, features, and complexion to announce her fulfillment of an ideal of womanhood that, throughout the 1920s, grew more closely aligned with consumerist demands, educational needs, and the continued celebration of service as the mainstay of the modern New Negro woman.

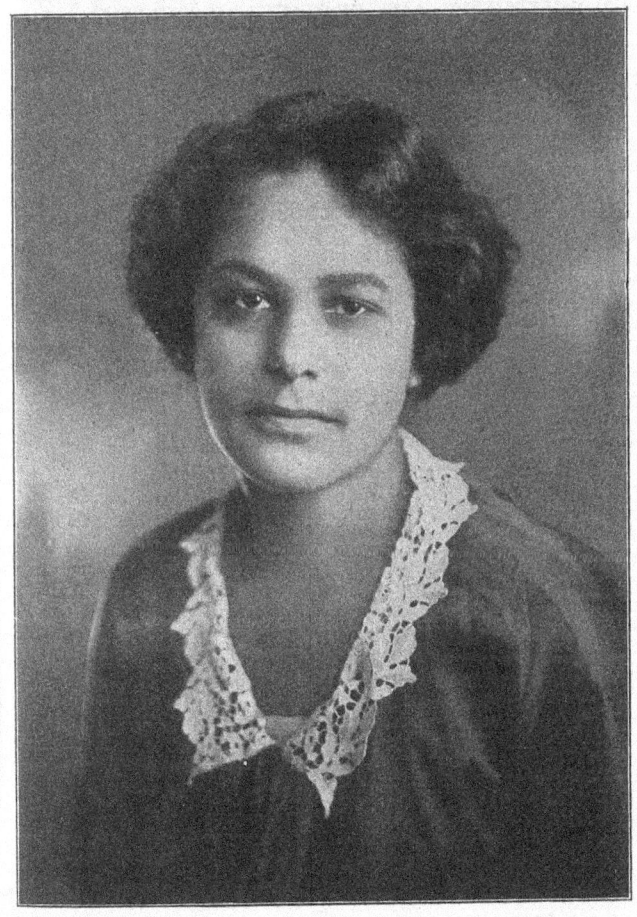

Figure 3.11. Clarissa Mae Scott, *Crisis* cover, July 1923. Courtesy of the Crisis Publishing Co., Inc.

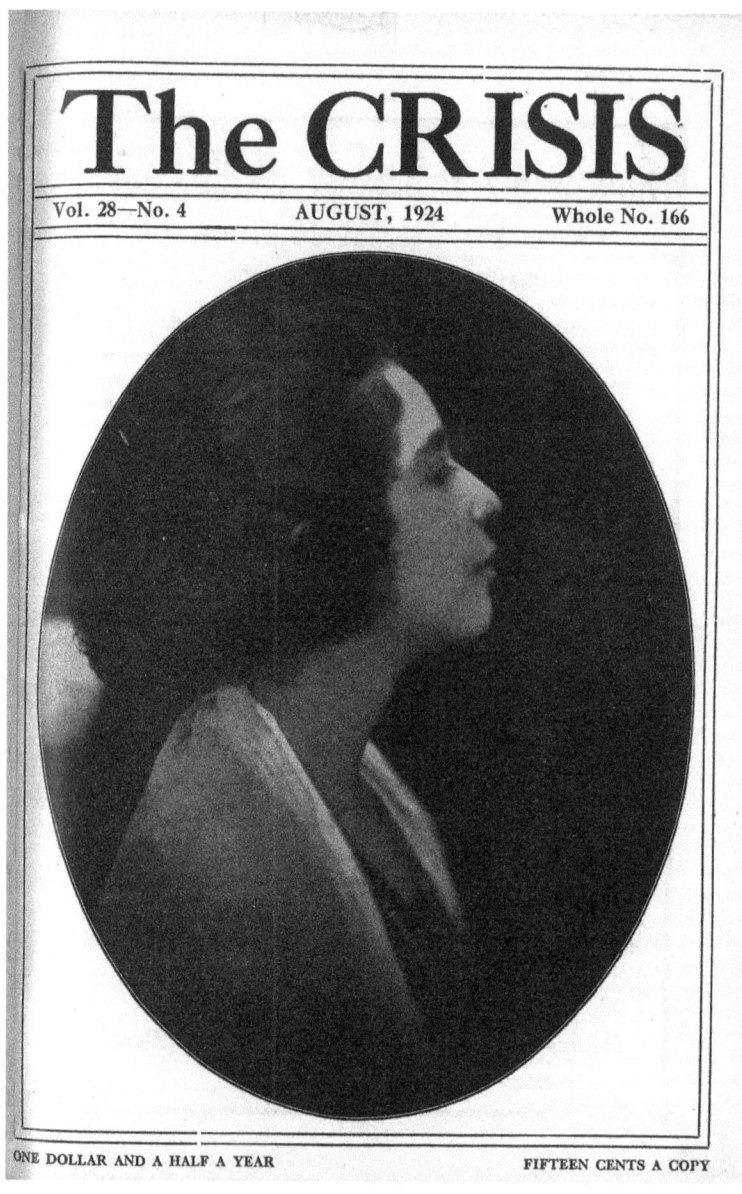

Figure 3.12. "Bachelor of Philosophy," *Crisis* cover, August 1924. Courtesy of the Crisis Publishing Co., Inc.

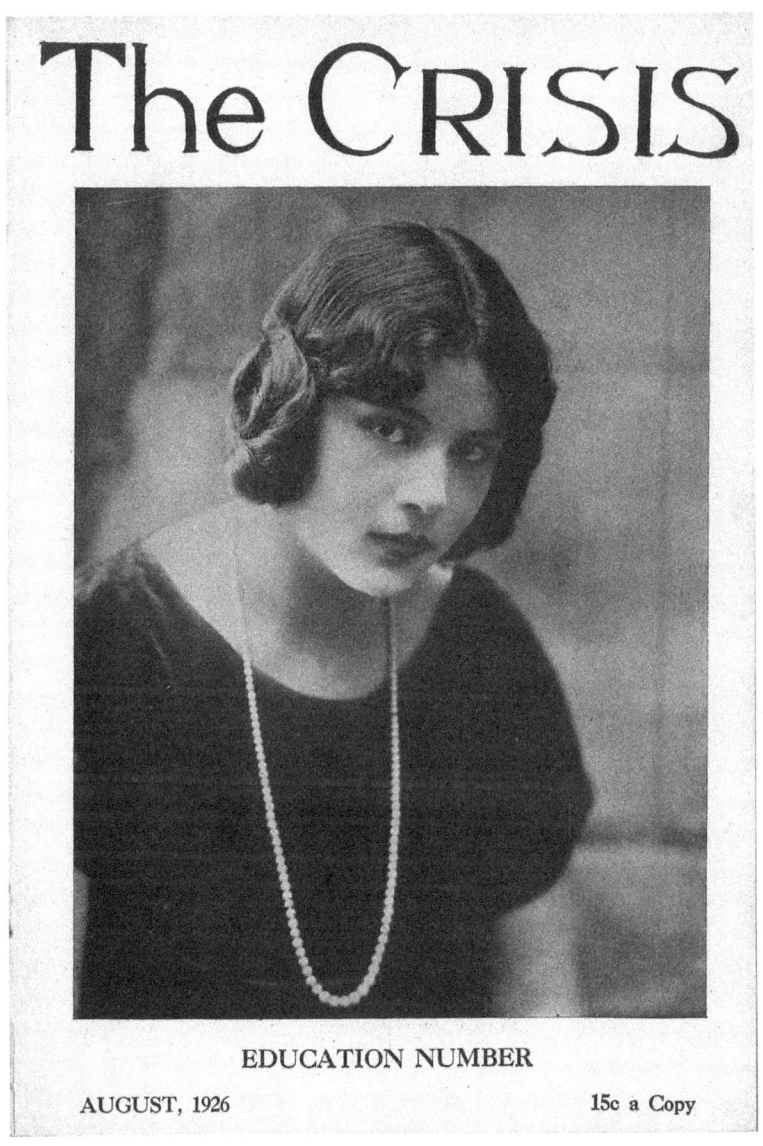

Figure 3.13. "A Bachelor of Music from Oberlin," *Crisis* cover, August 1926. Courtesy of the Crisis Publishing Co., Inc.

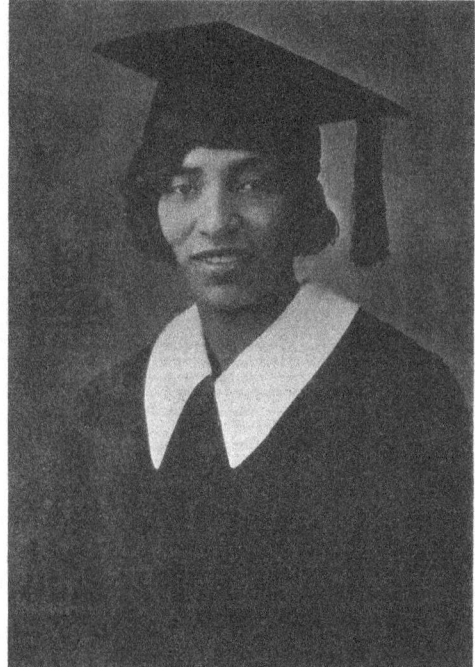

Figure 3.14. "A Salutatorian," *Crisis* cover, August 1930. Courtesy of the Crisis Publishing Co., Inc.

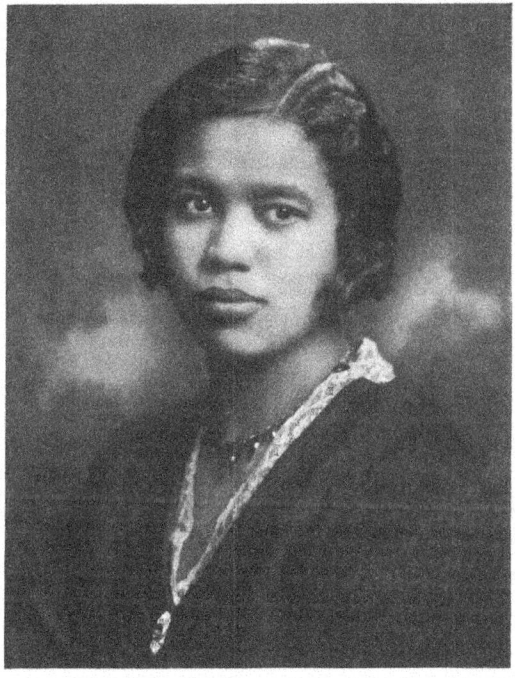

Figure 3.15. "A Western School Teacher," *Crisis* cover, September 1930. Courtesy of the Crisis Publishing Co., Inc.

Conclusion

By the late 1920s, Schuyler's directives to authors to produce literary representations of brown-skin types appeared well known and broadly implemented. A diverse set of examples drawn from Harlem Renaissance literary print culture reveals how a cross section of writers, poets, artists, and cultural commentators employed the motif of brown skin for reasons that surpassed being a simple reaction to publishing expectations and demands. By 1931, Schuyler drew a sharp, satirical view of America's fixations on color in a novel he entitled *Black No More*. The Harlem Renaissance author jeered not only at African American desires to attain "white" looks but also at the fashionable vogue of white Americans who, through cosmetic use and suntanning, were "enthusiastically mulatto minded."[111] However, the mulatto was not the only figuration of brown-skin womanhood.

From Madonna to mulatta to modern New Negro woman, the brown-skin type emerged as a popular literary and visual representations intended to celebrate modern racial identities as it rejected legacies of racist stereotyping seen to threaten the rise of the New Negro in the modern urban environment. So prevalent were these concerns that as often as new figurations of the brown-skin type appeared to positively assert women's modern status, they also worked to sublimate the popular view of the New Negro woman as a political subject and an autonomous citizen. When invoked by visual artists, photographers, writers, and poets in Harlem Renaissance print culture, the rhetoric of brown-skin types exposed a series of contradictions on New Negro women's modern status. On the one hand, representations of brown-skin types blurred the boundaries between adult and youthful women by feminizing girls and women in ways that offset generational differences between women; additionally, brownness worked to differentiate and erect barriers between women of different social classes and raced backgrounds. Encodings of women as brown-skin types consistently located, affirmed, and regulated the display of women's heterosexual, youthful, feminized, and fashionable beauty as primary in valuations of New Negro womanhood.

No doubt literature, art, and photography provided a broad range of gendered imagery from which to render brown skin's meanings, but other representations cast a different light on the era's crafting of the public identities of middle-class New Negro women. The chapter that follows turns to explore women's poetic expression of the 1920s, remaining attuned to the contradictions, celebrations, and anxieties that framed the making of brown-skin types. In the verses of thirteen New Negro women, powerful expressions of the alternate meanings of color in general and brownness in particular, erupt in the poetic gendered discourse on New Negro womanhood.

4

To a Brown Girl

The Poetic Discourse of Brown

Part I

    I love you for your brownness
    And the rounded darkness of your breast.
    I love you for the breaking sadness in your voice
    And the shadows where your wayward eye-lids rest.

    Something of old forgotten queens
    Lurks in the lithe abandon of your walk,
    And something of the shackled slave
    Sobs in the rhythm of your talk.

    Oh, little brown girl, born for sorrow's mate,
    Keep all you have of queenliness.
    Forgetting that you once were a slave,
    And let your full lips laugh at Fate!
    —Gwendolyn Bennett, "To a Dark Girl"

Poetry and the Women behind the Words

Penned by African American artist and poet Gwendolyn Bennett (1902–81), "To a Dark Girl" appeared in 1927 in *Caroling Dusk*, one of several important anthologies connected with the Harlem Renaissance.[1] Bennett, a twenty-four-year-old Columbia University graduate and professionally trained artist evoked neither Africa by name nor blackness as color to denote race in her subject. "I love you for your brownness," avows the speaker, at once assuming an intimacy with the "dark girl." Mediated by the qualifier "brownness," this expression of love for the dark girl encourages a vision of an array of brown complexions when picturing the female subject of the poem. In the minds of twenty-first-century readers, a tremendous diversity of brown shades and ethnic affiliations may well be conjured to situate this gendered body, but for readers of 1920s Harlem Renaissance poetry, the increasingly popular usage of "brown" likely helped shepherd connection with the dark girl as African American. This same audience probably encountered multiple and diverse representations of brown-skin women from a range of mass media publications that communicated ideas and images about the New Negro amid the continuing modernization of African America.

At the surface, Bennett's representation of the dark girl as brown is deterministic in drawing a connection between race and color. Yet, the poem works to dispel the narrow categorization of race as necessarily rooted in the fixed, biological, and chronologically aged-determined body: introduction to the dark girl as a "brown girl" mediates the need for further indices of race. At the same time, the poet troubles the youthful index of "girl" that becomes destabilized by the modern and womanly burden borne by the girl's brown body. Relying on the sociohistorical lens, Bennett sharpened the view of slavery as a particularly gendered experience. At the same time, she pointed to the persistent problematic of the brown girl that extended beyond her vulnerability to the physical, emotional, and psychic violence of the legacy of slavery; in doing so, "To a Dark Girl" pointed to the paradoxical and burdensome raced politics confronting the New Negro woman.

The poet—herself a young, educated, middle-class African American woman—underlined youth as central to her definition of this brown figure and emphasized the uncomfortable divide that this particular incarnation of New Negro women was expected to straddle. On the one hand, the threat of sexual objectification and misuse bears down on the dark girl; on the other, race collectivizing efforts emphasized the pathway to fulfillment through heterosexual, monogamous, and racially fated love for a male "mate" whose sorrow appears palpable despite the poem's focus on the brown girl. Still, Bennett's verse retained the centrality of the female figure, for it is she whom the poet loves. Endowing the dark girl with affection that is framed through brownness, the speaker renders the brown body as beautiful, thereby provoking, or even emboldening, the brown girl to claim her own beauty. In this way, Bennett offered one self-reflexive, decidedly modern mode for the brown girl to claim a glorious African past and "keep all [she has] queenliness."[2]

"To a Dark Girl" introduces several main strands in this chapter's analysis of women's subjective, individual, and collective negotiations with modernity through the poetic form. The poem's most vital importance comes from its common, rather than uncommon, expressive use of "brown": Bennett was one among many African American poets of the era to employ a visual language of brown when denoting modern or "new" identities of African American womanhood. Brown was used as a racial signifier by one of the most prominent poets of the era, Countee Cullen, who attracted broad acclaim in

1925 when his poem "The Ballad of a Brown Girl" was published in *Poetry*, an influential mainstream periodical. In 1925, Cullen also produced *Color*, a collection of verse that critics then and now judge as his finest work. No doubt Cullen was influential as a cultural producer of Harlem Renaissance poetry and as the editor of *Caroling Dusk*, and this invocation of color and brownness signaled a key trope in Harlem's literary production that endured throughout the period. While Cullen's use of brownness emphasized mixed ancestral heritage as African American, the employment of brown and brown skin in poetry at large engaged a diverse set of meanings. How women crafted various iterations of the brownness deserves particular attention for their capacity to capture, contest, and challenge notions of New Negro womanhood that according to the dominant agenda of the Renaissance were increasingly rooted in urban, middle-class values. For these reasons, Bennett's poem foreshadows some of this chapter's central concepts, arguments, and themes that help trace the production of brown-skin womanhood in women's poetic discourse.

Age, as much as class, shaped African American women's poetic expressions and helped buoy critiques that moved beyond the address of racist attitudes and practices to take up concerns less universally expressed among Harlem's literati. Women's poetry points to male chauvinism, gendered interracialism, and intergenerational conflicts over respectability as forces that delimited the fully autonomous creative practice of women. Whether these women personally believed in the ideologies they espoused or rejected the narrow middle-class dictates of sexual respectability to follow nonmarital, nonreproductive, or nonheterosexual passions is less central to my analysis than are the expressions themselves. With this view, it is also important to resist reading women's poetic voices as manifestations of freedom versus remonstrations against individual identity making. I study women's verse as evidence of the prevailing social, sexual, and cultural constraints facing New Negro middle-class women in 1920s urban America, particularly those involved in the literary production of the Harlem Renaissance.

What follows in this chapter is an exploration of a selection of writings of thirteen poets who all published in major anthologies and important literary journals. Largely Harlem-based and oriented to middle-class readers, these magazines include the *Crisis*, *Messenger*, and *Opportunity*, and the Boston publication *Saturday Evening Quill*. Together, women's poetry presents a textured compendium of the frustrations, expectations, and desires of middle-class New Negro women. Neither a collective movement nor an explicitly designed set of political expressions, this range of women's verse showcases the use of color as a poetic device and as a descriptor of African American complexions. More acutely, the employment of color in women's verse exposes some of the era's contested gender politics, while emphasizing the role of complexion in general, and brownness in particular, in determinations of women's beauty, social worth, and sexual respectability. This chapter is organized into two parts: first, it considers the women behind the words to offer biographies of these poets; second, it analyzes the poetry associated with middle-class notions of New Negro women with attention to the metaphoric use of brown. This popular mode illuminates the divide between women's public physical personas and their creative attempts to reconcile subjective views of self from some of the aging prescriptions of New Negro womanhood. To put these two strands into fuller context, it is helpful to consider the unique importance of poetry in women's cultural production of brownness within the larger context of Harlem's literary and arts movement.

"The Voice of My Own Experience"

Writing in 1972, Arna Bontemps, an African American male writer, reflected on the Harlem Renaissance and his role within the vibrant cultural movement. As he signaled certain key moments as marking its dawning and his "awakening," Bontemps underlined the poem "Brown Boy to a Brown Girl" as one that "sounded like the voice of my own experience." Reflecting on the poem written by Countee Cullen and published in *Opportunity* magazine in 1925, Bontemps explains, "I was enchanted."[3] Clearly, men also wrote and were moved by poetry and the use of brownness in poetry of the period; Bontemps's reflection underlines its accessibility to readers across gender lines. This chapter focuses on women's use of color descriptors, most notably brown and brown skin, to excise some of its unique meanings for and about New Negro womanhood.

Poetry played a major role in the Harlem Renaissance's commitment to representing the New Negro. Regularly featured in the major journals of the arts-based New Negro Renaissance, poetry was also showcased in the movement's influential anthologies. Not surprisingly, these collections were assembled by African American men. Predating Locke's *New Negro*, *The Book of American Negro Poetry* was compiled in 1922 by James Weldon Johnson, an older, well-established author. At the height of the Renaissance, the titles of anthologies engaged more metaphoric language, signaling the growing use of color to signify racialized identities. For example, in 1927 Countee Cullen, by then a renowned Harlem poet, edited the collection *Caroling Dusk*; its title evokes both light and darkness, suggesting the time and tone of the New Negro's relation to racial oppression. That same year, the well-connected and influential editor of *Opportunity*, Charles S. Johnson, produced another vital anthology, *Ebony and Topaz*; this time the collection's title more obviously enumerated the rich diversity of complexions among New Negro people as it romanticized hardy wood and jeweled tones to do so.

In at least one instance, the job of literary gatekeeping was upheld by a woman. In October 1919, Jessie Fauset, an established author and educated elite Philadelphian, joined the staff of the *Crisis* when Du Bois appointed her as literary editor. No doubt this was an important position. In 1940, as he reflected on the Harlem Renaissance, Langston Hughes enumerated Fauset, along with Locke and Du Bois, as one of "the three people who midwived the so-called New Negro literature into being."[4] Still, the overwhelmingly masculinist temper in Harlem's literary movement remains clear. In 1926, Fauset resigned from her influential post after being increasingly eclipsed by the attention paid to powerful male editors like Locke and Johnson and to the younger writers whom she helped mentor. In her foreword to Fauset's novel *There Is Confusion* (1924), Thadious M. Davis explains that male chauvinism, misogynistic attitudes, and "unspoken antagonism towards women" deterred their greater participation in the arts-based movement, particularly in these powerful roles.[5] Furthermore, Fauset's appointment was exceptional. News of her appointment appeared in the November 1919 issue in the magazine's regular feature, "Men of the Month." In profile, a photo of the new literary editor appeared between those of two men: N. H. B. Cassell, the U.S. representative for Liberia College, and the late John Merrick, the founder and president of the North Carolina Mutual Life Insurance Company.[6] The biographical sketch and photographic display of Fauset presented between these two men hinted at the coming decade's greater accent on women, as seen in the previous chapter.

The *Crisis* and other literary magazines including *Opportunity* and *Messenger* were important venues to feature the poetry of the New Negro movement. So too were shorter lived periodicals, namely the radical *Fire!!* and *Harlem*, a single-issue publication that was also edited by Wallace Thurman. Other magazines, including the Universal Negro Improvement Association's *Negro World*, catered to a more working-class audience—it also featured verse, and hosted a Women's page, titled "Our Women and What They Think."[7] No doubt, these magazines appealed to mixed and global audiences, yet Harlem's literati focused on attracting an audience of readers comprised of middle-class African American and white liberals. In addition to featuring the images and artwork produced by New Negroes, these periodicals employed African Americans as writers and editors. Magazines promoted fiction and poetry through regular publication and with annual literary prizes. No doubt magazines like the *Crisis* and *Opportunity* had serious financial backing, operating as the official journals of powerful organizations. The feature of women's voices in organizational journals and magazines was not new to the Harlem-based arts movement, but the modern publications assumed a very different tone, purpose, and audience from earlier efforts.

Women's poetry played a particular role in the reformist efforts of clubwomen beginning in the late nineteenth century. *Woman's Era*, the precursory founding magazine of the National Association of Colored Women widely featured a range of writing by women. While there is some debate over dating the first issue to 1890 or 1894, the magazine provided control over the making of representations of African American women by women themselves. *Woman's Era* holds the distinct honor as the first magazine owned and operated by an African American woman.[8] Anne Gere Ruggles and Sarah R. Robbins explore the meanings and manifestations of literacy in the woman's club movement of the late nineteenth century, underlining how *Woman's Era* engaged a "collaborative construction of [African American women's] own ideology of literacy" that redressed historic associations of women with degraded positions stemming from slavery. While *Woman's Era* worked to connect "educated and refined" women, it also assumed a broader focus than that of white women's clubs of the same era by engaging its "self-consciously reformist enterprise directly outward to whole society."[9]

Domesticity and education formed the magazine's key tenets. Under its founding editor, Josephine St. Pierre Ruffin, the magazine simultaneously drew on an "ideology of domesticity and . . . feminine anxiety about how to carry out at home responsibilities despite restricted opportunities for learning."[10] Essays, reports, minutes, commentaries, and poetry were used to uphold these ends. Yet, reading one woman-authored verse from 1896, we find hints at desire for a more public and less drudged existence. "The Poet," penned by Ida Evans Luckie, celebrated and lamented the poet's lot in life. "No mighty deeds of fame / Are thy bequest," she wrote. "But that thou gavest us / We prize not less." The poem continues to describe the poet's "remembering" their duty, resulting in their "turn[ing] away / From flowery paths wherein / We fain would stray" and returning to "life's dull task again / In fields where toiling ever / Bring weariness and pain."[11] The differences in women's modernized circumstances and modernist expression notwithstanding, Luckie's poem presages some of the contradictions between the demands endured and desires expressed by New Negro women during Harlem's Renaissance.

Throughout the 1920s, women's verse was published in the journals of powerful organizations and anthologies edited by prominent men. In general, these poems reflected the collective aims of the New Negro renaissance. Modernist poetry also granted a crucial artistic license to women; this form offered the potential to question aging middle-class prescriptions on respectability as women's verse broached some of the complex realities of New Negro women as modern women who lived, moved, and worked in various urban settings. Many poems were written by educated women. The heightened freedom of urban living that included their greater visibility within the public sphere, enhanced access to consumer goods, and the increasing embrace of modern gender norms and sex values translated into a diminishing celebration of voluntary work or the domestic sphere that so characterized older notions of respectable middle-class womanhood. If one were to look for "feminine anxieties" in women's poetry of the 1920s, one certainly finds far less concern over familial obligations in the domestic sphere than over femininity itself. At times, the domestic sphere appears stultifying; in other cases, it emerges as a positive space for women's freedom. Indeed, women who wrote used their domestic spaces to do so. For example, after resigning from the *Crisis* in 1926, Jessie Fauset sought employment as a reader for publishing firms. Recognizing that racist attitudes might well preclude her welcome in office spaces, Fauset volunteered to "work at home"—an option that no doubt promised a haven for Fauset and a less public commitment for white publishing firms. No such offer materialized.[12]

The diverse roles of African American women as historical agents, including their roles as cultural producers in the Harlem Renaissance, attracts significant attention in contemporary scholarship; that hard-won recognition is attributable to the dedicated work of pioneering scholars, including Hazel V. Carby, Barbara Christian, Anne DuCille, Deborah E. McDowell, Gloria T. Hull, Cheryl Wall, Erlene Stetson, and the late Claudia Tate. Still, as Venetria Patton and Maureen Honey explain, despite the inclusion of women's writings in new collections on the period's literature, "the gender ratio is still nearly two to one or greater—in favour of selections by men ... with the exception of Zora Neale Hurston (and perhaps Nella Larsen), women continue to be classified among the movement's minor writers."[13] The status of women as "minor writers" cannot be endorsed by their lack of productivity or engagement with the Harlem Renaissance, but perhaps reveals more about the gendered value given to poetry as an expressive form used by women. African American women published short stories, fiction, poetry, and plays that appeared in the era's prominent journals, periodicals, and anthologies, but few published single-authored works of creative writing. Patronage facilitated the work of writers, but patronage privileged men.[14] Gloria T. Hull finds it "not surprising . . . that during the Renaissance proper, only Fauset, Larsen, Bennett, and Hurston published fiction." Hull explains how women "kept themselves and were kept in their lyric sphere."[15]

In the realm of the creative, poetry as a genre was particularly important for this movement's purpose—it afforded gendered respectability to its creator.[16] While women poets of the period were respected and accepted as producers of Harlem Renaissance expression, their voices—while many—were scattered throughout the era's influential journals and showcased in anthologies, yet seldom emerged in single-authored collections, the landmark of poetic achievement. Hull argues that although poetry is perceived as a universal and classical form of expression when written by women, it is viewed "somehow a lesser form than when handled by men."[17] Elizabeth McHenry expands on this analysis, finding that during the New Negro Renaissance, "the quality of a woman's poetic expression was [seen to be] located in its emotion."[18]

Patton and Honey are joined by other feminist scholars in identifying "recurring discussions across both genders of migration, domestic servitude, motherhood, children, nature and passionate love."[19] Like other Harlem Renaissance poets, women's verse did not set new conventions regarding style or form. Writing in the tradition of the English Romantics, poets writing within the racially motivated aegis of the era found little resonance of oppression or submission to white dominance through their emulation of Romantic style in its lyric verse or central preoccupation with nature and love (rather than politically overt subjects). Embracing both the Romantic belief in "art and truth as connected," Harlem Renaissance poets found inspiration in Keats, Shelley, Browning, and other nineteenth-century poets as they conjured poetic landscapes of a racially divined paradise. As Maureen Honey shows, poets of the 1920s also married modern values to the Romantic tradition in evocations of the sensual body. Although Honey connects this appeal to primitivism, this chapter shows how women's poetic voices reflect values far more subjectively than mere capitulation to primitivist appetite; this is especially true when read through the lens of color.[20]

The Voices, the Verses, the Women

Thirteen women whose poetry appeared in the era's major journals and anthologies throughout the 1920s fuel this analysis of brown as a linguistic and visual metaphor of modern African American womanhood: Gwendolyn Bennett, Effie Lee Newsome, Angelina Weld Grimké, Helene Johnson, Anita Scott Coleman, Mae V. Cowdrey, Georgia Douglas Johnson, Clarissa Scott Delaney, Blanche Taylor Dickinson, Jessie Fauset, Virginia Houston, Anne

Spencer, and Alice Dunbar-Nelson. Selected primarily for the use of color as a race signifier, and of brown as a referent to women's gendered bodies, the poems by these women are mined from among a diverse cohort of poets whose individual experiences and subjective stances should not easily be subsumed under a rhetoric of collective classed and gendered expression, nor should their poetry be read as autobiographical simply because a woman's voice occupies the verse. I view women's poetic representations as partly reflective of the social realities and gendered concerns of modern, urban, middle-class African American women.

Frequently emerging from class-committed perspectives, these creative expressions sometimes crossed class lines as representations of beauty and sexuality highlighted how prescriptions on middle-class respectability conflicted with women's modern realities and public identities. At times, these poetic expressions suggest alternatives to the conservative demands of respectability attained through marriage, motherhood, and domesticity, and through service to the race as defined by men; at times, women's verse is seen to comply and even revere these expectations, while at other times they rest uneasily. These poetic representations of the era offer alternative understandings, or nuanced ways of viewing, popular historical narratives about race, gender, and sexuality during the 1920s. These poems reveal that many women employed the language of color to help define modern gender roles, sexual practices, ideals of beauty, and commitments to race politics and to men. Certainly, women's verse also disengaged from the use of color and brownness. Color's use appears less frequently in the poems expressing the more (or less) private concerns of self, fulfillment, and general poetic musing, suggesting that references to color and brownness were at once political and expected when representing Harlem's New Negroes.

Color or complexion emerges in degrees of importance in the personal lives of these thirteen poets, but for none more so than Dunbar-Nelson. Triracial in identity, Dunbar-Nelson's white ancestry prefigured most prominently in her light complexion and "reddish-blonde curls that darkened to red to auburn."[21] Throughout her life, the poet found color particularly troublesome to her private and public identity. Dunbar-Nelson's highly personal essay "Brass Ankles Speaks" recalled a southern childhood filled with disparaging chants, "Light nigger, with straight hair!" Estimated to have been written around 1929, Dunbar-Nelson submitted "Brass Ankles Speaks" pseudonymously, but at least one magazine rejected the story due to its controversial matter.[22] The autobiographical account chronicled the aspersions directed to "yaller niggers" as ones well known; the author claims that "every fair colored woman or man, girl or boy who reads this knows that I have not exaggerated." Above all, "Brass Ankles Speaks" identified not white racism but intraracial colorism as the painful problematic. In this story, Dunbar-Nelson explained how interracial sexual unions produced varying skin tones among "mixed-blood" offspring; in turn, these variances broached normalcy and acceptance within these communities; Dunbar-Nelson found the same was not true in broader African American society.[23] She wrote, "And the line of demarcation was rigidly drawn—not by the fairer children, but by the darker ones. I had no color sense. In my family we never spoke of it. Indian browns and cafe au laits, were mingled with pale bronze and blonde yellows all in one group of cousins and uncles and aunts and brothers and sisters. For so peculiarly does the Mendelian law work in mixed bloods, that four children of two parents may show four different degrees of mixture, brown, yellow, tan, blonde."[24] "Brass Ankles Speaks" reflected on Dunbar-Nelson's childhood in a "far Southern city," but as Gloria T. Hull, biographer and editor of the author's diaries, explains, Dunbar-Nelson found that this "kind of rebuff and persecution continued into a Northern college and her first teaching job."[25] Kevin Gaines considers the poet's status as a "race woman" of middle-class to elite standing to show how these were particularly "painful color tensions." Drawing on her journalistic writings and on the diary she kept beginning in 1921, a period described by Gaines as one of "financial and emotional stress," the historian underlines Dunbar-Nelson's sensitivities within and exclusions from social spaces that scholars often celebrate as ones that welcomed and sustained African American women. In at least one instance, Dunbar-Nelson viewed the beauty parlor as a "site of class conflict among black women."[26] In an August 1928 newspaper column, she critiqued how the space gave room to women to "drag their social ambitions into commercial life," resulting in "short shrift, poor service, and insulting discrimination" being directed at patrons of higher social standing than the operators who tended to them. Analyzing this account, Gaines concludes that in addition to dress, demeanor, speech, and hair, color was the dominant marker of class. He shows how the light-complexioned Dunbar-Nelson admitted to passing to receive service in a white beauty salon in Wilmington; despite the risk of being recognized as African American, this temporary passing allowed her to "momentarily escape the painful color and class tensions among black women."[27]

Class rather than color provides the first connector between these women, but socioeconomic status proved tenuous and varied. Largely from upper class or elite backgrounds was an older cohort of women, namely, Grimké, Georgia Douglas Johnson, and Fauset. Middle-class backgrounds defined the status of the remaining nine poets, although those classed identities were wide-ranging in character and origin. Middle class is a broad term; it includes

Bennett, who was born in 1902 in Giddings, Texas, to parents who taught on an Indian reservation and then moved to Washington, D.C., where Joshua Bennett studied law and Mamie Bennett, like many other African American women who realized the independence that beauty work promised, "trained to become a manicurist and beautician at a finishing school."[28] Also raised with middle-class comfort and opportunity were other young poets, Cowdrey and Scott Delaney, whose image appears in figure 3.13. In Germantown, Philadelphia, Cowdrey's mother was a social worker, her father a postal clerk and caterer; at Tuskegee, Scott Delaney benefited from her father's important assistantship to Booker T. Washington and traveled to New England, where, for seven years, she participated in middle-class college culture as a member of a hockey team, sorority, debating team, and the Christian Association at Wellesley College.[29]

At the time of their writing during the 1920s, other women were also decidedly middle class, acquiring such status through education or marriage or both. At least nine of these thirteen women were married at least once; others, namely Alice Dunbar-Nelson, married on three occasions, and others still remained single, including Cowdrey, Dickinson, and Grimké. Scant biographical information on Houston leaves her marital status open to question. One of the few women poets to enjoy economic security was Spencer, who wrote until her death at the age of ninety-three. Like many other creative women, Spencer worked for wages outside the home, holding a job as a librarian beginning in 1924. Due to her commitment to her work and to improving literacy, Spencer walked two miles to work during a boycott of local transportation. As a married woman, Spencer found emotional support in her husband—the first African American parcel postman in a white-dominated Virginia town—who not only built a "one room cottage" at the back of their house and at the edge of Spencer's beloved garden, but who also employed a housekeeper to allow more time for her writing. In the early 1920s, Spencer's husband welcomed her mother to join the couple and their three children in their Lynchburg home, offering the poet further support and freedom from domestic and childcare duties.[30]

Like other women who ascended to the ranks of the middle class, Spencer's origins lay in a working-class background. She was born in Virginia to parents of "discordant personalities: Sarah was the daughter of a former slave woman and a wealthy Virginia aristocrat, and Joel was of Afro-American and Seminole ancestry." In Martinsville, Virginia, Spencer's father, Joel Cephus, ran a saloon where the young Spencer spent much of her time; Cephus "always insisted that the little girl entertain male customers by parading up and down the long bar, charming everyone with her beauty."[31] Greatly disapproving of her husband's behavior and environment, Spencer's mother, Sarah, left her marriage and took her daughter to Bramwell, West Virginia. Sarah's employment as a cook for a mining camp engendered a great protectiveness over her daughter in the working-class white town. She placed Anne in foster care, where she befriended an older white girl and gained the acceptance of the mainly white townsfolk. Until the age of eleven, Spencer had no formal education; her mother deliberately kept her out of Bramwell's free school due to her worry about her daughter's association with a student population of "the children of miners."[32] In 1893, Spencer entered a boarding school in Lynchburg, Virginia, enrolling under her mother's maiden name of Annie Bethel Scales. Despite her humble beginnings and lack of formal education, Spencer continued on to graduate in 1899 as class valedictorian, married Edward Spencer, and together they built a decidedly middle-class life. Their home and garden in Virginia are now designated as a historic landmark.[33]

Marriage alone did not provide economic security or middle-class status for women, and only a few women were ensured freedom from waged labor. Coleman, a married mother of four, ran a boarding house in Los Angeles while she continued to write for publication throughout the era.[34] For others, marriage appeared to make little difference either by choice or by design. Women like Alice Dunbar-Nelson worked in journalism and teaching even though her marital status changed three times; others, like Helene Johnson, "took a lengthy hiatus from her writing when she married . . . and had to help support the family." Years later in an interview, Johnson recalled this economic need as real obstacle to her continuing to write after 1929.[35]

Divorce and separation were not unfamiliar to many of these poets. Stormy marriages affected Spencer, Bennett, Grimké, Helene Johnson, and Georgia Douglas Johnson, whose childhoods were influenced by single-parent households that sometimes followed volatile break-ups. These marital breakdowns had a meaningful effect for women's reinvention; for example, Douglas Johnson, a child of parents of mixed ancestry, George Camp and Laura Douglas, dropped her birth name Camp to assume the maternal surname Douglas and did so upon marriage to Henry Lincoln Johnson in 1903.[36]

Widowhood, separation, and divorce amplified women's continued economic dependence on men and sometimes heightened the already precarious economic security of women writers and poets of the Harlem Renaissance. In 1925, Henry Lincoln Johnson Sr. died, leaving forty-five-year-old Georgia Douglas Johnson to support herself and two children who were in their last years of education. Her full-time employment in various jobs included substitute teacher, librarian, and civil service positions where she found work as file clerk, immigration inspector, and labor inspector. Presenting obvious constraints on the time and energy left to pursue her creative work, the clear impediment to waged work outside the creative realm was recognized by the most eminent of her peers. In 1927, Du Bois nominated Douglas Johnson for the William E. Harmon Award for Distinguished Achievement in the field of Literature, identifying her in his letter to the Harmon Foundation as the "leading colored woman in poetry." As he described his twenty-year acquaintance with the poet, Du Bois attested to her "development" over the years; he explained that "she has succeeded by the hardest kind of application in the midst of every sort of distraction."[37]

Some months later that same year, Du Bois penned a far less favorable letter of recommendation to the Guggenheim Foundation. While he claimed Douglas Johnson as a "personal friend" and an "unusually interesting woman," Du Bois also characterized the poet as neither "a student nor systematic worker." His appraisal continued: "She is erratic, illogical and forgetful." Doubting her productivity after a year of study in Paris or "at home," he nonetheless conceded that "she is liable at any time or anywhere to turn out some little thing of unusual value and beauty."[38] It is not surprising that Douglas Johnson failed to win recognition in this competition given such an unflattering portrait. Although he wrote more positively of her talents on other occasions, this particular recommendation clearly shows a condescending view of one woman's talents. Replete with gendered assessments of work ethic and productivity, Du Bois neglects all mention of her household management, motherhood, and full-time waged labor, the latter of which was a dimension of her life that the poet could not so easily dismiss. She expressed her own frustration: "If I might ask of some fairy godmother special favors, one would sure be for a clearing space in which to think and write and live beyond the reach of the Wolf's fingers."[39] Despite the economic burden, widowhood brought freedom for Douglas Johnson as evidenced by her "Saturday Nights" in Washington, D.C., when she opened her home to a stream of New Negro literati whose energies and output circulated in urban centers beyond Harlem's geographic borders.[40]

Among the most crucial relationships formed by women poets and writers were those formed with other women. Through friendships and networks of support many women assisted one another on creative, personal, and financial matters. As Honey tells us, although women "were not always in positions to further each other's careers, women poets received emotional support from socializing together, reviewing each other's work, and having female role models."[41] Among the poets featured in this chapter, many actively cultivated friendships with other women and relied on the support of these close associations. These women included Helene Johnson, who was mostly raised by her aunt in Oak Bluffs, Martha's Vineyard. Johnson arrived in Harlem with her cousin, Dorothy West, and when parted, letters between them show a sisterly bond. The two women also formed a fast and enduring friendship with Zora Neale Hurston. The established older author opened her apartment to them while she was away for summer research in Florida.[42] In 1930, Hurston also employed Johnson to assist with typing and research, and for some reason neither Hurston nor Johnson made this known to Charlotte Mason, Hurston's infamous white patron, described by Johnson as "that mysterious woman, Zora's boss."[43]

Women also opened their homes to other women. Douglas Johnson accommodated Hurston in her D.C. home in a time of need. Douglas Johnson, the genteel socialite and literary hostess, formed friendships with other women, including poet and children's writer Effie Lee Newsome. This relationship benefited them personally and professionally as we may recall from the glowing review Newsome offered on *Bronze*, Douglas Johnson's second collection of poetry.[44] Douglas Johnson also formed a meaningful friendship with Alice Dunbar-Nelson who, as Hull explains, maintained a woman-centered social world "despite her [three] marriages." Hull describes her home base as "almost always a gynocentric arrangement involving her mother and sister." Between Douglas Johnson and Dunbar-Nelson, there existed a friendship close enough for the latter to playfully speculate that the poet's third and most mature collection of poetry, *An Autumn Love Cycle* (1928) had been inspired by a love affair.[45]

Despite these close circles of friendships, not all women found a ready place among other New Negro women associated with the Harlem Renaissance. For example, Cowdrey, whose modern and "unusually frank poetry" met encouraging reception through publication and award, remained "curiously distant from other black women poets who tended to know each other."[46] Honey speculates that disconnect can be attributed to timing. Honey considers how, after graduating from high school, Cowdrey arrived in Harlem in 1927, but at that time it was likely too late to forge important links. One year earlier, Fauset had resigned her editorial role at the *Crisis*, and Bennett left *Opportunity*: their respective roles as "midwife" and modern "mover and shaker" no doubt presented a significant change to the gendered order of Harlem's literati. Honey speculates further: "Once this fragile network fell apart [women poets] had a hard time holding onto their identities as poets."[47] Honey muses that this network of friendships between women might have offered Cowdrey the lifeline she needed; sadly, she took her own life in 1953.

Women assisted other women in ways that transcended the professional literary arena to address the material realities of modern womanhood. Dictates of dress, style, and fashion emerged in interactions between women. In 1921, Dunbar-Nelson recalled that her visit to friend Douglas Johnson became a lesson in style that met with the approval of the latter's domineering, class-conscious husband, Lincoln [Link] Johnson. In her diary, Dunbar-Nelson recalls: "[she] wanted to know how to put on hats, and I began to teach her. She really did not know how, and I made her practice again and again. Link seemed so glad that I was teaching his wife an essential thing that he suggested luncheon." Despite Link Johnson's pleasure at his wife's cultivation of this feminized display, and despite the fulfillment of her own desire to learn the correct way a wear a hat, Douglas Johnson did not sacrifice her creative self for style. Dunbar-Nelson's diary notes, "we ate his salad and slice pineapple, and everything, while Georgia showed me the manuscript of her new book."[48]

The expectation of women's fashionable and appropriate dress at the many public occasions in the literary social scene and within the city also appears to have been a concern for some women, especially when dressing for formal occasions. Helene Johnson's letter to Dorothy West, or Dot, as Helene affectionately called the novelist, conveys regret over the matter of clothing. Writing on March 2, 1931, Johnson was apologetic as she refused her cousin's request to exchange dresses for separate events they both planned to attend: "Dot darling, I don't know what to say about the dress. You see it's the only party dress I have, just as the beaded dress is the only party dress you have. It isn't as attractive on me as it is on you, but is all the formal dress I have." Obviously embarrassed at having to say no to her cousin, Johnson rationalizes the grounds for her denial on her own limited formal wear options; at the same time, she flatters Dot, perhaps truthfully admitting that the dress Dot was willing to exchange may well suit her better. Still, she defended her decision: "I think it just as formal as the beaded one." Questioning the appropriateness of the dress for the event West planned to attend, Johnson surmises: "Do you think you should wear a white taffeta dress like that unless men are going to be in a tux, and isn't this going to be a tea? If it's a formal party as that, your own little beaded dress will be quite the thing. You will look heavenly in that."[49]

As roommates, cousins, and friends, and as young, social women in Harlem's literary scene, Johnson and West likely shared and advised each other on matters of dress and style on other occasions; the letter's palpable regret and good knowledge of the other's clothing indicate this to be true. Johnson advised West further: "If you want something new, can't you pick up something at Klein's, or is it $?" As Johnson identifies a retail store opened to African American consumers seeking stylish clothes, she also considers the possible monetary limitations encumbering West from buying a new formal dress. Writing in 1931, she advises her cousin on creative recycling: "Has anyone seen your green chiffon with little lace jacket? I love that, it's so flimsy and feminine." Johnson expresses regret, fear of being selfish for not wanting to loan her dress, and a particular understanding of West's wants and desire, "I know how you feel about the tea & especially about the blonde boy."[50] The need and aspiration for fashionable clothing for social, and likely professionally linked, outings in heterosocial spaces further attests to the influence of broad cultural trends in modern urban culture on Harlem Renaissance women poets and writers.

Certainly, all women did not share these bonds of friendship and support. As well, the physical distance between those who lived and worked in Harlem, in Washington, D.C., and in Boston, as well as those from other urban centers and local spaces, reinforces understanding women's poetic expression as individual expression geared toward the collective cause of representing New Negro womanhood. Regardless of their points of origin, these educated and urban women articulated the constricting gendered and sexed politics of New Negro womanhood, doing so through the device of color. As the second part of this chapter moves to explore, women's poetic use of color and brownness exposes women's discordant relationships with middle-class conservative gendered ideals, sexual norms, and social roles accorded to New Negro women of the urban, northern middle class.

Women's poetry of the Harlem Renaissance frequently exposes desire for sexual autonomy that included freedom from the dictates of marriage, sexual partnership that coupled physical attraction with romantic views of love, access to consumer goods associated with modern womanhood and middle-class status, freedom of movement in the urban space, and freedom from motherhood. In the analysis that follows, I first consider Harlem Renaissance women's verse as expressions of racial ideology—what Hull has categorized as "obligatory race poetry."[51] I then move to explore the growing significance of color with particular attention to the gendering of women's bodies, identities, and social roles. Thematically organized to address concerns unique to modern, urban, middle-class African American womanhood, this analysis considers women's poetry about color, sex, beauty, motherhood, aging, consumerism, and brownness. Expressing individualist perspectives and collective gendered concerns, women's creative expressions highlight alternative understandings of modern or New Negro womanhood. That alterity starts with brown.

Part II

> I am not proud that I am bold
> Or proud that I am black.
> Color was given me as a gauge
> And boldness came with that.
> —Helene Johnson, "I Am Not Proud"

Representing the "Race"

In her 1929 poem, "I Am Not Proud," Helene Johnson (1906–95) seemingly defies the mandate of the Harlem Renaissance by denouncing prideful acceptance of racialized identity.[52] Within the pronouncement "I am not proud," Johnson's verse claims color as a gauge or social judgment that was provided for, rather than forged by, the individual. In this sense, "I Am Not Proud" positions color as central to the rubric of racial identity that claims characteristics such as "bold[ness]" as a necessary bolster against the social ordering of race/color identities; in doing so, it underscores the subjugation of African-descended people in 1920s U.S. society and culture. Johnson's rejection of blackness is less a denouncement of black as a positive color-based term to describe African American identities than it is a censure of white racism. The connection of race and colors as markers of binarized difference helped maintain the dominance of white, native-born Americans. In the poetic remaking of New Negro gendered identities, color played a significant role when crafting verse that squarely addressed the era's racial ideology. Although constrained by the movement's ideological demands and its masculinist imperative, women's "obligatory race poetry" highlights re-evaluations of the role of color in defining race at the hands of women poets.

"The Colorist" by Anita Scott Coleman (1890–1960) invokes imaging of God through the lens of color. "God is an Indian—He loves gay color so . . ." the poem begins. It continues to speculate on God as Irish, declaring, "He likes green color best." The Indian and Irish God both summon colors associated with natural and lively surroundings, yet when "The Colorist" paints God as white, the spiritual being appears distinctly male: "Saxon, stern and cold."[53] Finally, the poet considers God as African-descended:

> God is African—for night is robed in black.
> The twinkling stars are black men's eyes,
> The black clouds, tempests tell.
> While little seeds of flowers birthed are. . . .
> Tans and browns and blacks.[54]

Offsetting the bright gaiety of the Indian God, the Irish "green garments ofttimes dress," and, most drastically, the coldness of white ice or the ethereal "downy" softness of white clouds, Coleman engages with strength and mystery to characterize blackness. Blackness and night accrue positive accent by the "black men's" eyes appearing as "twinkling stars" that seemingly alit the "robed" darkness of night. Darkness appears as stormy in the "black clouds" whose tempestuous nature may well be connected not only to slavery's past and Jim Crow's present but also to the histories of miscegenation from the era of slavery to the era of the New Negro. Coleman celebrates the promise that follows troublesome times. Most powerful in its last stanza, the poet celebrates the flowering of the seeds of blackness as "tans and browns and blacks," thereby invoking a range of blackness under God's (African) "flowers."[55] Here the signifier of brown seemingly competes with avowals of blackness, but it simultaneously complements the less expansive color-coded identities of "tans and browns and blacks" that dotted the sightline and city-line of Harlem during the 1920s.

Gwendolyn Bennett's "Advice" (1927) considers the weighty demand of producing race poetry and employs color to articulate the poet's discontent. Bennett's youthful critique of the demands facing "young" New Negroes, appeared in *Caroling Dusk*. The poet writes:

> You were a sophist,
> Pale and quite remote,
> As you bade me
> Write poems—
> Brown poems
> Of dark words
> And prehistoric rhythms.[56]

The obligation to write "race poetry" is cast within ahistorical African syncopated verse; "dark words" are used to declare the poet as the writer of "brown poems." Similar to Coleman's reference to the white God in "The Colorist," Bennett uses "pale" as a metaphoric reference to color. In this case, it denotes emotional distance of pale bodies to "dark words" as they hope for "prehistoric rhythms" to entertain and satisfy consumerist appetites for primitivist representations of African-descended people. Scholars speculate that the "sophist" referred to Alain Locke who assumes the role of the "pale and quite remote."[57]

As a poetic device for advancing the racial inclusion of African Americans of all complexions, color also emerges in Cowdery's poem, "Lamps." Appearing in the *Crisis* in 1927, and winning that journal's poetry prize, Cowdery (1909–53) explores themes of racial inclusion and exclusion by likening racially defined people to lamps that appear identifiable by color. The young Cowdery writes,

> Bodies are lamps
> And their life is the light.
> Ivory, Gold, Bronze and Ebony—
> Yet all are lamps
> And their lives their light.[58]

The poet considers the challenges and privileges of these lamps and "some flames rise high above the horizon / And urge others to greater power / Some burn steadfast through the night," while "Others flicker weakly, lacking oil to burn / And slowly die unnoticed." Cowdery considers the problem facing Ebony lamps; the poet ponders,

> You and I are lamps—Ebony lamps.
> Our flame glows red and rages high within
> But our ebon shroud becomes a shadow
> And our light seems weak and low.[59]

The only solution for the "ebon shroud" that "shadows" or presents new darkness of unnatural making, is "to break that shadow / and let the flame illumine heaven." Here, the poet, like others of the period, employs color along with elements of light and shadow to qualify ebony or blackness within a positive framework. That racially defined color identity—here appearing as ebony—possesses positive elements of vitality and strength, but remains shrouded by the "shadow" of preconceived or externally formed ideas of blackness that weaken positive self-identity and claim to the New Negro identity.

Other poets drew even more expansive ideas of race by also drawing on color. Douglas Johnson captured the nation's long mixed-race heritage in her poetic rendition of the "True American." Appearing in the *Crisis* in 1927, the poet presents to America "your son, born of iron heel; / Black blood and red and white contend along this frame of steel."[60] In this poetic celebration of the "true" American, Johnson claims mixed ancestral heritage—Indian, African, and European—as a bulwark against racial prejudice. Within the urban, industrial setting of 1920s America, the poet urges the nation to face the real character of her citizen body; the poet avows, "From his commanding triple coign, all prejudices fade. / The ebbing nations coalesce in him and flow as one; / The bright shining rainbow sweeping back to God at set of sun."[61] In its last lines, the sonnet demands, "America, regard your son, The Cosmopolitan, / The pattern of prosperity, The True American."[62]

While Johnson's consistent gendering of the "true American" as male easily fulfilled the overriding masculinist ethos of the Harlem Renaissance, it nonetheless challenged rigid hierarchies of race by referencing the long history of what historian Gary B. Nash describes as "mestizo" America or the long history of racial intermixture as a foundational aspect of the United States as a nation.[63] Invocations of color—black and red and white—infer racial designation as African descended, American Indian, or white Euro-American, while at the same time emphasizing the role of God and nature in forming a rainbow coalition of these racially based identities. Despite her romanticizing the proximity of a truly integrated nation that appears consistent with the overall positive outlook of the Harlem Renaissance as a movement for political change, Johnson also provided a steely reminder of America's capitalist character as one inbred with racial dominance and white economic control.

While women's obligatory race poetry frequently cast as male the subject of such verse, other poems highlighted the particular burden of the era's gendered ideology on women. In "The Ordeal" (1925), Georgia Douglas Johnson, the most acclaimed women poet of the era (though certainly not the most radical), cautioned,

> Ho: my brother
> Pass me not so scoffingly
> I am doing this living of being black
> Perhaps I bear your own life-pack
> And heavy, heavy is the load
> That bends my body to the road.

As the speaker implores the New Negro man to acknowledge the work of the assumedly female African American burden-bearer, she reminds him that not only does she carry "his own life-pack," but she also does so while "keep[ing] a smile for fate."[64] While the poem reads as a testament to women's patience, forbearance, and support of men, the final lines reveal the poet's inclusion of self in the "ordeal" of racial struggle. In doing so, the poem accesses fate rather than individual choice as the answer to the ordeal.

> Intrepidly, I strive to bear
> This handicap: The planets wear

>The Maker's imprint, and with mine
>I swing into their rhythmic line;
>I ask—only for destiny,
>Mine, not thine.[65]

Despite this resignation to fate, and claim for protection of her brother at the expense of the woman subject of this poem, other New Negro poets also firmly rejected the fate of "being black" as an identity that fully shaped their lives. In the most intimate and personal realm of women's lives, the sexuality of African American women emerged as an ongoing public discourse. As previous chapters show, a largely male-dominated discourse venerated their biological roles as mothers, while elite and middle-class educators, reformers, and older professionals continued to emphasize respectable display, deportment, and sexual morality as important prescriptions of modern, middle-class womanhood. In light of women's growing freedoms within modern urban settings, these conservative gender ideals and sexual norms were increasingly outmoded. In the poetic expressions forged by African American women of varying ages, New Negro women revolted against these aging demands.

Women's poetry scrutinized the gendered double standard that permitted greater sexual freedom for men and moralistic judgment for women. In "The Mask," Clarissa Scott Delaney (1901–27) describes the woman subject of the poem appearing "so detached and cool" that her public mask reveals nothing of "the secret life within her soul."[66] The poem evokes a street scene to help the reader envisage a woman who appears fortuitous and brave and walks alone. On one occasion, she is "passed by on the street" by a "woman with a child"; another time, "she heard from casual lips / A man's name, bittersweet."[67] Here, several matters particular to single women in the urban environment come to the fore as Scott Delaney paints the portrait of a woman whose devaluation seems first embedded in her seemingly denied status as mother, and then later, with reminder of a lover's abandonment. No longing for either lover or child is expressed. The poem reveals the woman's mask as protection against already lost respectability. The casual nature of the street scene highlights the ease with which a woman could fall into sexual disrepute.

Women's poetry reveals little about desire for children or for attaining motherhood as a means to elevate or confirm one's status as woman. More frequently, poetic expressions reflect upon sexuality by highlighting a series of unfettered pleasures, unquenchable longings, and irreparable heartbreaks. At times fusing the emotional with the physical, these expressions reveal the serious limitations modern women faced in the sexual realm. These poems do not always frame the racial as central to the love/sex verse but as expressions of New Negro womanhood by Harlem Renaissance poets; understanding these scenes in the context of the social, cultural, and sexual histories explored in earlier chapters, women's poems on sex, love, and desire underscore the limits of modern women's sexual autonomy.

Sexual desire emerged in ways that positioned women's subjective desire as sometimes central and sometimes secondary to the love/sex scene set by the poet. Beauty appears a common connector between sex and love. Beauty is invoked to position women either as the subject of desire or to underline heteronormative understandings of sexual desire. In rare instances, it does both. For example, Fauset's "Touché" explores the contradictory longings of both female and male partner. As the female speaker of the poem considers her lover's adoration of her "black hair . . . so lustrous and rare," she finds that her male suitor upholds a vision of beauty that remains rooted in white aesthetics. Her male suitor murmurs, "Surely no gold locks were ever more fair."[68] When defined by the male figure, this poem positively avows African American women's sexual beauty through hair color and texture rather than fairness of skin. Still, the woman speaker of the poem believes she knows better. She insecurely translates her lover's nightly recital of these words as an attempt to convince himself of her beauty rather than to pay her a compliment.

As "Touché" progresses, the speaker of the poem considers her lover's holding dear a memory of "that girl of young manhood's dream." She probes for details on his past love, asking, "Had she blue eyes? Did *her* hair goldly gleam?" This veneration of the imagined white woman's beauty is offset once more when we learn that the female speaker of the poem also "knew a lad in my own girlhood's past / Blue eyes he had and such waving gold hair!" The contradictory race and color politics of this poem is complicated by the raced and gendered politics of the era that intimately connected New Negro women as expected partners to New Negro men. In this poem, one partner allegedly once held, or holds, lustful desire for a white partner; the other, avowedly, and shamefully, does so too. This competing and taboo desire ultimately provides no trusting foundation for the couple's romance. Most radical here is Fauset's overturning the privilege of choice in romantic love interest as solely the domain of men. In this poem, women too are moved by their own desire, and not necessarily comforted or convinced at male avowals of their beauty and social worth.

Another poem, published in the March 1925 issue of *Opportunity*, foregrounds the poet's emotional quest for freedom, doing so in the body of the brown girl. Her beauty and sinewy movement suggests both the possibilities and problematic of her raced, sexed body that is evoked through the dawning of spring. Multiple interpretations that range from self-love to sisterly support to same-sex love arise when reading "At April," but despite these various understandings, brown dominates in descriptions of the gendered body; the poet, Angelina Weld Grimké, writes,

> Toss your gay heads,
> *Brown girl trees;*
> Toss you gay lovely heads;
> Shake down your downy russet curls
> All about your brown faces;
> Stretch your brown slim bodies;
> Stretch your brown slim arms;
> Stretch your brown slim toes.
> Who knows better than we
> With the dark, dark bodies
> What it means
> When April comes alaughing and aweeping
> Once again
> At our hearts?[69]

The repeated descriptor of "slim" to describe the physical body, combined with the sensuous image of "downy russet curls" helps depict the feminized beauty of the brown female body, and perhaps too the mixed-race character whose brown complexion overrides "soft" hair as a signifier of race. Darkness also looms in the promise of spring. "At April" poses no joy to those with "dark, dark bodies." In sisterly collusion, the speaker confers knowledge that is both collective and private; there is no outsider vision into the sadness of the "brown girl trees": "who knows better than we," the speaker asks. The reader must take as given that the poetic "we" knows, and that that knowledge is sufficient. In another poem submitted in 1925 to Charles S. Johnson, editor of *Opportunity,* Grimké mused even more clearly on the divide between the brown womanhood's outward sensual exuberance and her inner conflict in a poem entitled "Brown Girl." "In the hot gold sunlight," the verse begins,

> Brown girl, Brown girl
> You smile
> And in your great eyes
> Very gold, very bright
> I see little bells
> Shaking so lazily.

The poet juxtaposes this happy freedom with the heavy plight that silences the brown girl's smile and makes her eyes "spill sunlight / over the dusk." "Close your eyes," the poet entreats, assuring her that "I hear nothing but the beating of my heart."[70] Similar to Gwendolyn Bennett's identifying with the brown girl, Grimké's poetic persona also relates to the brown girl as self. Both poems, "At April" and "Brown Girl," lay claim to the emotional challenges facing African American women in creating their own images of self that required no external endorsement, bolstering, or restoration to respectable order.

Same-sex sexual desire appears through a range of verse that reads the female-authored verse as the female speaker of poems that address or evoke a female love interest in erotic and sensual terms. Careful in their language and imagery, women who wrote about their passionate love for other women did so with the nuanced use of color. "You! Inez!," an unpublished poem by Alice Dunbar-Nelson and dated February 1921, avows love in vibrant colorful and softly feminized ways,

>   Orange gleams athwart a crimson soul
>   Lambent flames; purple passion lurks
>   In your dusk eyes.
>   Red mouth, flower soft,
>   Your soul leaps up and flashes
>   Star-like, white, flame-hot.
>   Curving arms, encircling a world of love.
>   You! Stirring the depths of passionate desire!

In this verse, the poet relies on colors disassociated from the human body and complexion. Only does the mouth possess color associated with the body, and there it assumes a rose red. "Orange gleams" and "purple passion" relay differently textured and sensual delights. The speaker's object of desire also has compassionate depth and acceptance of "a world of love" that supports and embraces this differently colored desire. Such use of color is also seen in Cowdery's poem "Insatiate," that, although appearing in the poet's collection *We Lift Our Voices* (1936), should not be overlooked. "Insatiate" tells of love and longing; the assumed female speaker of the poem describes all the sensual beauty that portends to fulfill her desire.

>   If her lips were rubies red
>   Her eyes two sapphires blue,
>   Her fingers ten sticks of white jade,

> Coral tipped ... and her hair of purple hue
> Hung down in silken shawl. ...

In this poem, Cowdrey draws the sensual appeal of color through rich jewel tones of lips, and brilliant ones of eyes; slender whiteness of hand and polished nails; and flowing mane of purple-hued hair. Like "You! Inez!," "Insatiate" relies on a colorful array of vibrant tones that help further demarcate these works as expressions of women's same sex sexual desire.

Other woman-authored, woman-speaker, woman sex/love object poems, including "A Mona Lisa" by Grimké, reflect a different use of color. Appearing in *Caroling Dusk* in 1927, "A Mona Lisa" moves with emotional and physical desire for the beautiful woman central to the speaker's desire. But in this poem, purples and coral and orange gleams and purples are absent; rather, the poetry relies both on the intimate associations of body and brownness, as well as brown's less ebullient tones.

> I should like to creep
> Through the long brown grasses
> *That are your lashes;*
> I should like to poise
> On the very brink
> Of the leaf-brown pools
> That are your shadowed eyes;

The speaker is prepared to immerse herself fully in "glimmering waters" and "sink down / and down / and down / ... and deeply down." Still, she fears being engulfed in a love that is unreciprocated: she worries, "Would my white bones / Be the only white bones / wavering back and forth, back and forth / In their depths?" In this poem's eroticized worry over unrequited passion, the enigma of "A Mona Lisa" is presented as the power of beauty to elicit longing in the other to the point that it threatens to overwhelm, engulf, and ultimately strip the brown body to stark white bone. Far less a pleasurable surrender to the sensuality of brownness, the speaker's desire is framed in tentative, troubled terms.

When described beyond abstract or passionate longing, women's sex and love poetry often privileged heterosexual expression that focused on African American men as love interests. When described by color or complexion, the African American male subject is frequently described as black, while many (though certainly not all) references to "brown boys" persist with the same primitivist associations ascribed to the brown-skin girl described in earlier chapters; at times, brown skin appears to mark effeminacy in boys and men.[71] In other cases, brownness asserts youthful joy. For example, Helene Johnson's nondescriptively titled poem, "Poem," uses the street vernacular of urban Harlem to descriptively celebrate,

> Little brown boy,
> Slim, dark, big-eyed,
> Crooning love songs to your banjo
> Down at Lafayette—[72]

The association of brownness with boyish youth, happy countenance, and musicality is offset by other color-coded images of African American manhood. In this poem, Johnson embraces the less respectable representation of New Negro manhood as the speaker celebrates the "eyes flashing," "patent-leathered feet," and "shoulder jerking" of its object of joyful appreciation. In the brown boy, the speaker finds "the real stuff" and avows connection,

> Gee, brown boy, I loves you all over . . .
> I'm glad I can
> Understand your dancin' and your
> Singin', and feel all the happiness
> And joy and don't care in you.[73]

While black and brown manhood fared well in relation to women's avowals of support and heterosexual love, desire and admiration, "yellow" appears an almost pejorative description of manhood. For example, Virginia Houston's "Troubadour" (1930) draws a less than positive image of a figure described as yellow. Depicted as "an unremembered, sorrowful man," the speaker declares at the poem's opening, "I do not like you / You strut about your ghetto streets / Revering no one, despising yourself." The reader finds the source the speaker's dislike of the troubadour and his own self-hatred as bound to his physical body. Color shapes the speaker's vision of the man; she says, "Your yellow skin, and reddened eyes / Are dull within your yellow face, / And your body is soft." Nothing of life seems to exist within the male yellow body. Largely drawn as "yellow," one line in the three-verse poem refers to this man's supposed predecessor: "an unremembered, sorrowful man" who appears as an enslaved African American man. This "scarred body and black face," the poem reveals, "gave his soul to make the songs" the troubadour, or yellow man, "distort[s] to a silly dancing rhythm." This juxtaposition of the masculine scarred body with blackness and the description of yellow manhood as soft and dull with a "narrow chest and pimpled skin" summon nothing of honorable strength in "black" African American manhood of the past. The troubadour's denial of heritage, and minstrel persona renders him a "mongrel" in the eyes of the speaker who finds no redemptive qualities in his being. Above all, the poet finds, "There is no beauty in you, / And I do not like you."[74]

Although yellow and brown were sometimes used to describe men in poems that assumed a heterosexual stance, the most powerful declarations of women's love for a man, or men, appeared when the male figure is encoded as black. Blackness, when most clearly evoked as "black," appeared in poems that attended to women's romantic relationships with adult men. For example, an unpublished poem by Anne Spencer (1882–1975) considers not the relationship of the black man to the African American woman, but her worth to him. Despite Spencer's activism, her poems rarely took on racial matters, although important exceptions exist as they evoke color to reference race. These poems include Spencer's powerful antilynching poem, "White Things" that appeared in the *Crisis* in 1923. This poem also soberly demonstrates the neglect of women in ideological considerations of the raced citizenry. "Black men are most men; but the white are free!"[75] Black men form the subject of Spencer's homage to degraded black manhood as it premises freedom on terms gendered entirely as male.

In Spencer's unpublished work, this gendering of color and positioning of women in support of men also emerges, as in "Black Man o' Mine." The poem's speaker begins, "Black man o'mine, / If the world were your lover / it could not give to you what I give to you." Never identified by color, the African American female lover speaks confidently of her commitment to the black man, whom she seeks to "hush and caress, . . . close to my heart."[76] Darkness is called forward in the next lines of the poem as the speaker appears to work to convince her black man that he is best served only by her.

> Then with your passing dark comes my darkest part,
> For living without your loving is only rue.
> Black man o'mine, if the world were your lover, it could
> not give what I give to you.[77]

While "passing dark" suggests the black man's departure or abandonment of the female speaker, the speaker rationalizes that the love she offers the "black man o' mine" will not be found elsewhere. "Black Man o' Mine" reads clearly as an expression of collective support in the era's charge of bolstering the New Negro man. The speaker offers emotional support and physical comfort to her lover and hopes he does not stray to find something, or someone, else more worthy of his affections.

Love and its loss remains a consistent theme in poetry of the Harlem Renaissance. Women underlined the problems of finding love in the urban environment. In Helene Johnson's short verse, "Futility," the speaker of the poet scoffs,

> It is silly—
> This waiting for love
> In a parlor.
> When love is singing up and down the alley
> Without a collar.[78]

Appearing in *Opportunity* in 1926, "Futility" captures, with brevity, the parameters defining and limiting women's sexual and emotional fulfillment. The domestic space of the parlor not only confines but also appears as an outdated space when compared to the heterosocial environment that increasingly defined urban life, work, and commercialized leisure. The "collar"-less love provides romantic appeal to the speaker, who seems to have already mentally abandoned the parlor for the street.

The domestic space was also represented as a captive one, and some women depicted their social roles within this realm as unsatisfying and monotonous. Alice Dunbar-Nelson's 1927 poem, "I Sit and Sew" highlights these confines. The speaker sits and sews when her "heart aches with desire" to appease the suffering of men who were battling at war. While supportive of men's military movements, the speaker does not assert any desire independent from the suffering of "the martial tread of men." Still, the repetitive lines "I sit and sew" emphasize the speaker's own judgment of her task as forming "this pretty futile seam." Most clearly, women's sideline role in supporting men's political identities as prideful and strong is rejected as a wasted potential; the speaker shouts her shocking truth, "You need me, Christ!"[79] By underscoring men's dependent need on women and a fated Christian dependence on women, Dunbar-Nelson's verse equivocates the problem of women's seeming lack of value. Women needed to insist on their worth by aligning themselves in support and love of African American manhood.

Helene Johnson's "Widow with a Moral Obligation" offers a bold view on women's sexual freedom when marriage ends in widowhood.[80] Although the status of widowhood infers the address of older women, widows were women of all ages.[81] Indeed, the widow in Johnson's poem appears quite young in sexual energy, if not in descriptions of body that materialize only through inference of expectant arousal. The widow's "moral obligation" to her husband restricts her freely making love with another. The speaker recalls sending her suitor away citing "shy[ness]" and "foolish" behavior as having made her "run away before." Assuming the guilt of a cheating lover, the speaker conjures an image of her late husband, seeing "his lips call / me something very vile." Despite this shamefaced "conscience / or a quirk in my head," the speaker beckons her suitor,

> Ah come again, my friend,
> I'll not be so shy.
> I shall have a candle lit
> To light you by,
> I shall have my hair unbound,
> My gown undone,
> And we shall have a night of love
> And death in one.[82]

Though not challenging the convention of marriage itself, "Widow with a Moral Obligation" underscores the role of marital status, and women's relationships to men, in defining their sexual roles and identities, desires and behaviors. For this widow, the grieving is over, and the sensual imagery of unbound hair and undone gown describe not the body in color and form, but in movement and, ultimately, in renewal.

"I Sit and Wait for Beauty"

Women's love and sex poetry underscored male assessments of female beauty, but the realm of beauty played a key role in defining women's social and sexual identities. African American women who fell outside the dominant rubric of feminized beauty expressed their poetic concerns over this physical standard in various ways. This final section explores women's poetic expression of beauty by considering beauty as natural phenomena and spiritual quest; beauty in positive claim to dark complexions, and beauty as consumerist, and often racist, idealization.

Partly the poet's charge to find and represent beauty, beauty emerges as spiritual aesthetic search. "Be not averse to Beauty or to Love," urged poet Helene Johnson in "Sonnet 1" (1931). The speaker proclaims the importance of both love and beauty endowing them with qualities of "truth" and "peace." In knowing beauty, the speaker warns, "Grow in awareness, delicate and keen. / But keep the tingleness of life and mold / Your way in Beauty, vigourous and clean."[83] This moral dimension to beauty, and its approximation to romantic love, also appears important to both subsistence and sustenance of living. The poet muses, "Beauty's the wine, and Love the loaf of bread. / They are the sacrament of Life, I think, / So eat your warm white bread and drink and drink."[84] Johnson's only reference to color as white appears in the sonnet's last line summoning various possible interpretations. These lines suggest the gendering of Beauty as female, and of Love as male. One provides the pleasurable intoxication of wine, the other the substantive and necessary bread to sustain life. The "warm" whiteness of bread is perhaps suggestive of interracial sexual union or dependence of white patronage on whom, ultimately, many Harlem Renaissance poets directly, or indirectly, relied.[85]

Beauty also appears as a spiritual journey in the poet's search to define the ethereal qualities of beauty. In her 1927 poem "Questing," Anne Spencer first urges,

> Let me learn now where Beauty is;
> My day is spent too far toward night
> To wander aimlessly and miss her place;
> To grope, eyes shut, and fingers touching space.

In this quest for knowledge, the speaker of the poem asserts the need for her proactive search as the darkness of racial subjugation shapes her daily living. Spencer alludes to classical figures and celebrations of beauty but does not rely on brown or black bodies, African queens, or physical descriptions of the beautiful body to provide concrete visuals of beauty. The speaker insists that she must "learn now where Beauty is," insisting "I was born to know her mysteries." At once claiming a rights-based understanding of beauty, the poet also invokes birthright as a claim to beauty; Spencer's musing is further tempered by the effort needed to acquire this knowledge of beauty.[86] The speaker reflects on the challenge of this claim and quest for beauty: "And needing wisdom I must go in vain: / Being sworn bring to some hither land, / Leaf from her brow, light from her torched hand."[87] Here, the central obstacle to women's access to beauty appears as African Americans' American status. While the last line may reference a figure from antiquity, or perhaps that of Marianne of the French Republic or the American Statute of Liberty, the gendered body's promise of freedom and liberty rang hollow for the descendants of Africa's forced migrants.

Cowdery's poem, "I Sit and Wait for Beauty," first explores beauty as the physical body, then accesses more abstract notions of beauty to complicate the speaker's search. The poem begins,

> Long have I yearned and sought for beauty
> And now it looks a futile race
> To strive to look for the marvel
> Upon so fair a face.[88]

Here, the use of "fair" to denote beauty assumes new connotations in the writings of African American women. While this poem does not rely on color descriptors of beauty, the double entendre of "futile race," and the application of this futility to "fair faces" to define beauty reveals the powerful rejection of whiteness as a single standard to measure women's beauty. Published in 1935, "I Sit and Wait for Beauty" appeared at the end of the era's celebratory claim of New Negro womanhood. Poets like Cowdrey who were active in the latter part of the 1920s found themselves still "sitting and waiting" for definitions of beauty that were independent of men's making or free from their comparison to white women.

Color provided one way for poets of the era to claim beauty as within the reach of African Americans. Anita Scott Coleman's 1929 poem "Black Faces" evokes black as beautiful. Its expression of the androgynous and erotic quality of beauty renders it an exceptional poem, while references to white desire supply overtly gendered notions of male desire. In deeply sensuous terms, the poet writes,

> I love black faces . . .
> They are full of smould'ring fire.
> And Negro eyes, white—with white desire,
> And Negro lips so soft and thick,
> Like rich velvet within
> Fine jewelry cases,
> I love black faces.[89]

Coleman also demonstrated this positive appraisal of blackness and beauty in her long poem, "Impressions from a Family Album." Published in the *Crisis* in 1930, the poem provides portraits of family members in sections titled "Grand-Pap," "Old Praying Sue," "Melissa—Little Black Girl," and "Jim—a Weary Traveller." Both female and male subjects assume normative raced and gendered roles: Grand-Pap as the patriarchal figure, Sue as the religious and faithful, Jim as the hard-working migratory man, and Melissa, the young "black girl," who rejects the beauty of the white doll given to her by a "kind lady." In the poetic rendition of Melissa, readers confront the power of beauty in defining beauty and difference as they encounter the child's early socialization to such values. Despite the doll's being "pretty and sweet" and "dressed up neat," the speaker of this section of verse senses a coldness to the doll, who, also made by God (or rather in God's image), still lacks something. The child finds that despite God's endowment of "long flaxen hair" and "blue eyes" to this white doll,

> the man that made you, didn't put any feel
> Inside your cold little breast.
> He left the feel out
> From your head to your heels,
> But he gave you blue eyes instead.[90]

A denigrating portrait of the white doll as an emblem of white womanhood, the white doll gains the consolation prize of "blue eyes."[91]

Coleman summons African American women's outsider status as the site of the white doll's coldness. She cannot understand the plight of the "little black girl" who challenges,

> Now suppose you were me . . .
> Oh . . . my doll-baby Rose . . .
> And you knew how it felt
> To be lonely and black
> And I . . . just sat on a chair
> And gave you a cold stare . . .
> Wouldn't you . . . give my head
> A hard whack . . . Just like that!
>
> Oh . . . oh . . . My dolly . . .
> My doll-baby Rose.[92]

The speaker's angry frustration transforms into indifference toward the doll's "cold stare." For white Americans who stared back at African American women in judgment, censor, and superiority, the little black girl challenges their vision that assumes, rather than knows, the identity of the black girl. Although never depicted, the "kind lady" who provides Melissa with the doll can be assumed to be white as this verse highlights how ideas and images of beauty, embodied in the "doll-baby Rose," were provided to girls with little encouragement for the individual's own crafting of beauty as self-image.

Beauty also appears in women's representations of youth, or rather its cultural counterpart, aging. Women writers and poets of the period overlapped two generations of women. Some were born during the end decades of the nineteenth century, while others were born in the first decades of the twentieth century. As much as the incidence of youth resulted in conflicting demands on younger women, older women faced the additional concerns over aging. Some women writers and poets lied about their age, making themselves sometimes six to ten years younger than their real ages; often in their forties at the time of these creative mathematics, these women included Georgia Douglas Johnson (1877–1966), the poet, Saturday night hostess, and literary socialite; Nella Larsen (1891–1964), the Guggenheim-award–winning novelist; Jessie Fauset (1882–1961), the *Crisis* coeditor and acclaimed novelist; and Zora Neale Hurston (1891–1960), who would join the young avant garde in challenging narrow dictates of Harlem Renaissance literature—these women all lied about their ages, doing so with seeming regularity.[93]

Perhaps this deceit about age had less to do with women's vanity of being perceived as old than it did with fears about their declining sense of productivity and accomplishment in the era of the New Negro. One particularly poignant view of women's self-assessment of aging and accomplishment emerges in the diary of Dunbar-Nelson. She did not lie about her age, but she did lay awake worrying about her failures as a middle-aged woman supporting a "household full of dependents" in whom she could not confide her financial worries.[94] In her diary she wrote, "I lay in bed this morning thinking, 'forty-six years old and nowhere yet.' It is a pretty sure guess if you haven't gotten anywhere by the time you're forty-six you're not going to get very far."[95] While later entries reveal Dunbar-Nelson's more positive views on aging as she entered her fifties, delighted to maintain her looks and energy, her diary entry at forty-six years old portrays a despondency and insecurity deeply connected to a gendered time frame for the attainment of economic and social success.[96] These gendered aspects of aging are even more revealing given Cheryl A. Wall's astute note that among the Harlem literati, "no men felt compelled to take years of his age."[97]

Concerns around aging and loss of beauty and vitality appear in several women's verses; this is not surprising in an era intent on celebrating the modern, new, and youthful. But women's poetry also presents empowering views of women as they aged. In "Welt," poet Georgia Douglas Johnson summons the view of a woman who knows she cannot "mend the fabric of my youth / That daily flaunts its tatters to my eyes." In looking ahead, she considers her current love affair, realizing that "I would go further while with you, / And drain this cup so tantalant and fair." Here, the speaker implies the love affair will take the last remnants of her youth as the metaphoric cup of love and sex "meets . . . parched lips . . . / ere time has brushed cold fingers thru my hair!"[98] The poet describes a willing trade; she articulates the practical and the passionate dimensions of mature sexual desire and welcomes the satisfaction of passion as still desired in life's later years.

Douglas Johnson also addresses gendered matters of age and youth in her poem "To a Young Wife." This time, the poet assumes a male voice in offering advice to a young wife. The speaker laments his marriage to one much younger than he, but empathizes with his wife's sexual energy:

> I am sedate while you are wild,
> Elusive like a sprite;
> You dance into the sunny morn
> While I approach the night.

Here, youth is privileged as joyfully unfettered. The limitation of marriage, and especially marriage to an older man, moves the speaker to set "free" his young wife. The speaker says, "Return and live those burning years . . . / And then, come back to me!"[99] Douglas Johnson, a middle-aged, married mother and eminent poet, appears to be an unlikely author of this poem, but like other creative endeavors, poetic expressions like these reflected more on the status of African American middle-class women in the 1920s than on the lives of the poets themselves. At the same time, the poet's third collection of poetry, *An Autumn Love Cycle*, positions age most prominently and hints that Douglas Johnson's poem "To a Young Wife" can be read as both a self-lament on aging as well as a positive claim to modern sexual values of dating and heterosociability as important methods for securing compatible and marriageable mates. The speaker's hope that his young wife will come back to him once she has experienced her freedom is less suggestive of naïve hope or male assumption of women's emotional ties to men than it is a declaration of women's independent living and youthful dating as essential apprenticeship to the later formation of happy and stable marriages.

Women's poetry also characterized beauty through the consumption of material goods. In "The Proletariat Speaks," Alice Dunbar-Nelson juxtaposes the desire for "beautiful things" with the harsh conditions of the urban workplace "whose grimed windows" offer only impoverished visions of the world.[100] "I love beautiful things," the speaker asserts,

> Carven tables laid with lily-hued linen
> And fragile china and sparkling iridescent glass;
> Pale silver, etched with heraldries,

> where tender bits of regal dainties tempt,
> And soft-stepped service anticipates the unspoken wish.[101]

Framed in the desire for household consumer goods, feminized by their fine making, this vision of women's consumer desire demonstrates that elegant taste could be held by one who sleeps in a "hot hall-room whose half-opened window / Unscreened, refuses to open another inch." The female speaker is not the dreamer of a home "pleasing and attractive" to children and husband, but rather seeks the sensual for her own pleasure.

> I love beautiful things:
> Soft linen shades and silken coverlet,
> Sweet cool of chamber opened wide to fragrant breeze;
> Rose-shaded lamps and golden atomizers,
> Spraying Parisian fragrance over my relaxed limbs,
> Fresh from a white marble bath, and sweet cool spray.[102]

In the three stanzas that declare the speaker's love for "beautiful things," beauty begins with natural beauty captured through the scent of "lilacs and roses and honeysuckle"; it then moves to the table setting, and then into the bedroom where the speaker imagines herself consuming not only "beautiful things," but also imagines a beautiful space that transcends the domestic familial world so frequently defined as the domain of middle-class New Negro women. As a member of the proletariat and occupying the periphery in her access to "beautiful things," the speaker nonetheless desires the goods she cannot afford; in this sense, she engages with the capitalist enterprise of modern mass consumerism. The poem closes with imagery of the speaker as she returns to the reality of the proletariat woman, whose urban, single, tenement or boarding living, provides few of the comforts described. In the end, the only matter the speaker can control is her own appearance, and that too is a challenge. The poem concludes:

> And then I rise
> To fight my way to a dubious tub,
> Whose tiny, tepid stream threatens to make me late;
> And hurrying out, dab my unfreshed face
> With bits of toiletry from the ten cent store.[103]

In addition to consumerism's role in constructing and denying the desires of the woman worker, African American women also demonstrated the powerful hold of their male counterparts to control all impulses for independent thought and expression. Much like the speaker in Dunbar-Nelson's "The Proletariat Speaks," who voices her desire through the capitalist lens that holds her captive to a life of waged labor, the speaker appearing in Anne Spencer's 1927 poem, "Letter to My Sister," makes clear the confined parameters for the performance of womanhood. Spencer is disdainful of the "gods" who administer praise, judgment, and instruction on women's very being. In dispensing her sisterly advice, the poet warns,

> it is dangerous for a woman to defy the gods
> To taunt them with the tongue's thin tip
> Or strut in the weakness of mere humanity
> Or draw a line daring them to cross.[104]

The curtailment of women's independent expression, movement, or challenge to male order angers the poet who finds it is "worse still if you mince timidly / Dodge this way or that, or kneel or pray." In this "Letter to My Sister," the poet warns that nothing will appease the gods, whose arbitrary delights dominate the world of women. The speaker warns her "sister," "If you have beauty or none, if celibate / Or vowed—the gods are juggernaut, / Passing over. . . . over. . . ."[105] Consistent with many other female-authored expressions, and reflecting what Darlene Clark Hine describes as a "culture of dissemblance" as African American women's purposeful imposition of sexual silence to assert respectability,[106] the poet counsels her sister to

> lock away her heart, then quietly
> And lest they peer within
> Light no lamp when dark comes down
> Raise no shade for sun.[107]

Here, light and dark are reinterpreted to access the positive meanings of darkness so affiliated with descriptions of complexion that do not primarily rely on color. In this case, darkness provides protection and cover to deflect the criticism of womanhood based on ideals of beauty, sexuality, or displays of femininity that defy submissive acceptance.

The relationship between beauty and consumerism and sex and color helped shape the public identities of African American women as modern, urban, and progressive emerges most powerfully in Blanche Taylor Dickinson's 1927 poem, "Revelation." Divided into two parts, the poem places the young African American urban woman at center stage, though not as the speaker of the poem.[108] It begins with the young woman's oblivion of her racial difference:

> She walked along the crowded street
> Forgetting all but that she
> Was walking as the other girls
> And dressed as carefully.
>
> The windows of the stores were frilled
> To lure femininity,
> To empty the pocketbooks,
> And assuage queen vanity.[109]

Here, the street provides sanctuary to the modern African American woman who can forget her status as other through clothing and dress. Still, the poet remains critical of the barrage of consumerist messages seeping through shop windows, and attuned to the financial investment necessary to not only assuage vanity and desire but to also bolster the confidence of the young African American woman. The poem continues,

> And so my walker liked a dress
> Of silver and of gold,
> Draped on a bisque mannequin
> So blond and slim and bold.

The woman walker purchases the outfit that dresses the body of the "bisque" female mannequin. The poem continues to capture the walker's acquisition of the dress. At home, the walker's applies makeup and dresses in an orderly, ritualistic fashion:

> She took the precious metal home
> And waved her soft black hair;
> Powder, rouge and lipstick made
> Her very neat and fair.

However, a harsh revelation emerges. Despite her purchase of the same dress that adorned the "blond and slim and bold" bisque mannequin, and regardless of the marcelling of her hair, and using cosmetics to refine her looks, the walker faces the mirror to find

> Her vain dream slipped away. . . .
> The mirror showed a brownskin girl
> She hadn't seen all day![110]

"Revelation" engages with the consumerist construction of womanhood through the accoutrements of urban feminized beauty. Whereas clothing and dress assured the walker's dignified walk among other women, they too were "carefully" dressed, underscoring the dictates of feminized dress for American women in the modern urban setting. The dream of being seen as beautiful, or at least equal to the other woman who also moved through the cityscape, is foiled upon seeing her own reflection. Here, the "brownskin girl" assumes the quality of ordinary African American womanhood defined in difference from whiteness as the brown skin. As we have seen in mass media representations of the 1920s, this use of "brown skin" to describe the African American women as beautiful signaled the use of cosmetics to attain this claim to respectable beauty, but Dickinson's poem showed the false promise of brown-skin womanhood as an equalizing or democratizing force. Women's brown-skin beauty seemed to rely on consumer products, fashionable dress, stylish hair, and men's attentions rather than on positive self-imaging that was crafted independently from dominant views of beauty that still relied on a single standard. The poem ends by underscoring the importance of women's positive self-imaging. No doubt the poet's intention was to critique the walker's final view of herself as "dark-eyed, thick-lipped, harsh, short hair": the poem's final line recognizes, "But Lucifer saw himself, too, fair."[111] A series of distorted notions of moral and racialized beauty, of goodness and light, depict the walker as more beautiful than she can visualize. "Revelation" underscores the power of image making by those "fair" and in power. Like many poems analyzed in this chapter, "Revelation" critiqued the narrow gendered dictates of beauty, color, and sexual expression, finding brown beauty as a useful and powerful metaphor to both indict the dominance of white aesthetic standards and to claim a modern view of racialized beauty as modern, feminized, and respectable.

Conclusion

Women's poetic expression shows the use of brown as a poetic device to help express a series of concerns that were unique to modern African American women. Their status as both educated and urban women helps fix their identities as middle-class producers of the Harlem Renaissance, although that status was more tenuous than their male counterparts. Although widely published in major literary print venues that reached interracial audiences, women rarely received the same degree of support as their male peers. Friendships and networks between women played a crucial role in sustaining and honing their creative efforts, and some men also supported the efforts of women. Some women won wide acclaim, while others labored more quietly. Despite these differences and others, all thirteen poets in this study used color-inflected language in ways that were specifically gendered. Reading women's poetry through the lens of brownness and color shows how class associations, youth and aging, sexual desires, reproductive circumstances, and career aspirations formed the chief interests of these New Negro women.

Respectability as a central tenet of middle-class womanhood was renegotiated in women's poetry of the 1920s. In different ways, women critiqued the middle-class, masculinist, and aging dictates on the expected trajectory of the lives of girls and women; the very act of public writing and art making as racial protest revealed that marriage and motherhood were not their sole interests, particularly when defining womanhood. To a large extent, these women rejected domesticity as their primary domain: as they articulated desire and need to move freely in the urban public world, their poetry reflected on color and on brown-skin beauty as a growing ideal. Some poets celebrated brown beauty but also pointed to the double standard that kept women circumscribed to lives of judgment and control by white standards, by African American men, and by middle-class dictates of respectable conduct that ran counter to the realities of urban living. The language of brown is also seen to provide pleasure and freedom to identify with self and with other women in ways that were both loving and sexual (though not always necessarily both). Various iterations of brown as a poetic trope helped to articulate sexual desire in passionate, nonthreatening ways. At other times, the brown skin appears to be a warring body, caught between object and subject status, as the poet appeared to wrestle with older conventions and modern values. In sum, women's poetry articulated gendered values, sexual attitudes, and social practices inconsistent with the movement's idealization of New Negro womanhood and frequently challenged that ideal as outmoded, stultifying, and sexist. Their poetic representations on aesthetic and feminized beauty, on sex, love, and marriage express the weary impatience with these demands and suggest gendered values more modern than the dominant racial ideology of New Negro womanhood during the Harlem Renaissance.

This oscillating representation of modern brown-skin womanhood emerged, with exotic appeal, in the second novel of the most eminent race leaders of the era. W. E. B. Du Bois's novel *Dark Princess: A Romance* (1928) also drew on the narrative device and racial imaging of New Negro womanhood through an optics of color that positioned brownness as central to its representation of an Asian Indian princess as a woman of brown complexion. The following chapter explores the use of brown as it examines the literary representation of New Negro womanhood as constructed through the masculinist, middle-class, and extraordinarily influential eyes of Du Bois. His literary creation of the dark Asian Indian princess as a woman of brown complexion highlights further the paradoxical form and character of brown-skin beauty as a racialized, middle-class ideal that was at once both traditional and modern.

5

Browning the *Dark Princess*

Asian Indian Embodiment of New Negro Womanhood

> First and above all came that sense of color: into this world of pale yellowish and pinkish parchment, that absence or negation of color, came, suddenly, a glow of golden brown skin. It was darker than sunlight and gold; it was lighter and livelier than brown. It was a living, glowing crimson, veiled beneath brown flesh. It called for no light and suffered no shadow, but glowed softly of its own inner radiance.
>
> Matthew pulled himself together and tried to act sensibly. Here—in Berlin and but a few tables away, actually sat a radiantly beautiful woman, and she was colored.
>
> —W. E. B. Du Bois, *Dark Princess: A Romance*

In his novel *Dark Princess* (1928), W. E. B. Du Bois introduces to his readers to Kautilya, an Indian princess whose brown complexion facilitates the first connection to Matthew Towns, the narrative's African American male protagonist.[1] In a Berlin café, just as his ache for the "soft, brown world" of African America renders him "utterly, terribly lonesome," the self-exiled young man first sights the "dark princess." As Matthew longs "to clasp a dark hand . . . to kiss a brown cheek . . . to see warm, brown, crinkly hair and laughing eyes," the "glow of [Kautilya's] brown skin" appears as an innate exuberance that "called for no light and suffered no shadow, but glowed softly of its own radiance." So compelling was this "wildly beautiful phantasy," the omniscient narrator reveals several pages later, Matthew would "never quite recapture the first ecstasy of th[at] picture."[2]

Kautilya's brownness excites and confuses Matthew. Like the author who created him, Du Bois's hero envisions the Asian Indian princess through masculinist, Western, and African American eyes. To Matthew, Kautilya appears to be a "golden brown" that is "lighter and livelier" than the familiar brownness of his "soft, brown world." Perceiving Kautilya as "colored and yet not at all colored in his intimate sense," the well-dressed, educated young man nonetheless "assume[d] sympathy" at the "mere sight of her smooth brown skin."³ As competing emotions of racialized loneliness and gendered male desire drive this scene, Kautilya's brownness commands attention. Amid the Orientalist underpinnings and overt tones that partially shaped Du Bois's rendition of the Indian princess, this chapter finds it is precisely this brownness that encourages connection of an African American man to an Asian Indian woman in this work. This allegorical tale of Afro-Asian unity Du Bois subtitled simply *A Romance*.

This chapter continues to explore brown-skin womanhood's emergence in Harlem Renaissance literary print culture by turning to book-length fiction to study the sustained use of brown by a single author. Certainly, Du Bois, as an eminent race leader, secures a unique place in any assessment of Harlem Renaissance fiction, but his novel *Dark Princess* is equally distinctive for its focus on an interracial romance between an African American man and an Asian Indian woman—both of whom are described as brown. The author's use of brown as a narrative device and as a linguistic metaphor to describe the complexion of an Asian Indian female character and an African American man unmoors "brown" from narrow boundaries of race, place, and gender; this reading complicates the historicizing of the gendered brown skin as a motif employed by Harlem's writers, poets, and artists to represent New Negro women. As the novel moves between three continents—western Europe, North America, and South Asia—it helps expand the vision of the public worlds occupied by modern "raced" women. This analysis is particularly interested in showing how Du Bois's representation of the dark princess as a woman of brown complexion helped mediate familiar and unfamiliar constructions of "race womanhood" in 1920s America.

Focusing on the representation of an Asian Indian princess as a brown-skinned character, this chapter first considers how her depiction as bejeweled, feminized, and brown fulfilled and defied readers' expectations. It then turns to focus on brown complexion as a narrative device employed by Du Bois to assert unity between the "darker races" by studying brownness as a mutable racial marker that simultaneously evoked ideals of New Negro womanhood while invoking traditional gendered representations of Asian Indian womanhood. Throughout the novel the princess confronts and resolves a series of personal, political, and social trials—these negotiations can be viewed as processes that help soften the lines that demarcated women of the "darker races" as black or brown; in doing so, the character's brown skin, while never losing its racial designation as Indian, achieves a closer the connection to New Negro womanhood. In assessing the dark princess's embodiment of characteristics commonly emblematic of the middle-class New Negro woman, the analysis to follow explores the ways that, in writing his character as a brown woman, Du Bois simultaneously reinscribed, and at times challenged, rigid class- and color-based parameters that helped define the era's gendered notions of race womanhood.

Dark Princess: A Romance

Dark Princess tells the story of Matthew Towns, a bright, young man disillusioned by ill treatment and limited opportunities in the United States. Matthew opts for self-exile and sets sail for Europe, lamenting, "I cannot and will not stand America any longer." At a Berlin café, Matthew encounters Princess Kautilya, whose physical demeanor both excites and motivates him to chivalry. After defending Kautilya from the aggressive and unwanted male attention of a white American, Matthew discovers Kautilya's royal lineage and organizational efforts with the "Great Council of the Darker Peoples"—a radical group preparing to counter global white dominance through interracial, internationalist cooperative effort. Kautilya recruits Matthew's assistance as the council's African American representative, for despite being represented by "all the darker world . . . the darkest"—the African-descended—remained absent from the council. Despite the Egyptian council member's parochial perspective on Bolshevism, and the Japanese representative's expressed concern over the "ability, qualifications, and real possibilities of the black race in Africa and elsewhere," Matthew returns to the United States with renewed purpose and energy.[4] A series of misadventures follow. After liaising with a Garveyite figure named Perigua, Matthew is saved from perpetuating Perigua's violent scheme of bombing a train carrying a Ku Klux Klan member when Kautilya miraculously appears.

The plot foiled, Matthew is sentenced to prison, but freed a few years later with the scheming help of Chicago politician Sammy Scott and his assistant, Sara Andrews, who hide their own designs for Matthew's future. Later, Matthew enters a mutually loveless marriage with Sara, an emotionless, light-skinned mulatta. Consumed by the quest for power, security, and material wealth, Sara manipulates Matthew's burgeoning political career by selling his vote to the highest bidder. Disgusted by Sara and by his own weakness, Matthew verges on the brink of compromise and corruption when Kautilya appears miraculously to save him, for a second time, from disaster. Kautilya has resisted her own descent into a loveless, arranged marriage in loyalty to Matthew and in order to protect her crown and kingdom. Finally, Matthew and Kautilya acknowledge their deep spiritual and physical bond, and Matthew abandons Sara to enter into an adulterous relationship with the princess. The lovers share a brief period of intense happiness and then solemnly realize they must both continue their quest to unite the darker races. After this separation, Kautilya summons Matthew to his mother's home in Virginia where he discovers that the Indian princess has given birth to his son, Madhu. The novel closes with a display of pageantry and the claiming of the couple's son as "Maharajah of Bwodpur" and "Messenger and Messiah to all the Darker Worlds." Through their union, Kautilya and Matthew produce the messiah who will assumedly lead the "people of the darker races" to glorious freedom from white dominance. Madhu's royal lineage and African American heritage confirm Matthew's belief, expressed early in the novel, in the possibility of "slaves . . . becom[ing] men in a generation."[5]

Reorienting Orientals in Harlem Renaissance Literature

Debuting toward the end of the Harlem Renaissance's peak years, *Dark Princess* puzzled and disappointed Du Bois's supporters and readers who, although forgiving in their assessments, found the mixture of eroticism and racial propaganda strange and difficult to comprehend. *Dark Princess*'s complex and fantastical plot of an interracial romance that moves among three continents left reviewers nonplussed or disappointed. They puzzled over the novel's "amazing mixture of fact and fantasy," even as the *New York Times* noted its "queerest sort of mixture," which provided "enough material . . . for several novels."[6] Judging *Dark Princess*'s plot "flamboyant and unconvincing," the *Times* reviewer affirmed Alain Locke's more diplomatic assessment of the novel as "not wholly successful."[7] In his study of *Novels of the Harlem Renaissance*, Amritjit Singh offered first scholarly attention to *Dark Princess*, and relied on the language of brownness in his description of Kautilya as an "imperious and elegant brown beauty."[8] Appearing later in 1976, Arnold Rampersad's in-depth assessment of *Dark Princess* characterized the novel as a "queer combination of outright propaganda and Arabian tale, of social realism and quaint romance."[9] In calling attention to matters of style, genre, and literary politics of the era, these pioneering assessments also hint at expectations and understandings of Harlem Renaissance literary representations of raced people as African American as well as the curious representation of raced women as Indian. Considering its agenda of representing the New Negro, it is not surprising that within the range of artistic visions that contributed to dynamic expressions of African American life, society and culture, Harlem Renaissance literature included few representations of Indian women.

Du Bois troubled middle-class dictates of sexual respectability further in constructing a tale of a miscegenated union between an African American man and Asian Indian woman. In the period's fiction, interracial romances or sexual interludes were mostly limited to tormented tales against passing, the fetishism of African American women by white men, or the failed or nearly failed unions between whites and African Americans as in Jessie Fauset's *Plum Bun* (1928) and Nella Larsen's *Passing* (1929).[10] Yet, the modern discourse on African American middle-class marriage supported interracial unions, although such advocacy largely articulated a resistance against racist antimiscegenation laws by underscoring individual civil rights denied to African Americans. Celebrating modernity's mores of sexual intimacy and pleasure, African American advocacy of interracial unions surrounding romantic love, and unions based on principles of companionship and partnership, Du Bois used the fiction of *Dark Princess* to display the potential power of Afro-Asian unity in resisting white dominance. By uniting two people of the darker races whose color, rather than race, defines their mixed-race union, Du Bois subverted the typical view of miscegenation as structured by African American and white sexual alliances.

Orientalist fascinations of the 1910s and 1920s may have framed readers' understandings of the Asian Indian princess, and at times even may have fueled the author's representation of the exotic feminine other. Edward Said's influential and powerful study defined Orientalism as a series of dominant Western discourses and "discipline[s] by which the Orient was (and is) approached systematically, as a topic of learning, discovery, and practice."[11] To white Western readers and scholars, Orientalism provided a series of "dreams, images and vocabularies" taken as ready knowledge of the East.[12] With his study beginning in the mid-eighteenth century and moving into the post-Enlightenment period, Said exposes the static boundaries of this knowledge while highlighting how these formulations reveal less about the Orient or the East than they do about values, identities, and concerns of the Occident or the West.[13] In Said's *Orientalism,* the Eastern colonial subject is nearly always a male who, in subjugation, assumes effeminacy associated with the gendered position of women.

Said is not guilty of neglecting gender but rather, as Valerie Kennedy asserts, gender "forsakes him."[14] Kennedy highlights Said's brief descriptions of women as "usually the creatures of male power-fantasy. They express unlimited sexuality, they are more or less stupid, and above all they are willing," pointing out that they offer no historical analysis of the role of gender in either constructing these images, or in forming resistance to them.[15] Some of the sharpest critiques of Said's Orientalism show how this forsaking of gender advances the acceptance of Orientalism as entirely male both in production and reception. In addition, incisive critiques from scholars including Homi Bhabha redress the problematic of seeing Orientalism as a dominant and unified discourse by highlighting heterogeneity, hybridity, and mimicry as key components to skew understanding Orientalism as singular in dominance, dissemination, production, and response.[16] In assessing these responses, postcolonial scholar Gayatri Spivak invokes the language of brownness while critiquing British colonial efforts in India of "white men saving brown women from brown men" and questions why, in the imperialist movement to abolish *sati* or "widow burning," "one never encounters the testimony of women's voice consciousness."[17]

In addition to excising the absence of women's voices in Orientalist discourse and practice, other feminist scholars emphasize both the historicity and "heterogeneity of the imperial moment."[18] As Valerie Kennedy, Lisa Lowe, and Reina Lewis demonstrate, white Western women, as travelers, missionaries, and writers, also participated in the Orientalist enterprise and their works pose different and crucial questions regarding gendered relations to power and production.[19] Finally, Said's binary modeling of "Western strength and Eastern weakness" also proves unsatisfactory to scholars as it underscores "what is believed to be radical difference."[20] For Kennedy and other feminist scholars, this binary modeling "reproduces a similar opposition in terms of gender," thereby eclipsing "complex and variable relationships" held by women in relation to Orientalism, and by extension to all other discourses of power.[21]

Within the literary genre of Harlem Renaissance literature, Oriental or Asian characters, male or female, remain unusual with one notable exception. Latnah, an Arab character in Claude McKay's *Banjo* (1929), is described by Amritjit Singh as "a female roustabout, and within her Oriental aloofness, she is as much a beach bum as any of the male characters."[22] In addition, Vijay Prashad highlights the reach of Orientalist discourses in shaping African American visions of race. Drawing on Fauset's *Plum Bun* (1928), a novel about "passing," Prashad discusses the female protagonist, Angela Murray, as "bear[ing] no special love for blackness."[23] Yet, when attending a lecture on race, Prashad shows how Angela's vision of race is affirmed more positively when "she sees an East Indian in [the African American male speaker]."[24] Angela perceives the seated speaker's possession of "curious immobility, gazing straight before him like a statute of an East Indian idol" as evidence of "some strange quality which made one think of the East."[25] To Angela, the "odd, arresting beauty" of the speaker's physical body helps imbue more positive assessments of raced people even as her perception of an African American man as Indian decried phenotypic attributes commonly associated with the African American body.

As Prashad demonstrates, this "vision [was] born partly from U.S. Orientalism but also partly from the strong wave of solidarity for the anticolonial struggles in India that swept parts of Black America."²⁶ Prashad's attention to the heterogeneous influences of Orientalism to create images of the "odd, arresting beauty" of the East is also tempered by the growing transnationalistic discourses and African American struggles for race equality. While these interconnections are developed later in this chapter, here it is important to note how, for African American writers and readers, Orientalist imaginings provided not merely a ready set of understandings of Indian people as colonial subjects but also as race-proud activists.

Others too invoked the image of Buddha but claimed Afro-Asian embodiment in different ways. "On Being Young—a Woman—and Colored," published in the *Crisis* in 1925, a young African American Radcliffe graduate contested older values that confined her youth, her womanhood, and her African American identity. She "decid[ed] that something is all wrong with a world that stifles and chokes; that cuts off and stunts; hedging in, pressing down on eyes, ears and throat. Somehow all wrong." Marita O. Bonner's expressive lament realizes that she, as a woman, must wait for change. Rather than resigning in acceptance, Bonner finds inspiration in the Buddha. She decides that sitting and waiting for change shall not be frenzied, burdened, or "weighted as if your feet were cast in the iron of your soul." Rather, Bonner opts to be "quiet; quiet. Like Buddha—who brown like I am—sat entirely at ease, entirely sure of himself; motionless and knowing, a thousand years before the white man knew there was so very much difference between feet and hands."²⁷ As Bonner ponders, if Buddha is female, she, like Fauset's Angela Murray, finds inspiration in the Buddha's brownness, dignified display, and patient forbearance. Appearing in the *Crisis* in 1925, Bonner's essay no doubt was familiar to Du Bois. Three years later, in the pages of *Dark Princess*, he would also evoke the representation of the Buddha but to very different effect.

Departing from these examples, Orientalist representations most frequently devolve onto a sensualized mise-en-scène evoked by room furnishings such as Oriental carpets, Chinese vases, and Japanese kimonos. Such examples exist within *Dark Princess*. Du Bois sets the sensual scene of postcoital sleep and awakening to a stormy Chicago day in Matthew's "attic nest."²⁸ Here, Matthew ministers tender affections to Kautilya as he "arranged the golden glory of the Chinese rug around her, tucking in her little feet."²⁹ Kautilya's Orientalism seems complete when, between sleep and sex, she calls her lover's name, and it is not Matthew. "'Krishna,' she murmured." Matthew is not upset upon hearing another man's name, but rather "his mind went racing back through the shadows and he whispered back, 'Radha.' And again they slept."³⁰ The African American male protagonist, so in tune with his Asian Indian female lover, happily engages in Orientalist invocation of the Hindu paradigm of divine love and partnership. Later, upon her second wakening, Kautilya "sat up suddenly with a little cry of joy, throwing aside the great white Chinese rug and swathing herself in the silk of the white mandarin's robe that lay ready for her."[31] This scene positions Kautilya as the movable object in an Orientalist feast of sensual delights. She is wrapped and tucked by Matthew, but finally, on her own accord, moves swiftly to ensconce herself in Orientalist accoutrements. For readers, this ready set of Orientalist images assumedly inspired a fraught familiarity with Kautilya, yet likely also endorsed the raciness of this love/sex scene as a characteristic understanding of all things Oriental.

Despite his broad vision, Du Bois did not escape creating Kautilya through Orientalist eyes. But, as Bill Mullen and Cathryn Watson argue, Du Bois's "Afro-Orientalism" differed significantly from that produced by white imperialists, travelers, and writers. "Afro-Orientalism," Mullen and Watson claim, "may best be understood as the complex effort to undo a form of white supremacy—Orientalism—which Du Bois understood threatened black Americans as well as Asians."[32] Mullen sees both potential and pitfalls of Afro-Orientalism as a heterogeneous discourse on race by raced people. He describes how "practitioners... have self-consciously used historical materialist and Marxist methods to avoid the pitfalls of culturalist and raciological thinking," and include Du Bois, who throughout *Dark Princess* "both knowingly and unconsciously deployed Orientalist ideas and tropes that dramatize the peculiar and unique contradictions of his position as a black Western intellectual crisscrossing the hemispheric color line."[33] This already problematic positionality is further complicated by Du Bois's other sex identification. As the racialized male Western Other writing the female Asian Other, *Dark Princess* presents a complex interplay of racialized ideologies surrounding gender, sexuality, and nationality.

For 1920s audiences, the most known representation of Asian Indian women likely derived from the odious production in the 1927 inflammatory tract *Mother India*. Authored by U.S. "historian" Katherine Mayo, *Mother India*'s publication on three continents and its vicious attack on visions of Indian self-governance provoked heated response. While she based her claim of "objectivity" on her three-month research visit to India, this neutrality is easily challenged by the gross exaggerations and lurid judgments of India and of Asian Indian people. Mrinalini Sinha describes these representations as so abhorrent that they inspired "international controversy" and prompted protests in New York, San Francisco, London, and Calcutta.[34] Sinha also shows how Mayo's declaratory statement in the introduction to *Mother India* that her text was not "connected with official life" of any "Briton or Indian" was later proved false by Mayo's own "political blunder of later acknowledging her tremendous indebtedness to the British government" in writing *Mother India* as evidence of its pro-imperialist mission.[35]

Mayo's depiction of India's people as unfit for self-rule emerged within the midst of a growing nationalist movement in India, and in wake of Mayo's own activism in advancing anti-Asian exclusionary rhetoric in the United States. In representing the lack of Asian Indians' fitness for self-governance, Mayo drew on logic akin to paternalism by castigating the "slave mentality" of Asian Indians.[36] She stated: "inertia, helplessness, lack of initiative and originality" bound the Asian Indian "soul and body" to slavery. In addition to admonishing Hinduism as a primitive religion that bordered on the ridiculous in its ritualistic practice, Mayo also underscored, or rather highlighted, cultural "norms" as confirmation of Asian Indian inferiority.[37]

At the center of Mayo's critique of India was the wide aspersion against Asian Indians as sexually obsessed. Mayo viciously indicted the male penchant for pubescent girl-brides who, after enduring early pregnancies and dangerous birthing practices, were summarily disposed of upon the death of older husbands. Mayo's *Mother India* portrayed a country in grave need of white civilization as savior and ignored the efforts of contemporary Asian Indian feminists for legislative change to protect young girls from early marriages.[38] Gender and sexuality proved so important to Mayo's description of India that two of the text's five parts attended to gender relations. After exhausting her diatribe on debased sexuality, Mayo, according to Sinha, "could not resist the temptation of maximizing her case against Indian self-rule by including a miscellaneous grab bag of Indian social ills. Yet it was the 'bomb' about Indian sexual practices [that] remained the heart of her argument."[39] As Sinha demonstrates in her incisive introduction to a reprint of selections from *Mother India*, the representation of women through the dual lens of sexual debasement and primitive birthing practices helped position the status of Indian women as pivotal to the emerging nationalist discourse.[40] The gendering of nation as female in response to *Mother India* underscores how notions surrounding race womanhood played a central role in crafting new political representations and public identities in aid of collective efforts to represent race, nation, and citizenship.

While perhaps not a direct conversation with *Mother India*, *Dark Princess* challenges the view of Asian Indian women as illiterate, dependent, and impoverished even as it evokes an Orientalist fantasy. Yet, *Dark Princess*'s representation of Kautilya as an independent, regal, and activist woman reveals less about Du Bois's musings on Indian womanhood or his limitations in forging a counter-Orientalist image, than they do about his classed and gendered notions of "race womanhood." Du Bois's endowment of the Indian princess with color and characteristics commonly synonymous with ideologies of New Negro womanhood underscores his celebration of gendered notions of classed raced identities. At once expansive and restrictive, notions of race womanhood assume meaning through the novel's deployment of brown as a visual language to describe gendered race identities in 1920s America.

Du Bois's invocation of the dark Indian princess may also have deterred readers who may have found the character inaccessible in its departure from readily understood representatives of African American women, especially as anticipated sexual partner to the New Negro man. In discussing the novel for late-twentieth-century readers, literary critic Claudia Tate mused that the interracial love affair was perhaps the fictional element that most perturbed readers. Tate assessed: "Privately, they seem to have regarded *Dark Princess* as a dirty old man's fantasy that should never have been published."[41] In her introduction to the 1995 reprint of *Dark Princess,* Tate considers more closely the misfit connection between literary sexual representation and race literature by judging the lukewarm reception to *Dark Princess* as "historic preference for representing collective social arguments rather than personal desire in black literature."[42] In guiding contemporary readings of the novel, Tate connects the personal to the political: "when we place this novel alongside Du Bois's major autobiographical, sociological, historical and creative works, it allows us to reconstruct many of Du Bois's private feelings, beliefs and longings."[43]

The appearance of darker-skinned female characters in Harlem Renaissance literature displaced the representation of women as middle-class mulattoes, but did not always successfully dislodge gendered notions of womanhood from these representations. As early as 1911, in his first novel, *The Quest of the Silver Fleece,* Du Bois featured Zora, a dark-skinned African American woman, but as Claudia Tate argues, Zora's darkness was questionable. Describing Zora as dark, Du Bois also characterized her as a "dull-golden" mulatta, which Tate deems as possible evidence of Du Bois's own attraction for brown or light-skinned women or expression of his own feminized, biracial self. Tate argues: "By using as uplift symbols ideal dark women who are, in actuality, golden-hued, [Du Bois] undermines his own argument on black exceptionalism. Kautilya's portrait exacerbates this problem."[44] Here, I part ways with Tate. Rather than exacerbating the gendered hierarchies of color that privileged light-skinned women, Kautilya's brownness works for two seemingly paradoxical reasons. Kautilya's brownness does not outstrip reverence of African American womanhood precisely because she is not African American; simultaneously, brown was increasingly employed as a descriptor of a particularly classed expression of African American complexions. In "coloring" his protagonist, Du Bois selected brown complexion—an identifiable, malleable, and mediating complexion—as the index of the raced woman's body. In representing the brown woman as one ideal of respectable race womanhood, Du Bois retained the primacy of longer-standing middle-class ideals of racial uplift and activism; at the same time, he channeled an amalgam of modern values on sex and desire to rework sexual pleasure as a vital and complementary component of New Negro womanhood.

Sex, Love, and Modern Marriage

The sexual respectability of brown womanhood is challenged and upheld in the novel. Marriage occurs long after sexual consummation; when the union is solemnized, it retains its deeply erotic connection while clearly conforming to ideals of modern middle-class marriage.[45] Revisionist thinking on modern middle-class marriage entailed the embrace of "sexual intimacy, greater freedom and privacy for the couple, and women's equality." As historian Cristina Simmons explains, this ideal was endorsed by African-descended people and whites, but important differences existed; the "needs and context" of African American living are key to this understanding. Simmons points to "the racist sexualisation they faced, the need for group cohesion, the claims for equal citizenship rights and economic marginality" as important factors that led to "less emphasis on sex and privacy and [marriages that] incorporated wives' paid work" into respectable unions. When compared to the more "companionate marriages" that defined the modern marital unions of whites, middle-class African Americans appear more frequently invested in "partnership marriages."[46]

Anastasia Curwood, who underscores the turbulence of married life, draws a less favorable picture of marriage between middle-class New Negroes during the interwar years. Uplift, respectability, and community activism played important functions in the married lives of New Negroes between the wars. However, Curwood underlines how rapidly changing sex values and gender roles were destabilizing forces that imbued women and men with vastly different understandings of their appropriate public and private roles, ultimately sparking conflictual relationships between married couples. Drawing on films, magazines, academic studies, and the personal papers of New Negroes, including a vast correspondence between her grandparents, Curwood argues that women's waged work created "real conflict" between married partners. Curwood provides a window to view the ongoing conflicts between a sample of couples and argues that rapidly changing class and gender ideals kept them aiming at a "moving target."[47]

Certainly, the views of both scholars offer important understandings of marital relationships during the interwar era as private/public affairs that were nuanced in reality and effect; accepting that heterosexual married couples of the middle classes faced the enhanced expectation to uphold respectability, we can readily recognize that marriages were personal relationships that couples negotiated, although not always on equal grounds and not necessarily free from outside influence and external pressures. Respectability also appears a more onerous burden for New Negro women. For example, one of the era's most respectable New Negro men, W. E. B. Du Bois was a "priapic adulterer." In his two exceptional biographies on Du Bois, David Levering Lewis first brought to light suggestive and hard evidence of Du Bois's "serial affairs," explaining that several of these entanglements were "the equivalent of parallel marriages."[48] Despite Nina Du Bois's becoming "practically invisible by the late twenties," Du Bois's marriage endured for over fifty years as Nina remained "the official and everlasting Mrs. Du Bois until her death released him."[49] No doubt the stark view of Nina Gomer Du Bois as the "invisible" long-suffering wife is troubling, but as Gary L. Lemons explains, Nina Du Bois left no record for historians to construct a fuller vision. Lemons shows that despite Du Bois's later characterization of this marriage as one of duty, obligation, and intellectual incompatibility, he acknowledged his failures as a husband.[50]

Published in the same year as *Dark Princess*, in an essay entitled "So the Girl Marries," Du Bois reported on the marriage of his only daughter, Yolande Nina Du Bois, to the Harlem poet Countee Cullen.[51] The essay appeared in the June edition of the *Crisis*, two months after the grand affair. Lemons argues that it is "an important text to examine how DuBois' public, woman-identified voice contradicts the private one, articulated through a much more male-identified, hegemonic discourse."[52] In an essay where the mother of the bride features little, Du Bois reflected on her steady influence during their daughter's teenage years. "Mother stuck to her job," he wrote. "I've always had the feeling that the real trick was turned in those years, by a very soft-voiced and persistent Mother who was always hanging around unobtrusively."[53] Years later, on the occasion of his wife's passing, Du Bois reflected on his own shortcomings as a husband to Nina. "I was ranging away in body or in soul and leaving the home to my wife. She must often have been lonesome and wanted more regular and personal companionship than I gave."[54]

With understandable reluctance, scholars have troubled over the exposure of private affairs on the eminent race leader and derive various stances on the relevance of adultery to their estimations of Du Bois and his work. It is a difficult matter particularly for those who acclaim his feminist stance: Hazel

V. Carby's critique of *The Souls of Black Folk* proves instructive as she points to Du Bois's "multifaceted identity" in making sense of his complete "failure to imagine black women as intellectuals and race leaders." She frames her analysis by arguing that Du Bois "described and challenged the hegemony of the national and racial formations in the United States at the dawn of a new century . . . in ways that both assumed and privileged a discourse of black masculinity." Carby cautions against normalizing sexism by excusing such behavior under the umbrella of historical patriarchy; she reminds us of the platform that forms center stage when studying Du Bois: "In the public arena, as an African American intellectual and as a politician, Du Bois advocated equality for women and consistently supported feminist causes later in his life."[55] Still, in a book that studies the private lives, public representations, and written expression of women of the Harlem Renaissance, it is difficult not to reflect on the potential impact of extramarital affairs on the personal and professional lives of New Negro women. This is particularly true when we encounter women like Fauset and Georgia Douglas Johnson at points in their lives when professional struggles and economic crises loomed in the shadow of the most powerful figure in the community with whom, at various times, they shared intimacies.

Rather than speculate or ruminate on the consequences of these affairs, let us return to the idealized marriage in Du Bois's fiction to draw a final characterization of its representation of modern marriage. Kautilya and Matthew's marriage sustains the more dominant "white" embrace of eroticism and sexual pleasure and reinforces the partnership role of women to men; moreover, the modern interracial couple remains committed to a radical racial politics of dismantling white racial oppression across the continents. In *Dark Princess*, the romanticized marriage between Matthew and Kautilya never forsook its responsibility to the broader struggle for civil rights—in many ways it relied on that connection for its action and success.

The Color of Race and Ethnicity in White America

Written during the closing years of the 1920s, *Dark Princess* reveals the complex intersections and competitive discourses, practices, and beliefs about raced people in the United States. The dual forces of triumphant anti-immigrant sentiment and Jim Crow's continued exclusion of African Americans from the body politic marked color, in conflation with race, as a renewed divide. Color, as a category to define race difference, though not new to the first decades of the twentieth century, rose in social practice and parlance due to important changes in census data collection, scientific ideologies, and literary representation. As color identification drew on long histories within African American communities, this renewed focus melded with and morphed older, pre-established ideas about skin tone, especially in the aftermath of slavery, and later in response to the entry of "new" immigrants. Beginning in 1882 and ending in 1924, the color of these new immigrants played a significant role in their eventual total exclusion from U.S. shores.

Beginning in the post-Reconstruction years, census records furnish evidence of the rising importance of color in reformulations of the "the color line [as it] steadily became more rigid."[56] In "Fractions and Fictions in the United States Census of 1890," historian Martha Hodes shows how this census, the first and only to provide four categories to enumerate African Americans, forged notions of "whiteness . . . [as] an impassable divide."[57] Hodes examines how, as fractions of whiteness, categories of "black," "mulatto," "quadroon," and "octoroon," "ultimately worked not to illuminate, or even to acknowledge, the history of sex between people of African ancestry and people of European ancestry but rather to mark Americans of African descent in efforts to exclude them from the nation in the aftermath of the destruction of racial slavery."[58] Hodes also points to the use of "colored" to sometimes include Chinese, Japanese, and "Civilized Indians," and highlights how earlier censuses (between 1850 and 1880) "continued not to ask for each person's 'race' but rather for 'color,' a term that betrayed reliance on perception rather than any truly measurable feature."[59] The interchangeability of categories of "race" and "color" in this census record demonstrates both the subjective judgment in assessing "color," as well as the era's unreliable and unsatisfactory racial categorizations that the U.S. government endorsed in representing the nation.

For the small numbers of South Asian immigrants who entered North America between the late 1800s and 1920, color as a visual marker of race and ethnic identification also proved problematic. Asian Indians immigrants, broadly classified as "Hindoos" (although adhering to Sikhism, Islam, and Hinduism), remained mostly small in size, male in composition, and largely located on the West Coast. Although accounts vary in absolute numbers, by 1920, between 6,500 and 6,800 Asian Indian men worked on the railways, as well as "in the lumber fields of Washington and the agricultural fields of California."[60] Small compared to larger numbers of "other Asians"—namely Chinese, Japanese, Korean, and Filipino settlers—Asian Indians did not escape racial animosity. Sometimes called "niggers" because of their dark complexions, Asian Indians were more frequently maligned as "Orientals."[61] Late-nineteenth- and early-twentieth-century racist stereotyping against Asian people was vicious. These crude judgments ranged from casting them as deviant heathens and submissive coolies to sweated labor and hysteria-inducing "yellow peril." These aspersions were especially directed toward Chinese immigrants as the Asian group of earliest arrival and exclusion. Racist stereotyping also provided a composite for constructions of Asian people as perversely different from native-born, white Americans, and stoked further attacks on Japanese, Koreans, and Asian Indians that culminated in the 1917 "Barred Zone" Immigration Act that ended almost all Asian immigration.[62] South Asians, or probably more correctly, Asian Indians, were often caricatured as turbaned, bearded, and brown. To the nativist-minded, they appeared much like other Asians in their distinct unassimilability to modern white America.

During the first decades of the twentieth century, in California's Imperial Valley, the mostly male Punjabi population formed intimate bonds with women of circumspect color. In her study of Mexican-Punjabi marriages, Karen Leonard emphasizes the role of ethnicity as both "persistent and flexible" and points out that identities forged from ethnic association "are continually constructed and reconstructed by individuals and society."[63] As Mexican women and Punjabi men negotiated their married and familial lives, Leonard shows how these were not merely unions for land, nor did accession on the part of Punjabi men always prove a central motive for marriage. Although California's Alien Land Law of 1913 and its subsequent amendments made it impossible for "aliens ineligible for citizenship for leasing or owning agricultural land," these marriages fulfilled an even greater mutual need and desire for stable romantic alliances and familial formation.[64] Leonard also shows how California's antimiscegenation law, though formally forbidding interracial marriage, relied on more subjective assessments. The historian explains: "the clerk had to fill out the same word for the man and the woman. For the Punjabis and their intended spouses, clerks sometimes wrote 'brown,' sometimes 'black,' and sometimes 'white,' depending on the applicants' skin coloring and on the county."[65] This assessment of difference (or for hopeful couples, sameness) once again highlights the period's unfixed definitions of race, the specificity of place in determining color, and the conflation of the two as visual assurance of raced identities.

By the mid-1920s, white America ranked and rejected certain white people as unfit for U.S. residency and citizenship, while claiming others as native. Brown complexions held some potential to work to the opposite effect. It helped create inclusive and internationalist visions of people of color that remained flexible to the bodies and identities it described. In 1928, Du Bois's invocation of brown gendered identities in *Dark Princess* reflected his decades-long interest in expanding conflicting, unsatisfactory boundaries of race.

Du Bois and the Race Concept

Du Bois (1868–1963) dubbed his own life's narrative as an "autobiography of a race concept."[66] Throughout his long and illustrious career as social scientist, educator, editor, novelist, journalist, and race leader, Du Bois questioned the "race concept" critically and earnestly to find "not just the meaning of race but . . . the truth about it."[67] Between the late 1890s and the publication of *Dark Princess* in 1928, Du Bois's careful consideration of race demonstrates a critical and innovative thinker whose views were nonetheless partly shaped by the science, scholarship, and culture of his era. The diminishing validation of racial science and the rise of social scientists as professional "race experts" granted this space for the creative and innovative reclassifications of race, and perhaps even alternatives to race itself. Du Bois's reliance on color to capture the fantastical romance of the *Dark Princess* reflects both his creativity as a fiction writer and his efforts to circumvent reliance on definitions of race that he questioned with curiosity, concern, and commitment throughout his long career.

At the vanguard of his era, Du Bois rigorously questioned the foundations of race truths as they shifted throughout his lifetime. In his analysis of Du Bois's "evolving understanding of what he called the race concept," Joel Olson situates Du Bois's thinking on race into three broad periods: 1897–1906, 1906–30, 1930–63. This periodization helps situate Du Bois's thinking on race as a consolidation of study, reflection, political commitment, and personal experience rather than reinforce any notion that Du Bois uncritically reaffirmed essentialist and racist views of race.[68]

In 1897, at the age of thirty, Du Bois first questioned the "real meaning of race" in his inaugural address to the American Negro Academy. The newly minted sociologist and Harvard Ph.D. explored the limits in defining race by late-nineteenth-century standards. Titling his address as "The Conservation of Races," Du Bois found that "when we thus come to inquire into the essential difference of race we find it hard to come at once to any definite conclusion." Critiquing the boundaries of scientific classifications as unsatisfactory, inconsistent, and untenable, Du Bois argued that scientific judgments of "the grosser physical differences of color, hair and bone go but a short way toward explaining the different roles which groups of men have played in Human Progress." For Du Bois, the "badge of color" proved as problematic in categorizing raced people as did other physical standards. Du Bois drew out these contradictions: "color does not agree with texture of hair, for many dark races have straight hair; nor does color agree with the breadth of the head, for the yellow Tartar has a broader head than the German."[69]

Du Bois underscored shared physical, experiential, and psychic bonds as an index of race identity, defining race as "a vast family of human beings, generally of common blood and language, always of common history, tradition and impulses, who are both voluntarily and involuntarily striving together for the accomplishment of certain more or less vividly conceived ideals of life."[70] At once a sociohistorical view of race in its advocacy of shared experience, Du Bois complicated, but did not entirely refute, scientific concepts in his celebration of "common blood" and acceptance of "the final word of science, so far, is that we have two, perhaps three, great families of human beings—the whites and Negroes, possibly the yellow race."[71]

As scholars consider the long trajectory of his intellectualizing on race, these early assertions appear more consistent with essentialized views of race than with the sociohistorical model that marked his later thinking. Arguably, this overlapping of ideas delineates one of the very processes of intellectual change—key notions are questioned and tested before being fully repudiated. Moreover, as Bruce D. Dickson Jr. argues, "because the view [Du Bois] accepted left no room for a simple rejection of racial distinction, they demanded a confrontation with identity in terms that were assertive and 'racial' at the same time."[72] Kwame Anthony Appiah goes further, arguing that Du Bois "never finally accepted what he came gradually to grasp intellectually— namely, that there was no scientifically recoverable notion of race."[73] But, as Joel Olson demonstrates, and Du Bois admitted in *Dusk of Dawn* (1940), this early inability to unwed scientific views of race from the sociohistorically defined did not characterize his full thinking on the race concept that markedly matured between the 1930s and 1940s.[74]

In his fictional work, the narrative device of color that appears throughout *Dark Princess* emphasizes Du Bois's creative and intellectual efforts to circumvent a dependence on the era's dominant mode of racial classification that fluctuated between race and color designations. At its most fluid, brownness in *Dark Princess* works as a mediating device to offset notions of bodily color as a fixed marker of raced and ethnic identity rather than as a signifier of difference. As much as brown confers raced identity, brownness also resists restrictive definitions of race in its transracial and cross-gender applicability: indeed, both Matthew and Kautilya are brown. Brownness further advances oscillating notions of race as brownness or complexion; it frequently appears of the body, but not necessarily fixed to, or even defined by it; and brown entirely defines the body. For example, when first envisioned as a brown woman, Kautilya appears at the moment of Matthew's disconnection from and longing for America's "brown world." Here, Kautilya's brownness requires no definition other than brown: despite his surprise, Matthew recognizes brownness out of the local space and place of African America; brown just is. In this universalizing vision of color, Du Bois relies on the male viewer, in this case, the male other, to validate the brownness of the female Other.

Du Bois's movement to a more inward study of race, though not of gender, appears in the profoundly influential *Souls of Black Folk*, published in 1903. Problematizing the psychological dimensions of raced identity, Du Bois's identification of "double consciousness" at the turn of the century resonated then, as it does today, as one of the most powerful paradigms for subjectivizing ideas of race identity. In this text, Du Bois generates a complex view of race that highlights the unique psychic reality of African Americans. The theory of "double-consciousness" underscores how essentialist ideas crucially—and sometimes cruelly—define and limit the social reality of African Americans as "two warring ideals in one dark body."[75]

In *Souls*, Du Bois also expands notions of race by invoking classifications based on color. Defining "the problem of the twentieth century [as] the problem of the color line," Du Bois connects racial oppression as the shared heritage of "the darker to the lighter races of men in Asia and Africa, in America and in the islands of the sea."[76] In 1914, Du Bois revised this thesis finding that "the Problem of the Color Line in America instead of being a closing chapter in past history is the opening page of a new era."[77] By connecting the localized problem of virulent nativist and racist sentiments that shaped U.S. society and culture in the first decades of the twentieth century to those experienced by nonwhite people in Africa and Asia, Du Bois recast the "color line" as a "world problem"; in doing so, he advocated for international unity among the "colored people" as necessary to dismantling white global dominance.[78] As Du Bois continued to refine his considerations of the "race concept," his turn to a broader internationalism, like other African American thinkers and doers of the era, engaged a more worldly sense of racial collectivity.[79]

Women's organizational efforts were further influenced by the discourse of pan-Africanism and the enhanced sense of internationalism among African Americans activists and intellectuals of the interwar era. One group formed by women found Du Bois's language of "darker races" relevant to their organizing efforts. In 1922, eighteen elite and activist women came together, partly in protest of their segregation within the long-established International Council of Women, to launch the International Council of Women of the Darker Races (ICWDR). Their leader, Tuskegee educator Margaret Murray Washington, explained their motivations as a response to the "felt . . . need of doing a definite piece of work" for the cause of "our strong fine women everywhere."⁸⁰ Modest in size and never growing beyond forty-one members, the group was active in key women's organizations like the NACW and in mixed-gender civil rights groups, namely the NAACP. The ICWDR highlighted women's common bond of gender as uniting them in their exploitation as both women and as women of the "darker races." Still, questions remain about the degree to which that difference was also understood when shaping the discursive common bond between women of the "darker races." One critique by clubwoman Mary Church Terrell underscored the material reality of African Americans living in a segregated nation where complexion or class status offered little reprieve. In 1940, the light-complexioned clubwoman published her autobiography and identified the "double-handicap" of race and sex. Drawing on a speech she made to the United Women's Club in 1906, Terrell reflected on the efforts of African Americans trying to find accommodation in her hometown city of fifteen years, one that she noted with irony was dubbed "The Colored Man's Paradise," Washington, D.C. Clearly it was not an easy task. She concluded that "Indians, Japanese, Chinese, Filipinos and representatives of other dark races can find hotel accommodation as a rule, if you can pay for them. The colored man or woman is the only one thrust out of the world of the hotels of the national capital like a leper."⁸¹

Material conditions mattered to the ICWDR. The group focused on researching and studying the conditions of women of color in a global context, but the ICWDR remained limited in scale and scope. Michelle Rief and Lisa Matterson show how the organization underscored the transitional character of women's organizing in the 1920s. Older notions of racial uplift and women's civilizing moral mission is evidenced in the ICWDR's slogan, "Better Homes, Better Schools, Better Churches and a Better Country," yet they also embraced more expansive perspectives of racial oppression in building their study and critique of imperialism under the rubric of gender.⁸² Although the ICWDR forged few real connections and little concrete action developed from its meetings, historian Lisa Matterson emphasizes the group's importance as a precursory women's organization that was fixed on "undermin[ing] American racism within larger global processes of racism, imperialism, and eventually decolonization."⁸³ By the 1930s, non-elite, working-class African American women emerged at the forefront of efforts to unite Asians and African Americans, suggesting that socioeconomic class provided a more clear connection between these groups. Still, the persistence of descriptors of "dark people" in activist language of the later decade underscores the deepening view of white dominance as a global oppression.

Afro-Asia and Du Bois

Between the publication of *Souls of Black Folk* in 1903 and *Dark Princess* in 1928, Du Bois looked attentively to Japan, India, China, and other Asian nations, and in doing so complicated his early interrogations on "race, nationhood, capitalism, labour, gender, imperialism, culture [and] colonialism."[84] As Bill Mullen argues, this intellectualizing "taxed both [Du Bois's] expertise and at times political judgement," yet, in assessing Asia's "place in the modern world," these ruminations facilitated his developing insistence that only "the union of the darker races [can] bring a new and beautiful world, not simply for themselves, but for all men."[85] In several important studies, Mullen shows that Du Bois aligned the political and economic concerns of African and African-descended people with Asia "well before it was fashionable to do so."[86] Introducing his first collection of Du Bois's writings on Asia, Mullen situates "Du Bois perceived globalization, national interdependence, and multiple ethnic diasporas as ineluctable elements of the modern world" as an avant garde stance that remains "both the least appreciated of his political career and the one perhaps most central to its leftist trajectory."[87]

Yet, Du Bois was not the sole proponent of a black transnationalistic discourse during the Harlem Renaissance or the first to envision political, social, and racial connections between African America and India. "Du Bois was not unique in looking longingly across the Pacific," argues historian Gerald Horne, pointing to the longer "linking of Africans with Asians [a]s an important priority for [African American] radicals."[88] Long in the making, these Afro-Asian connections played a significant role for African American intellectualizing and agitating to forge a "'colored' global community."[89]

During the late nineteenth century, "a variety of social reformers began to articulate analogies between the injustices of colonial India and the United States." Nico Slate shows how this discursive connection between African Americans and Indians was premised on the "juxtaposition of emancipation and empire." As it prefigured caste oppression in India with racial oppression in the United States, Slate underscores how this association "revolved around the tension between two at times contradictory pairs of analogies." Underscoring a lack of linearity, Slate's study exposes how "connections between Indian and African American freedom struggles were as varied as the struggles themselves."[90] World War I proved a pivotal turning point for encounters between African Americans and Indians. Sudharsan Kapur shows how the emergence of Mahatma Gandhi on the Indian political front in 1915 stimulated anew and deepened the politicized connections between the two groups from those forged in the previous decade by reformers like Booker

T. Washington.[91] Slate also considers wartime to be a crucial period for the initiation of a "colored cosmopolitanism" among race leaders, intellectuals, and activists in diverse freedom movements; as colored cosmopolitans, they explored more fully the meanings of color and freedom.[92] The arrival of Gandhi followers in the United States in 1915 further marked this newly charged alignment of Indian nationalism with the movement for African American civil rights. Kapur shows how, by the early 1920s, prominent African American leaders like Marcus Garvey met with Gandhi's followers in efforts to ally the Universal Negro Improvement Association (UNIA) with Gandhi.[93] Nico Slate finds that among male leaders, Du Bois "articulated most eloquently" a colored cosmopolitanism that sought to move India to its "crucial role ... [in] encourag[ing] transnational solidarities between oppressed people."[94] Gerald Horne emphasizes how the lengthy and complex relationship between African America and India included a sharp critique of economic markets and political systems; a shared sense of grievance based on race and color proved a salient connection in America's "virtual equation of dark sin with bondage."[95]

Underlining the historical claims to a shared history of racial subjugation under white rule, Gerald Horne shows how "richly braided relations" were forged between "Black America and India." And Horne reminds us, "influence did not solely travel in one direction; nor was it physical."[96] African American and Asian Indian connections were also reciprocal and comradely in nature. One such friendship developed between Du Bois and Lala Lajput Rai, an Indian nationalist. In 1916, Rai exiled himself to the United States where he and Du Bois forged such a fast friendship that when writing *Dark Princess* Du Bois shared with him a draft and solicited the advice of his Indian friend.[97] In 1927, writing from India, Rai also solicited help from Du Bois as he prepared to write a response to Mayo's *Mother India*. In a letter dated October 6, 1929, Rai asked for "recent literature" and "telling pictures on the cruelties inflicted on your people by the whites of America."[98] In 1928, during a protest in Lahore (now in Pakistan), Rai sustained a beating by the British police that, two weeks later, resulted in his death. Du Bois honored Rai in a letter to the editor of a militant journal in Lahore naming him a martyr to the cause of the "free colored nation." Rai never read the final version of *Dark Princess*.[99]

In the years that followed Indian independence (1947), African Americans continued to look to India, at times evoking ancestral connections as Asiatic people. As the late Manning Marable shows in his recent biography of Malcolm X, the radical leader and other members of the Nation of Islam, colloquially known as Black Muslims, "preached that whites were devils and that Black Americans were the lost Asiatic tribe of Shabazz, forced into the slavery in America's racial wilderness."[100]

As early as 1907, Du Bois made similar connections, musing that India was "the land, perhaps whence our fore-fathers came, or whither certainly in some prehistoric time they wandered."[101] In the decades that followed, Du Bois maintained India's connection to the African diaspora and to antiracist activism. By 1955, the meeting of African and Asian-descended delegates at the Bandung Conference in Indonesia signaled the formal expression of Afro-Asian solidarity. Reporting on Bandung's proceedings, Richard Wright noted the extraordinary delegation from "twenty-nine free and independent nations of Africa and Asia" as "ex-colonial subjects, people whom the white West called 'colored' peoples." Wright, who began his career in the 1930s and continued to write until his death in 1960, invoked the language of color to describe the Bandung meeting. He reflected, "Only brown, black, and yellow men who had long been made self-conscious, under the rigours of colonial rule, of their race and their religion could have felt a need for such a meeting."[102] Despite this invocation of color, Wright positioned the shared histories of racial domination and economic exploitation between African and Asian-descended people—rather than merely skin tone—as the central motivation for this united action in Bandung.

Still, "colored cosmopolitans" of the post–World World I period grappled with more complex understandings of "freedom" and "colored." These words, as Slate argues, "not only have distinct histories and competing dreams but also have the ability to hide these differences."[103] Du Bois offered a more expansive view of "colored" people while at the same time eliminating the telegraphing language of race. His assessments of global geopolitical and economic change invoked the language of color by identifying that the majority of "exploited peoples were colored, yellow, brown and black."[104] "Yellow" and "brown" Asia appeared particularly crucial for joint contestations against white Western dominance.

In *Dark Princess*, Afro-Asian unity found expression in both essentialist and antiessentialist readings of race that situated color as a visual cue to raced identity. Yet, in his nonfiction work, other unseen markers of race shaped Du Bois's reflections. Evocations of "common blood"—appearing as early as 1897 in "Conservation of the Races"—found expansive expression in *The World and Africa* (1947), where Du Bois argued that "Dravidian Negroes laid the bases of Indian culture thousands of years before the Christian era."[105] This blackness, Du Bois argued, had not been subsumed under Aryan domination; rather, "the culture of the black Dravidians underlies the whole culture of India, whose greatest religious leader is often limned as black and curly-haired." Du Bois asserted that the Buddha "was imagined in the Negroid type" highlighted color as "proof of their origin."¹⁰⁶ Dissimilar to other evocations of Buddha, discussed earlier in this chapter, Du Bois's reference to the Buddha equivocated shared ancestral heritage rather than Orientalist appeal of dignified forbearance. This intellectual mapping of Afro-Asian ancestry, worked out in later years, found early expression in *Dark Princess*.

"Common blood" and shared ancestry appear in the tale of *Dark Princess* through the lens of color. At once affirming essentialist notions of race as fixed to the body, color works to unite two continents of "people of the darker races." Indeed, early in the novel, Kautilya considers her own ancestry in light of Matthew's claim of blackness and suggestion of her own. Kautilya does not claim blackness, but embraces a South Asian heritage of "mixed blood" through the "essentia[l] . . . testi[mony] in a hundred places" of "our black and curly-haired Lord Buddha."¹⁰⁷ Still, Du Bois moves beyond these essentialist reifications of "common blood," as does Kautilya, who, perhaps like Du Bois, realized the limitations of this evidence. She surmises, "enough of that. Our point is that Pan-Africa belongs logically with Pan-Asia."¹⁰⁸ Du Bois also privileged the psychic connection between African and Asian-descended people, and went further than simply asserting a "badge of color" to figuratively unify the "darker races." As Matthew tells Kautilya, "Black blood with us in America is a matter of spirit and not simply of flesh." In like manner, Kautilya strives to make India more palpable to Matthew. She describes India in ways both familiar and foreign to Matthew: "Man is there of every shade and kind and hue . . . the drama of life knows India as it knows no other land, . . . for stark poverty and jeweled wealth; for toil and song and silence—for all this, know India. Loveliest and weirdest of lands; . . . home of pain and misery—oh, Matthew, can you not understand? This is India—can you not understand?" Rather than knowing, Matthew feels the land. He replies to Kautilya, "No, I cannot understand; but I feel your meaning."¹⁰⁹

Much like the character he created, Du Bois referenced his own spiritual connection to Africa. Although he had not visited the continent until 1924, Africa figured prominently in Du Bois's pan-African expressions and political commitments. Like Matthew, Du Bois feels rather than knows; Du Bois describes his "African racial feeling" as "constitute[ing] a tie which I can feel better than explain."¹¹⁰ This connection, Du Bois concludes, derived from the "social heritage of slavery" that, when likened to the capitalist economic order of Du Bois's Western world, "puts the majority of mankind into a slavery to the rest." In looking to India as a nation of "people of the darker races," Du Bois bluntly encapsulates the problem: "European exploitation desires the black slave, the Chinese coolie and the Indian laborer for the same ends and same purposes, and calls them all 'niggers.'"[111] In refining his ideas of race and color, Du Bois's romanticized notions of Afro-Asian connections, through body and spirit, departed from biologized divisions of raced people. Through the representation of Kautilya as a brown-skinned woman, this connection attained its greatest significance.

Browning the *Dark Princess*

Undoubtedly one of the most influential African American men of the era, Du Bois crafted the dark princess largely through Matthew's eyes. From the perspective of the fiction's male protagonist, Kautilya's brownness, while attractive, first appears as different from other brown complexions. At first sighting, Kautilya is defined as "golden brown." Her brownness strikes Matthew as "lighter and livelier" than a seemingly ordinary brown complexions that Harlem Renaissance readers mostly certainly would have understood as African American. In rendering his consideration of Kautilya as "colored and yet not at all colored in his intimate sense," Matthew nonetheless "assume[d] sympathy" at the "mere sight of her smooth brown skin."[112]

Brown works not only as a referent to complexion and racial identity, but also metaphorically traces Kautilya's journey from princess to worker to mother. For much of the novel, Kautilya and Matthew are separated as each pursues his or her assumed role in the global fight for social justice. While Matthew's quest facilitates his return to African America and buoys his commitment to "the darker peoples who are dissatisfied," Kautilya's journey is structured to suspend her royal ancestry and to permit her vision into the lives of African American folk in her work as "servant, tobacco-hand [and] waitress."[113] Kautilya is essentially "browned" through living the drudged reality of countless African American working women. With prideful humility, Kautilya recounts the misery of these jobs to Matthew after their long separation. Horrified, Matthew moans, "Mud, dirt, servility for the education of a queen," to which Kautilya responds, "And is there any field where a queen's education is more neglected? Think what I have learned of the mass of men!"[114] From her first appearance as the bejeweled princess intent on organizing the darker races to her voluntary transition as lowly worker browns her as a racial equal to African American women.

Kautilya also faces perils familiar to African American women whose employment as domestics often inserted them into situations dangerous to their sexual safety and personal well-being. Particularly vulnerable in the position as a live-in domestic, Kautilya recalls, "Then came the thing of which your mother has warned me, but which somehow I did not get sense to see coming, until in the blackness of night suddenly I knew that some one was moving in my room; that someone had entered my unlocked door."[115] In this moment, Kautilya endures the peril of unwanted sexual advances from her master; a legacy of slavery, this sexual violence and threat of rape formed an all-too familiar suffering for African American women.[116] Kautilya sleeps with an unlocked door; her initial failure to protect herself, coupled with her inability to "sense" danger, highlighted the differential history of experience between the privileged Indian princess and the oppressed African American working-class woman. Based on the prior counsel of an African American woman—Matthew's mother—Kautilya becomes aware of this danger and wards off her aggressor with "a dagger which the grandfathers of [her] grandfather had handed down to [her]."[117] Here, Asian Indian and African American womanhood intertwine and triumph against white male dominance. Although it is not clear why Kautilya sleeps with a "long, light dagger with its curved handle and curious chasing," or if, in being handed down to Kautilya, its primary purpose was religious, symbolic or protective, Kautilya wields it skillfully, and a weapon that conjures masculine use saves her from harm. The defeat of white male sexual violence—a historic oppression for African American women—occurs through Afro-Asian unity of generational counsel by Matthew's mother and the inheritance of a material artifact that deters and defends.

Kautilya's ability to defend herself occurs only through the process of her browning. In opposition, when Matthew first meets Kautilya in a Berlin café, a loud, white American is harassing her. As he watches the man approach Kautilya, "a cold sweat broke over Matthew" although she has seemingly made herself prey by sitting alone in the public space. He wonders, "After all, who—what was she? To sit alone at a table in a European café." Matthew watches, and inwardly applauds, the princess's dignified dismissal of the man. When the white male aggressor follows Kautilya and reaches to touch her, Matthew's "fist caught him right between the smile and the ear." Kautilya later admits that women should not publicly venture unescorted, although "white women may, but brown women seem strangely attractive to white men, especially Americans; and this is the open season for them."[118]

The gendered divide of color comes into sharp focus in several ways. In expressing her surprise at this defense of womanhood, "It never happened before that a stranger of my own color should offer me protection in Europe. I had a curious sense of some great inner meaning to your act—some world movement."[119] Here, Matthew defends the dark female body by invoking traditional ideas of male protection historically denied to African American men during slavery. Matthew's prevention of the white man's grasp of the dark woman's body inverts the white paranoia of white women being touched in ways that sullied their womanhood. Indeed, Matthew's self-exile to Berlin—the setting of this scene—is prompted by his denied admission to study obstetrics. When pressed, the dean explains to Matthew the impossibility of "a nigger doctor delivering [white women's] babies."[120] Despite these race-based exclusions and humiliations of African American manhood, an impeccably dressed Matthew walks into the Berlin café "kn[owing] he would be served politely and without question."[121] While Kautilya shares this same privilege in service, the gendering of her brown body as a woman unescorted exposes her to dangers not shared by Matthew. Here, Du Bois reinforces traditional gender norms of male protection and female dependence, but as racialized others these movements highlight dignified female repose and prideful male action.

Kautilya's browning culminates in her final role as mother. As demonstrated earlier, Du Bois's representation departs from other representations of modern African American womanhood, especially those crafted by female writers. Certainly, Du Bois's representation of the child born to Kautilya and Matthew evoked the political union between Africa and Asia and the birth of a new world order in the male boy body that appears "golden brown." However, by engaging this reproductive trope, Du Bois reasserts conservative gender roles for women at odds with female-authored representations of New Negro womanhood. Du Bois also succumbs to further conservatism by depicting childbirth as women's work. Underscoring the irony of his desire to study obstetrics in the United States, and his perceived unsuitability to attend to the bodies of white women, Matthew does not witness or even have knowledge of Kautilya's pregnancy. At their final reunion, Matthew, enraptured by "the flash of great jewels nestling at her neck and arms" and "a king's ransom l[ying] between the naked beauty of her breasts," does not instantly see the "naked baby that lay upon her hands like a palpitating bubble of gold, asleep."[122] The peacefulness of the child, valued as gold, offset by the rich sensuality of Kautilya's adornment, fully romanticizes the pregnancy and childbirth as a natural phenomenon from which women, unaided by men, emerge as sexualized, radiant beauties.

Early descriptions of the princess and of India engage the fantastical land and body as romantic, ancient and bejeweled. Indeed, Kautilya is no ordinary woman; she is a princess and is captured as such in the text.[123] Our introduction to Kautilya reveals her royalty through her feminized body ensconced in jewels and luxurious fabrications; as Matthew notes, "There was a hint of something foreign and exotic in her simply draped gown of rich, creamlike silken stuff and in the graceful coil of her hand-fashioned turban.... There was a flash of jewels on her hands and a murmur of beads in half-hidden necklaces.... How came this princess (for in some sense she must be royal) here in Berlin?"[124] Du Bois reaffirms the jeweled imaginary of India to the extreme when the crown jewels, carried by Kautilya, go missing. The gems fall into unscrupulous hands but are rescued by a royal aide who, under orders from the princess, promptly returns them not to her but to Matthew. Here, Du Bois uses the jewels to symbolize India's mythic, resplendent past; their loss signals the debasement of ancient heritage under white colonial rule. In their return to Matthew, the jewels lose some of their exotic meaning as African American manhood secures the potentially lost treasure of India. No doubt Du Bois intended to depict the sharing of the gems as a sign of Afro-Asian unity; yet, as African American manhood triumphs in the role of protectorate, the gendered Oriental body, symbolized by the gems, not only needed but also sought out male protection and possession.

Femininity appears as a constant thread in all depictions of Kautilya. As she journeys from princess to worker to mother, Kautilya retains her femininity, paralleling the value of this gendered ideal to depictions of New Negro womanhood. From the outset, Kautilya is described as "slim and lithe, gracefully curved"; she is "always carefully groomed from her purple hair to her slim toe-tips." At first, Kautilya's femininity troubles Matthew, who worries that "perhaps he shook hands too hard, for her hand was very little and frail,"[125] although, as the novel progresses, Kautilya proves her strength and Matthew overcomes this view of the feminized as fragile. Yet, femininity remained the core representation of womanhood. Though described as a tall and majestic woman, Kautilya remains feminine and small enough that, on their reunion, Matthew "caught her to him so fiercely that her little feet left the ground and her arms curled around his neck as their lips met."[126] Kautilya's femininity and diminutive size reinforce Matthew's strength, virility, and masculinity. Underpinning traditional gender roles while simultaneously disrupting the boundaries of interracial sexuality and racialized ideals of beauty, Du Bois's feminization of the dark princess reflected the era's idealization of heterosexual, companionate love and women as feminized creatures happy to be swept off their feet.

While Kautilya never loses this much-touted aspect of womanhood, Du Bois is careful to differentiate between stylized femininity and seemingly innate feminine grace. Matthew's assessment of the princess captures this sentiment; he muses, "She was carefully groomed ... and yet with few accessories; he could not tell whether she used paint or powder." Not only does Kautilya use cosmetics, clothing, and jewels to enhance—rather than to define—her beauty, she also "never seemed in the slightest way conscious of herself. She arranged nothing, glanced at no detail of her dress, smoothed no wisp of hair.... She had no little feminine ways; she used her eyes apparently only for seeing, yet seemed to see all."[127] Consistent with the tenets of good grooming and respectable dress, Kautilya represents modern race womanhood with its updated and savvy use of consumer products such as makeup and tasteful accessories. Here, Du Bois refined his ideal of feminized race womanhood while mocking excessive use of cosmetics, feminized behaviors, and growing consumerist grooming concerns. Free from fussing over her dress, blatant display of cosmetic use, and manipulation of men through sexualized eyes, Kautilya's femininity, like the land free from white foreign colonial rule, appears "natural."

Kautilya's character also defies easy characterization as the colonized Indian woman. Her aides bemoan her independent spirit, viewing her as a "well-meaning but young and undisciplined lady."[128] Kautilya's confidence in Matthew seems reckless to her male aides as she entrusts him with a letter "to encourage treason.... [among] American Negroes." They lament Kautilya's visit to Moscow, where not only did she accrue "new European independence" but also became "inoculated ... with Bolshevism of a mild but dangerous type."[129] Referencing the Bolshevik Revolution, and his growing hopes for its promise to challenge white Western dominance, Du Bois subverts traditional gendered representations of race womanhood and assumptions about Asian Indian womanhood by depicting Kautilya's young and independent spirit. Like her aides, Matthew curiously glimpses an independence of another sort. He notices that Kautilya, "after fumb[ling] at her beads brought out a tiny jeweled box. Absently, she took out a cigarette, lighted it, and offered him one. Matthew took it, but he was a little troubled. White women in his experience smoked of course—but colored women? Well—but it was delicious to see her great, somber eyes veiled in hazy blue."[130] In this scene, Du Bois's employment of "beads" and a "jeweled box" romanticize and highlight Kautilya's Asian-ness. Yet, it is surprising when out of the jeweled box Kautilya draws a cigarette—a symbol of young, rebellious New Negro womanhood associated, by Matthew, with white womanhood. Indeed, "flapperdom" and modern womanhood signaled growing independence for American women of diverse class, ethnic, and racial origins, but the idealized "race woman" reinforced good manners and high moral standards, a "'cultured' appearance, and Christian character."[131] At once modern and traditional, Western-minded yet distinctly Asian, Kautilya's independence is foregrounded as she defies Matthew's perception of "colored women." However, in this instance, we also see the veil shielding Kautilya's true understanding of independence; through smoking, she absorbs and practices an independence enjoyed by white Western women.

Although both provocative and alluring to Matthew, the hazy blue veil is eventually lifted.

Returning to the first scene of the novel and the passage that introduced this chapter on the browning of the dark princess, Du Bois disrupts the very notion of complexion as a bodily construct as denoted by Kautilya's color appearing "veiled beneath the flesh."[132] Du Bois's evocation of the likely familiar trope of the veil was no doubt intended to also facilitate the ability of readers to "assume sympathy" with the unfamiliar figure of an Asian Indian woman. Toward the end of the novel, the metaphoric unveiling of Kautilya's brown body reflects her developing relationship to African American womanhood and to autonomous self-definition. After a long estrangement from Matthew, and rejection of male suitors who seek her hand in marriage for exploitative reasons, Kautilya reappears to Matthew "unveiled and uncloaked before him."[133]

Following the couple's physical consummation, the figurative veil is lifted, and in Kautilya's sleeping face Matthew notices "something had gone of that incomprehensible beauty of color" that "made her [on first meeting] the loveliest thing in the world." Matthew is filled with desire to see Kautilya's eyes that "he had never forgotten since first he looked into them, eyes that were pools at once of mystery and revelation, misty with half-sensed desire, and calm with power. He wanted to see her eyes again and see them at once with the high consciousness of birth."[134] Her eyes no longer misty or mysterious, Kautilya loses the royal glow of her brown complexion as she gains womanly strength and wisdom. The deveiling of her brown body permits sexual self-actualization and autonomous personal consciousness.

Still, a converse reading of the same passage highlights a heterosexist and phallocentric view of women's sexuality in its rendition that only at a man's hands does a woman become a woman and that womanhood is based on male perceptions. Kautilya, like other women, loses both mystique and beauty once potential lovemaking is made real. In a rare moment of self-doubt, Kautilya, late in the novel, questions the meaning of her sexual deveiling: "Oh, Matthew, Matthew! Did he know just what she had done and how much she had given and suffered? Did he still hold the jewel of her love and surrender high in heaven, or was she after all at this very moment common and degraded in his sight? ... She who had crossed half the world to him, fighting like a lioness for her own body. Where was she now in the eyes and mind of the man whom she had raised in her soul and set above the world?"[135] Of course, Du Bois proves his hero worthy of Kautilya's love by showing Matthew's anguish over their separation: "he needed the rubbing of a kindred soul—the answering flash of another pole. His loneliness was not merely physical; his soul was alone."[136]

Du Bois shows that Kautilya—like India—grapples with her movement from traditional princess to independent brown woman. Late in the novel, Kautilya reveals her past to Matthew, telling him of her childhood betrothal to a crown prince. When she becomes a young, virginal widow, Kautilya is spared the unfortunate plight of women who follow husbands to the grave as sensationalized by accounts of *sati* such as in Mayo's racist diatribe in *Mother India*. While Du Bois invokes Orientalist expectations of Indian womanhood and culture, he also defies them by sparing Kautilya such a fate. But, Kautilya's independence weighs heavily on her. Unmarried and pregnant with Matthew's child, she contemplates her rejection of cultural tradition: "She had violated every tradition of her race, nearly every prejudice of her family, nearly every ideal of her own life. She had sacrificed position, wealth, honor and virginity on the altar of one far-flaming star. Was it worth it? . . . . What if she did have to pay for this deep thrill of Life with submission to white Europe, with marriage without love, with power without substance?"[137] Through Kautilya's mental anguish, Du Bois underscores the complex plight of Asian Indian womanhood and, by extension, modern race womanhood. Du Bois's romantic idealism also saturates this passage as he questions the social rules that structured marriage, duty, and propriety. Kautilya's sexual activity prior to marriage, her relationship with a married man, and single motherhood may have scandalized Renaissance readers, especially in light of Du Bois's own sneer at seemingly transgressive indulgences. However, within the text, Du Bois defends this union through the deep, spiritual bond they share and the brownness of their bodies that unites them. Du Bois defends their miscegenated union, describing Kautilya and Matthew as a "beautiful couple, unusual in their height, in the brownness of their skins, in their joy and absorption of each other."[138] Reflecting the antimiscegenation hysteria of the period, this interracial and adulterous union raises the ire of the community whose castigations of the couple as "niggers" dismay Matthew. Yet, this aspersion confirms the concerns over miscegenation and its legal punitive definitions cared little about people of color who crossed the race line but not necessarily the color line. While Matthew's brownness comes sharply into focus and while gender as a relational category addresses all sexes, an analysis of Matthew as a brown man exists outside the scope of this present study. Indeed, the nonmarital and miscegenated love affair appears essential to Kautilya's development. It is through this test of courage that Matthew returns to her to claim her hand in marriage and his child as heir to Kautilya's realm of India. Kautilya, like India, needed to risk all to attain gendered independence as a woman and through marriage and motherhood gain sexual and emotional fulfillment.

Conclusion

As a work of fiction, Du Bois's *Dark Princess* offers a unique lens on the complex and changing notions on race, immigrant ethnicity, gender, class, and sexuality in its representation of the New Negro woman as the dark princess. As narrative device and racial metaphor, brownness exposes multiple points of entry to interpret its meaning in relation both to Du Bois's creative expression and to the broader intellectual, political, and social climates abounding in 1920s America. At times, the use of brown to signal color-based solidarity to modern readers relied on Orientalist understandings and evocations of Asian Indians as Other. Yet, Du Bois's internationalist outlook and his ongoing intellectualizing about race and color as biological, cultural, and political identities somewhat offset the Western male hegemonic embedded in these exoticized representations.

Furthermore, *Dark Princess* situates the local and national as important sites for the performance of modern womanhood's beauty, activism, and support of the African American male partner. At times, this rendition of brown-skin womanhood appears more closely aligned with nineteenth-century, middle-class ideals of respectability than with the tempered radicalism of the New Woman. To judge this conservatism solely as masculinist in construction and dissemination ignores its broader appeal, application, and assertion among New Negro women. Women, too, embraced, celebrated, and worked to further inculcate values of respectable womanhood along these older standards, but such endorsement was neither uniform nor equivocal as we have seen in transitional women.

Thus far, my analysis has explored New Negro womanhood and the rise of a brown-skin ideal as consumerist idealization, artistic rendition, literary trope, poetic invocation, and propagandistic fiction to claim Afro-Asian unity. The final chapter continues its exploration of the modern discourse on brown beauty in African American print culture, turning to the findings of interwar social scientists. As they arose as new authorities on race matters in the years between the two world wars, these professional academics eclipsed the role of writers, artists, and poets as cultural authorities on matters of race. The New Negro arts movement fell to the great economic Depression of the 1930s and harsh critique of its failure to bring about tangible or lasting change to the status of African Americans. While economic disaster compounded the already limited opportunities open to African Americans, government intervention in New Deal programs offered limited reprieve to unemployed youth. The problems facing the younger generation were compounded by the failure of efforts in the previous two decades. Wartime participation, race-proud rhetoric, artistic productions, labor unionization, protest movements, and urban riots did not bring about lasting economic or political change. In light of these disappointments and in the shadow of economic desolation, African America witnessed ongoing strife and uncertainty.

As the era of the New Negro closed, a new political activism arose among African American scholars who augmented the parameters of respectable protest beyond the organizational aims of long-standing middle-class groups like the NAACP and the National Urban League. Between the Depression and World War II, sociological theories gained heightened importance to redress the problems of race in America. Among the numerous, well-funded studies conducted during this period, three important works found that brown skin wielded a heightened cultural currency among African American youth. Transcending the literary imaginary, artistic rendition, and poetic musing, the discourse of brown-skin beauty appeared, in different regions of the nation, to fulfill social ideals on race, sex, class, and gender. Coming of age on the eve of the modern civil rights movement, a cross section of African American youth emphasized the power of brown.

6

Sociological Discourses on Color, Class, and Gender, from Depression to World War II

> The growing racial consciousness has fostered certain ideas concerning the Negro's physical character. The idealized picture of the Negro is presented in newspapers and magazines as not that of a black man or woman but of a brown man or woman with modified Negroid features. To the darker members of the lower classes, it provides an ideal which influences wishes concerning themselves, their marriage partners, and their children. To the middle class, the majority of whom are brown, it provides a means of racial identification. Even the upper class, with a large proportion of members of fair complexion accepts it with a variation towards the lighter shades.
> —E. Franklin Frazier, *Negro Youth at the Crossways*

In his 1940 study, *Negro Youth at the Crossways*, sociologist E. Franklin Frazier observed the powerful imaging of African American identities around an "ideal of Brown America."[1] Circulating broadly in newspapers and magazines, these images testified to the importance of physical looks as one significant force in shaping social attitudes and values among cross sections of African America. At first glance, Frazier's finding that the brown ideal was embodied in people with "modified" facial features and light-brown complexions underlines that some degree of mixed ancestry was essential to being defined as brown. However, in his book-length study of young African Americans, Frazier proved that the parameters of the brown skin ideal relied far less on the subject's connections to white ancestry, particularly in any immediate degree of relation. In his study of youth in Washington, D.C., and Louisville, Kentucky, Frazier underlined that a clearer correlation existed between complexions and class: he exposed the association of brown skin with middle-class status. Frazier's study of youth in two border-state communities found that the ideal of brown skin was accessible and desirable to African Americans of all social rankings. According to the eminent Howard University sociologist, dark-skinned lower-class African American youth aspired to brown-skin status through judicious marriages that were likely to produce brown tones in their offspring; at the same time, members of the largely light-skinned "upper class" accepted brown complexions although they preferred the color's "lighter shades." The long-held, contentious, and regionally determined equation of class and color now appeared as an exercise in mediation: brown skin was an acquisition and an asset when negotiating class mobility in a modern setting.

Other social scientists conducted studies and found remarkable the resonance of brown complexions, and some, like Frazier, drew similar conclusions on the connections between class and color. Sociologists Charles S. Johnson and Charles H. Parrish—both of whom, like Frazier, were African American—also noted brown's importance among youth in the period that followed the New Negro's demise. As these three scholars studied a broad cross section of youth in cities of border states and in rural areas of the Deep South, their findings trace the idealization of brown skin across a range of locales. These three sociologists found old hierarchies of light, medium, and dark-skinned complexions roughly translating into elite, middle, and working-class identities. Surveying female and male youth, these sociological studies found that when measured against ideals associated with brown complexions, girls and women encountered greater problems. Exposing the social settings, economic structures, and historic conditions that fueled this socialization based on color, these three scholars also intimated that the social values accorded to brown skin tones were sufficiently powerful to eclipse historic intraracial colorism.

The following analysis engages with three sociological studies conducted and published between the late 1930s and mid-1940s. *Negro Youth at the Crossways*, published in 1940, explores the relationship between social institutions, culture, and personality formation in two communities—Washington, D.C., and Louisville, Kentucky. Among the matrix of forces to influence youth personality, Frazier found that assessments of color as complexion frequently intertwined with those of class. Attitudes on color figured frequently and prominently to privilege a brown-skin ideal. In 1941, sociologist and former editor of the Harlem Renaissance literary journal *Opportunity*, Charles S. Johnson, published his findings on youth adjustment and personality formation in the eight counties of the rural South. Titled *Growing Up in the Black Belt*, Johnson studied the significance of complexion-based attitudes and values in the personality formation of African American youth; like Frazier, Johnson observed how youth bestowed the most positive aesthetic and social values onto brown-skin complexions. The most focused study on the social value of color emerged in the 1944 doctoral work of Charles H. Parrish, who published his findings two years later in the *Journal of Negro Education*.

"Intra-Group Notions about Color Classes" proved that color names were not merely descriptive identities of complexion; rather, the names given to dark, light, and brown-skinned people represented social stereotypes. Parrish concluded that brown complexions attracted the least critical and least stereotyped assessment.

Sociologists of the interwar era were mostly men. None worked to complicate the gendering of social values attached to color, nor to acknowledge the underlying sexism in assessments on brown complexions, but that is not altogether surprising given our modern understandings and knowledge on gender. This silence about the gendered burden of color emphasizes the deeply rooted acceptance of the secondary position of women in U.S. society. Chauvinistic attitudes that might or might not have erupted in the studies are not excused. Such instances remain difficult to prove as ones that necessarily display the exceptional sexism of men as individuals. Still, it is important to stay mindful of masculinist forces precisely because hegemonic practices and beliefs refract great illusions of their natural and eternal contours; they are repeatedly validated, reinforced, and naturalized. The social discourse of brown skin held great capacity to define a physical standard for interwar women's public identities. The ideal broke with older class conventions of respectability to applaud beauty and sexual attractiveness to men as racial achievement. By the 1940s, this ideal was validated by mass media representations.

As leaders, African American male sociologists held significant influence on racial matters. They held authoritative institutional positions and won commissions for important government-funded studies. The prestige of these men should not discount the vital work that women performed in contributing to their successes. For example, single-authored works, namely Frazier's *Negro Youth* and Johnson's *Growing Up*, drew upon the labor of vast teams of mixed-sex researchers and advisers whose individual accomplishments might be less well known. For example, Ophelia Settle Egypt, a social worker by training, also made significant contributions to sociological research on African American life and culture. In addition to working with Frazier in *Negro Youth*, Egypt worked at Fisk University as the chief field interviewer for Charles. S. Johnson's major study, *Shadow of the Plantation* (1934) and *The Negro College Graduate* (1938). Egypt left Fisk for Howard University, where between 1939 and 1949 she was assistant professor in the School of Social Work at Howard.[2]

A key paradigmatic shift occurred among the social sciences during the interwar period with the unmooring of race from biological classifications. This debunking of racist science—a long dominant feature of white Western intellectualizing about race—occurred across the social sciences and opened up new perspectives on color and race identity, including those built on popular, precalculated conceptions of sex, gender, class, and complexion. Scholars looked for the influence of color and race on personality, a concept of growing importance between these decades. As they sought to destabilize white dominant views of African Americans as a homogenized mass, these studies examined the construction of "Negro" practices, values, attitudes, and identities within their own communities. Rather than claim or demonstrate that African Americans displayed or inherited certain characteristics due to skin color, these studies postulated that social attitudes about complexion helped define stereotypes of individuals and the personalities of their subjects. As it completes its study of a brown-skin gendered ideal, this chapter offers close readings of these sociological texts to reveal the enhanced weight of consumerist values in shaping the racial liberal discourse around brown complexions from Depression to war.

Print Culture, the Popular Press, and the Rise of Racial Liberalism, from Depression to War

The ascendancy of social scientists as race experts and cultural commentators during the interwar period did not eclipse the long-standing role of the popular press in the fight for racial freedom and justice. The heyday of New Negro publishing clearly ended with the Depression. Eighty newspapers folded. Even the *Chicago Defender*, the nation's leading weekly, suffered a significant loss in circulation, but it rebounded, survived, and thrived in the decade that followed.[3] In 1941, a second great migration, triggered by Executive Order 8802, presented new opportunities for African Americans and ethnic people in wartime industrial work. The growth in jobs and incomes among urban African Americans drove new consumer dollars into various economies and appreciably expanded the audience for African American newspapers. Indeed, the 1940s was a prosperous decade for the black press. Between 1940 and 1946, circulation figures rose from 1,265,000 to 2,120,000.[4]

The most important weeklies to circulate on the national market were the *Pittsburgh Courier*, *Chicago Defender*, *Baltimore Afro-American*, and *New York Amsterdam News*.[5] Radical newspapers also addressed their constituencies. The *New Negro World* followed its 1920s predecessor, *Negro World*, the pan-Africanist newspaper of the Universal Negro Improvement Association (UNIA). James R. Stewart succeeded Marcus Garvey after the leader's death in London in 1940, and that same year, the new leader established the *New Negro World* in Cleveland. Despite its modest distribution (an estimate of fifteen hundred copies per issue), the newspaper circulated among African-descended people in Chicago, Cleveland, Detroit, and New York, and among others in Canada, Costa Rica, Cuba, and South Africa. Until it folded in 1944, *New Negro World*'s internationalist vision kept readers informed on radical and alternative political responses erupting in diverse struggles against imperialism, colonialism, and Western white capitalism.[6] Other newspapers expressed more conservative and regional interests; a weekly from tidewater Virginia, the *Norfolk Journal and Guide* commanded an impressive following; in the South, *Atlanta Daily World* attained a rare success as a daily publication. Mainstream news coverage also featured international events while maintaining attention to African-descended people.[7] It reported on Italy's invasion of Ethiopia in 1935 and on the Berlin Olympics in the following year when eighteen African Americans participated. One athlete, Jesse Owens, won four gold medals and the unofficial title of "the fastest human being." Media coverage presented Owens as a heroic embodiment of American democracy, although racial political realities were much more fraught and complex.[8]

At the outbreak of World War II, the African American press was a key institution in the growing demand for equal rights. In early 1942, the *Pittsburgh Courier* initiated a powerful protest based on a letter from James G. Thompson, a twenty-six-year-old cafeteria worker at an aircraft manufacturing plant in Kansas. "Being an American of dark complexion," Thompson wrote, a series of questions "flashed" through his mind; he shared them: "'Should I sacrifice my life to live half American?' 'Will things be better for the next generation in the peace to follow?' . . . 'Is this the kind of America I know worth defending?'"[9] As Thompson called critical attention to the nation's role in upholding its creed and commitment to democracy, the letter writer presaged Gunnar Myrdal's unequivocal finding that racial discrimination stymied the function of democracy in the United States. Thompson's challenge gained support; one month later, the *Pittsburgh Courier* "adopt[ed] the double 'VV' for a double victory," showcasing a new masthead design to promote the "Double Victory" campaign. On February 7, 1942, the *Pittsburgh Courier* vowed to fight fascism abroad and racism at home by exposing discriminatory policies in recruitment and hiring practices related to the war. The campaign garnered vast support. Advice columns, letters, and essays critiqued exclusionary policies in the armed forces and named practices and hostilities against enlisted men to champion democracy at home. These written pieces were complemented by "an avalanche of photographs" of African Americans "flashing a V with each hand." Photographs provided evidence of support across the nation and in action. Community and church leaders, well-known personalities, and ordinary people indicated their support for the campaign with the "VV" sign. Patrick Washburn finds, "The pictures always were posed, and they quickly became monotonous but the message was clear: Many blacks like the Double V."[10]

Photographic imagery supported the Double V campaign, prompting support from the public in actions that ranged from buying war bonds to accessorizing clothing. Hairstyles also took the shape of "VV" and women modeled "the doubler" as patriotic show. Woman's beauty also moved to the forefront to support democracy on two fronts. Mabel Burke of Chicago took center stage as the first "Double V Girl of the Week," which featured on March 28, 1942. White Americans also supported the campaign. On August 22, 1942, the *Courier* celebrated two women as "girls of the week." The photograph captured the full smiles of two women, standing side by side. Dressed in the full uniform of the American Women's Voluntary Association, Anita Lewis was presented to readers as "one of the many white women who hate practices of discrimination and prejudice." Lewis, "one of the most ardent fighters in the all-out war for democracy for all," stood shoulder to shoulder with Barbara Gonzales who, according to the newspaper, embodied "all the glamour of youth." The press did not need to announce Gonzales's race as it described the success of a "smart" woman who won a scholarship to "one of the most exclusive schools in New York."[11]

Other newspapers also championed the cause, and Double Victory evolved into a powerful media campaign that sharpened awareness of the exclusionary racial politics in the U.S. armed forces, and discrimination in hiring in defense plants and wartime industries supposedly protected by the Fair Employment Practices Committee (FEPC) against racial and ethnic discrimination. The widespread newspaper campaign came under the scrutiny of the federal government. It banned the *Pittsburgh Courier* from military bases and closely watched other publications for seditious claims against the government; no such charge was found or made.[12] Despite the militant voice of the African American press, newspapers largely endorsed integrationist goals and upheld traditional views of citizenship that could be linked to this strict censure, although other factors helped explain this position, including the assertion among moderate race leaders of shows of unity during wartime.[13] When race riots broke out in Harlem, Los Angeles, and Detroit in the summer of 1943, the press treated the violence between working-class urban people and their conflicts over unemployment, housing, and racial harassment as distracting from the war effort.[14] The Double Victory campaign ended in 1943.

While newspapers dominated the interwar and wartime press, specialized and literary magazines continued to circulate but with a different reach and influence. Only one magazine connected to the Harlem Renaissance survived.

The *Crisis* endured, although it too faced precipitous declines during the Depression: NAACP membership fell; by 1932, the magazine's circulation plummeted to 10,000 subscribers, an all-time low. A decade earlier, at its apex, circulation figures approached 100,000 in 1920; throughout the decade, the magazine averaged 62,417, although some issues were more popular than others. By February 1933, the *Crisis* was under stricter control of the NAACP, which had become an underwriter of the publication.[15] Differences between the NAACP executive board and Du Bois strained matters further. By 1930, Du Bois's editorials reflected a radicalized political stance.[16] And by 1934, Du Bois believed that progress "lay in the use of self-segregation against the fact of imposed segregation."[17] This espousal of voluntary segregation and endorsement of separatist racial economies represented a sharp departure from the moderate, integrationist ideology that shaped the NAACP from its origins. Provoking sharp criticism from the civil rights organization and refusing to compromise, Du Bois resigned on May 31, 1934.[18]

The new editor, Roy O. Wilkins, believed in a "move away from the magazine's lofty, ebony-tower approach . . . [to] broaden its appeal, audience, and circulation."[19] Under Wilkins, the magazine supported New Deal programs; it also advanced a consistently moderate, middle-class, and consumer-oriented vision that supported the NAACP's integrationist directive. Commenting on the Roosevelt administration in 1940, the editor judged its record as "spotty." While granting distance between the ideal and the reality, Wilkins deduced that the "most important contribution of the Roosevelt administration to the age-old color line problem [was] its doctrine that Negroes are a part of the country and must be considered in any program for the country as a whole." Despite his original intent to downplay lofty intellectualism and connect more with working people, the *Crisis* editor, Roy Wilkins, reaffirmed class difference, arguing that "for the first time *in their lives*, government has taken on meaning and substance for *the Negro masses*."[20] His language belied the view of a classless racial collective. At the same time, education persisted as a mainstay of the magazine, but with a different emphasis. Beginning in 1937, the *Crisis* introduced a new feature: an annual bibliography of scholarly publications related to African-descended people. Compiled by Arthur B. Spingarn, the listing foregrounded the value of scholarship to the magazine's liberal interracial audience and encouraged the broader readership of scholarly works.[21] It ran until 1968.

New Deal liberalism facilitated a significant change in white attitudes. After 1937, as Alan Brinkley explains, New Deal liberalism "developed only modestly as a program . . . [but] it continued to develop as an idea." One key development was its shifting of white views on race. By this time, commitments to restructuring the capitalist economy faded as New Dealers grew more firmly invested in the government's role in stabilizing and "growing" the economy. Alan Brinkley argues that the "idea and reality of mass consumption" made white liberals recognize its central place in the American economic and cultural order. "It is not surprising," Brinkley concludes, "that political thought began to reflect the consumer-oriented assumptions as well."[22] White liberals interested in race were racial liberals. They attributed the "race problem" to weaknesses in the economy, the physical segregation of African Americans from whites, and the consequential failing of white morality.

Peter J. Kellogg explains, "It was in the liberal community that white opposition to racism developed earliest and basic white attitudes were shaped." Specialized magazines geared toward liberal white readers, notably the *Nation*, the *New Republic, Common Sense*, and *Survey Graphic*, were "the most prominent forums of liberal discussion."[23] In 1942, *Survey Graphic* published a special issue, "Color: The Unfinished Business of Democracy." It showcased the works of intellectuals, race leaders, union organizers, economists, sociologists, artists, and writers to challenge, question, and overturn the relevance of color to the democracy on a global scale. The magazine's first part was devoted to "Negroes, U.S.A. 1942"; its second part, titled "The Challenge of Color," considered the war's influence on empire subjects in Latin America, the Caribbean, Asia, Africa, and western Europe, exposing color as an antiquated association that held real economic effect. One article, "At the Crossways of the Caribbean," noted a distinction between people judged as "colored" and people of color. Eric Williams stated, "the colored group occupies a peculiar position . . . they are not 'middle class.' They lack the property for that. The real petty bourgeoisie in the islands are East Indians, Chinese, Portuguese, and in some cases, Negro farmers. The colored group are a functional, salaried class."[24] The economic historian who, in 1962, would become the first prime minister of the Republic of Trinidad and Tobago, showed how diverse colonial patterns of settlement—the historically forced, indentured, or voluntary movement of nonindigenous people into the region—remained a salient force in the economic and social status of diverse Caribbean people. White readers and others, exposed to the broader historic realities of race, class, and white supremacy, found powerful inducement to a new racial liberalism that rejected assumptions of people's intrinsic morality, talent, and social worth as based on race.

Between the 1930s and early 1940s, racial liberals increasingly believed that economic reform could improve the conditions of African Americans; monetary success translated into class mobility; logically, greater interracialism followed; this would lead to the ultimate defeat of race prejudice.[25] Interracialism was essential for building tolerance among whites and to end the "damage" inflicted on African American people by segregation and other discriminations based on race. Hundreds of interracial committees formed throughout the North and some places in the South. African American thinkers, leaders, and scholars were also racial liberals. Frazier, Johnson, and the scholar Charles H. Parrish were among those social scientists who embraced "a new emphasis on empiricism, environmentalism and cultural relativism" to offer a "model of forward-looking liberal thought."[26] Most famously, E. Franklin Frazier endorsed a "class-driven worldview," but other African American sociologists embraced the politics of New Deal economic reform as a means to genuine progress.[27]

Critics of this liberal consensus underscore the formation of policy formulated by white understandings of African American material demands and political desires. Additionally, deeply patriarchal assumptions on race, gender, and class were embedded in racial liberalism. Ruth Feldstein studies the shift away from biological views of race to the rise of psychological understandings of race and its interworking with theorizations on personality and gender roles. Between the New Deal and the Cold War, Feldstein finds a rising discourse on "damaged personalities [that] propelled race more forcefully on the liberal agenda." While working to overturn racism, these views nonetheless "deflected attention away from systematic racial inequalities." Feldstein shows how liberal social scientists used psycho-social theories to explain race issues within the context of culture, environment, and social institutions. Practitioners ultimately racialized women as mothers by presenting African Americans as "matriarchs" and whites as "moms"; ultimately, women as mothers were responsible for the failings of family and community. This framework brokered an "intimate connection" between gender conservatism and racial liberalism.[28]

The feature of women in mass-media imaging confirms the development of gender conservatism alongside expanding interpretations on race. For example, as the *Crisis* continued to feature middle-class, college-educated women on its covers, it also presented images of women in industrial wartime workspaces. Megan E. Williams shows how this imagery of African American women reaffirmed beauty and glamour as key preserves of racial thinking. When depicted as "actively engaged in war production work," darker-skinned women were featured, as in the case of Beryl Cobham (April 1942) and Ida Mae Smith (May 1943). In September 1944, the portrait of a lighter-skinned industrial war worker, Aurelia Carter, portrayed an "inactive glamour girl." Carter's face was not shielded in a heavy industrial helmet, nor was she bent at work: she appeared pretty, smiling, and not working.[29] The positive imagery refracted through the image of glamorous and hard-working women appealed to readers. Between 1942 and 1946, the magazine's circulation expanded from 20,000 to 59,950—the latter figure clearly reflecting the expectancy of postwar African Americans.[30]

The 1940s was an era of significant development of civil rights activism on the home front. In 1941, A. Philip Randolph, labor organizer and former editor of the *Messenger*, called upon African American workers to join in a mass protest against the U.S. government with a planned March on Washington. Randolph's call to direct action garnered mass support from unionized and pro-union workers, but the NAACP and other race moderates opposed the protest as civil disobedience. The March on Washington movement, as it came to be known, was planned during "a time of opportunity." Robert Korstad and Nelson Lichtenstein explain, "high-wage, high employment economy, rapid unionization, and a pervasive federal presence gave the black working-class remarkable self-confidence."[31] Robin D. G. Kelley tempers this outlook, finding that among working-class people, a "sense of hope and pessimism, support and detachment" existed.[32] The open threat of an all-African American, worker-oriented march scared the federal government, which forestalled the action. In 1941, President Roosevelt issued Executive Order 8802, which banned discrimination based on race and ethnicity in employment in all government-sponsored wartime industries. Randolph's call for direct action also coincided with the formation of the interracial political organization, Congress of Racial Equality (CORE). Older groups like the NAACP expanded, growing from less than fifty thousand to almost half a million between 1940 and 1946.[33] The NAACP was quickly becoming "less of a protest organization and more of an agency of litigation and lobbying."[34] These and other important changes impinged deeply on African American sociologists who studied those African American youth standing "at the crossways" of racial progress. Coming of age during the Depression, African American youth moved to the forefront of sociological focus.

African American Sociologists

Scholars dub the period between the 1890s and 1945 as "the golden age in the sociology of blacks in America."[35] Two seminal sociological works mark the era: Du Bois's *The Philadelphia Negro* (1899) and St. Clair Drake and Horace Cayton's *Black Metropolis* (1945). These comprehensive studies focused on discreet communities as they studied the effects of modernization and urbanization in the social organization of African Americans. Scholars pinpoint a "second wave" of this golden age after 1930. African American sociologists in both periods paid "explicit attention to social conditioning as a primary causal force for the dilemma confronting African Americans," but sociologists of the later decades went beyond the main effort to present their subjects as moral and culturally equal to white Americans as an unspoken goal of social reform.[36] By the late 1930s, New Deal liberalism altered this agenda, making reform more pronounced; given the New Deal reliance on intellectuals and scholars in government functioning, sociologists and other social scientists materialized as "experts" on race relations.

Frazier, Johnson, and Parrish emphasized the improvement of social organization and the advancement of African American culture by calling attention to segregation as a cruel hindrance. These scholars, and others like them, highlighted social and historical factors—rather than innate biological deficiencies—as causal forces of disorganization within African American communities. As they promoted an assimilationist paradigm, these scholars strongly hinted at the need for nationwide integration. Robert Ezra Park was a key figure in the Chicago school of sociology who helped define modern social science. Park's concept, the race relations cycle, postulated that social contact between racial and ethnic groups resulted in a series of progressive reactions, namely competition, conflict, accommodation, and assimilation. Both Frazier and Johnson studied under Park to become his most celebrated African American students. They learned to analyze data that was highly qualitative and pertained to urban living. As a sociology Ph.D., Parrish also engaged Park's theory, focusing on its end point: assimilation.[37]

African American sociologists of the post-1930 period envisioned a somewhat "natural" social reform emerging from their studies on African American society and culture. Scientism, dominant during the interwar era and spilling into the war years, rejected activism as the role of the social scientist by celebrating objective methodologies and apolitical stances as disciplinary hallmarks. No such protracted agenda emerged until after the post–World War II period and the "return to normalcy." Daryl Michael Scott shows how interwar scientism granted "legitimacy to cultural dissent in race relations" by providing "cover to racial liberals who quietly labored to subvert the social system."[38] Under scientism's cover, these three men advanced Park's view that change depended on a genuine transformation of attitudes concerning race. Focused on African American subjects, these three sociologists rejected older reform-based, moral uplift efforts, and presented their academic findings as "objective information and useful categories of analysis."[39]

Race pride infused the work of social scientists during the interwar era to construct a sociological discourse on the brown-skin ideal. As Daryl Michael Scott demonstrates, race pride occluded any projection of the African American personality as "damaged" or otherwise pathological. Unlike activist social scientists of later decades, the interwar scholars "ensured they would not return a scathing moral indictment of segregation for the damage it inflicted on the black psyche." Rather than advancing arguments of damage and self-hatred, interwar and wartime social scientists postulated that African Americans had relative control in their constructions of ideas about themselves. In segregated spaces, Scott finds, Frazier and Johnson "argued both against black self-hate and for the rise of a brown ideal."[40]

By the late 1920s, the study of race in social psychology, anthropology, and sociology shifted to examine race prejudice. Social scientists embracing this paradigmatic turn investigated discriminatory prejudice arising at the individual level. The origins of race prejudice were found in personal maladjustment that suggested that such conflict could be overturned. Social sciences melded with psychiatry's focus on personality and individual social (mal)adjustment.[41] According to Scott, this fusion "marked a dramatic turning point in America's intellectual climate" as humanistic social sciences "began to locate the origins of individual pathology in social, cultural, and interpersonal relations."[42]

As the study of race prejudice slowly eclipsed the study of race in interwar social science, color discrimination offered one way to consider how and why different personalities held discriminatory views. With particular focus on youth, Frazier, Johnson, and Parrish described the historically rooted and sociocultural ways that color shaped both the individual and their communities to expose the bases of race prejudice and its effect on African American personalities.

"Studies of Negro Youth"

In 1937, so great was the concern over African American youth that the American Youth Commission, a division of the American Council on Education (ACE) commissioned a series of research projects to investigate the effect of racial prejudice on African American youth. "Studies of Negro Youth" commissioned four major research studies and published these findings between 1940 and 1941. A final volume entitled, *Color, Class and Personality*, summarized the findings in 1942; in this work, Robert L. Sutherland, director of the project, collated social scientific findings on the status of youth across regions that included eight counties in the rural South, two southern cities, two urban centers in border states, and two small and two large northern urban centers. Multidisciplinary in approach, the studies were conducted by anthropologists, psychologists, and sociologists to address the problems facing youth in diverse regions of the nation. One reviewer, Robert E. L. Farris from Bryn Mawr College, applauded the series for rigorous study "carried on by competent and experienced research men" who helped produce a "fund of organized knowledge [that] does its part to advance science."[43]

The new social scientific data emphasized the increasing maturity of the discipline as readers encountered empirical data—rather than literary exposé—to comprehend the race problem. Those like Farris found "the most sound and original . . . contributions . . . in the details of some of the research volumes," but other reviewers were less impressed.[44] Writing for the *Crisis,* James W. Ivy "reluctantly reported" that having read "all of the published series" he found "these ponderations simply state the obvious." Ivy uncovered nothing particularly new in research that found the development of youth "measured against two yardsticks of economic insecurity and race relations."[45] Others applauded the "especially timely" nature of these studies. Howard University professor Inabel Burns Lindsay considered proposals for change offered in the 1942 summary volume written by Sutherland. One "practical measure" Lindsay found unsatisfying was the need for a change of stereotypes. Sutherland explained that stereotypes were the key way "by which the white majority frequently identify all Negroes," but Lindsay was unmoved. She argued such change "involve[s] attacks on deeply embedded cultural patterns" that "would yield very slowly, if at all."[46]

More promising, Lindsay found Sutherland's recommendation directly addressed employment opportunities for youth. She agreed with Sutherland's findings that "demand[ed] that the [federal] government, as the largest employer, set sound and democratic personnel practice which will ensure the welfare of thousands of Negro youth." Lindsay urged readers to explore the "full value" of the series by reading each of the four volumes; she judged Sutherland's report in *Color, Class, and Personality* "of such importance that it ought to be on the list of every professional social worker."[47] Manet Fowler of Columbia University also assessed the multidisciplinary importance of the series; Fowler determined, "To anthropologists, as well as to Americans concerned with the efficiency of their nation, material should be of especial moment."[48]

"Studies of Negro Youth" included two sociological and two anthropological studies, the latter conducted by Allison Davis and John Dollard, and W. Lloyd Warner, Buford H. Junker, and Walter A. Adams. Proponents of the "class and caste" school, these scholars compared the nation's racial order to a caste system and the subordination of African Americans as fixed and unchanging.[49] In *Color and Human Nature,* Warner focused on Chicago and found a contradictory appeal in cosmetic advertising that placed "higher social value upon Caucasoid features" and "aggressive advoca[cy]" of "race solidarity." Particular "appeals to race pride" in African American print media emerged in "colored dolls and children's books with handsome Negro characters." The anthropologist also found a caste system that disparaged the advances of dark-complexioned African Americans, recalling "much talk about the 'beautiful brownskin' girls of our race."[50] In her review of the series of ACE studies, Lindsay concluded that they "all agreed that the Negro in the United States occupies a caste-like position in relation to the white majority."[51] Two ACE-commissioned sociological studies, Frazier's *Negro Youth at the Crossways* (1940) and Johnson's *Growing Up in the Black Belt* (1941), roundly rejected the permanence of second-class citizenship by accenting the role of class.

Negro Youth at the Crossways

In his ACE-commissioned study, *Negro Youth at the Crossways*, Frazier declared his objective to "determine what kind of person a Negro youth is or is in the process of becoming as a result of the limitations which are placed upon his or her participation in the life of the communities of the border states."[52] Frazier focused on Washington, D.C., and Louisville, Kentucky, as two cities in "border" states. Despite the limited development of slavery in both places, and the common perception of border cities as havens due to increasing urbanization, voting rights and practices, and access to education, segregation persisted in characterizing race relations in both areas.[53] Compared to the Deep South, the relative success of these states in securing somewhat amenable social, economic, and political conditions for African Americans presented a rich site to study the effects of race prejudice.[54] Although differing in size and scale, both locales were important commercial and communal centers. Frazier was also a product of the border states. His roots as a Marylander and his longtime affiliation on the faculty at Howard University in Washington, D.C., undoubtedly played some role in his scholarly perspective of this region.[55]

Frazier approached his study of youth personality by positioning culture, class, and sociohistorical forces as interconnected phenomena. His interpretation of culture rejected the view of white anthropologist Melville Herskovits, who argued that African Americans retained, transmitted, and expressed African cultural traditions.[56] Frazier believed that although one could speak of a distinctly African American "culture," that culture derived from a troubled history of the New World: the Middle Passage, enslavement, emancipation, and migration to urban centers forged central points in this development of culture. Frazier found these historical events central to the "minority status" of African Americans and the consequent social disorganization of families and society. Frazier also argued against framing culture as a holistic entity; he believed that "an exclusive focus on culture undermined the struggle for social and economic equality."[57] Frazier emphasized the important connection between class and culture. Like others in this second phase of the "golden age of sociology," Frazier advanced an assimilationist paradigm, but he argued that cultural assimilation, the final step in the race relations cycle, "could not proceed without a concomitant economic and social assimilation." According to Johnathan Scott Holloway, it was within this framework that Frazier underscored clear links between social and economic forces and culture.[58]

In his examination of youth personalities, Frazier studied the "social and cultural context in which that personality takes form." Employing nine field researchers—young college students and trained interviewers—as assistants, Frazier and his team gathered extensive data in case studies, demographic facts, and oral interviews.[59] In the two regions, these young social scientists interviewed a cross section of 145 girls and 123 boys, between nine to twenty-three years of age, with the majority falling between fourteen and nineteen.[60] To study the impact of social institutions on the personality formation of youth in these border states, Frazier divided the work into two parts. The first examined "Factors Affecting the Personality of Negro Youth." Each of the next seven chapters addressed a different social force, namely, community, family, neighborhood, school, church, employment, and social movements and ideologies. The book's second part, "Negro Youth," consisted of the only two cases studies in the text; it showcased Warren Wall and Almina Small to represent youth "at the crossways." Discussions of color appear most frequently in the chapter that addressed social movements and ideology. Responses and ideas concerning complexion are also found in other chapters, including those that address education, family, and church.

Like other sociologists of the period, Frazier rejected biological notions of disposition. Instead, he focused on the "social and cultural context in which the personality takes form."[61] *Negro Youth at the Crossways* configured personality problems as products of the social environment. Described as "social pathology," Frazier evoked terminology common among this era's social scientists to describe a host of problems in a predominantly urban context. While fraught with moralistic, scientific, and reformist overtones, "social pathology" and the less moralizing term "social disorganization" were not used to condemn the individual.[62] Rather, as Fred Matthews demonstrates, some sociologists like William Isaac Thomas "stressed that a 'disorganization' of social norms did not automatically mean that individual members of the society underwent a parallel personal disorientation."[63] The identification of "social pathology" assisted in the utilitarian work of sociologists to assist in social change.[64]

Frazier pinpointed social isolation as one grave consequence of segregation. He argued, "Since the Negro is not required to compete in the larger world and not assume its responsibilities and suffer its penalties, he does not have an opportunity to mature." Furthermore, segregation caused invidious problems within the community as "living within a small world . . . he may easily develop on the basis of some superficial distinction a conception of his role and status which may militate against the stability of his own little world."[65] Emergent among the "superficial distinction[s]" used by African American youth was color. Frazier observed the ways youth perceived themselves and others by interrogating and making clear that social values were affixed to skin color.

Attitudes concerning color often associated color with class status; for girls and young women these appear particularly austere. As he described the limited opportunities available to lower-class youth, Frazier found a paucity of opportunities available to the dark-skinned girl, who resided at the bottom of the social ladder. Through academic or athletic effort, the lower-class dark-skinned girl could attain social mobility, but Frazier found that "such 'success stories' are not common." In contrast, the lower-class girl of "somewhat lighter complexion" met a better chance of social ascendancy, "especially if she displays the talent or cleverness which will enable her to marry a prosperous business or professional man."[66] Frazier observed that cross-class marriage was not an option for the dark-skinned woman. The lack of social mobility through marriage for lower-class dark-skinned women hints at a perceived lack of aesthetic and sociosexual worth surrounding this gendered cohort.

Lighter-skinned women, whom wealthy men seemed to desire most, also faced challenges in securing marriage partners of means. Unlike the dark-skinned woman, who must "outstrip her schoolmates in studies . . . or in athletics," the woman of "lighter" complexion must utilize something akin to "womanly charms" to attract men. Like her darker-skinned sister, she too needed to cultivate her marriageability through "display [of] talent and cleverness [that] enable[s] her to marry." The reference to exhibition, the artifice suggested by the language, and the use of "cleverness" hint at the art of allure and seduction. The historical stereotypes of the Jezebel remained affixed to women of lighter complexions, and often mixed ancestral backgrounds. Although color prefaced the discussion of women's marriage to wealthy partners, the complexion of these well-off men did not appear in Frazier's observations. This omission echoes the era's gendered double standard in the perceived imbalance of the importance of color between the sexes.

Despite his efforts to resist representations of African Americans as pathological, at times, Frazier's descriptions reinforced stereotypes of women. As he examined the familial role in children's socialization on color, Frazier considered the example of a fifteen-year-old "black" girl from Louisville. He described the girl's unhappy home life, seeking to pinpoint the reason for the "child of dark complexion" becoming so embittered toward her family that she "may also engage in aggression toward those in the outside world." The "boisterous" young woman was known to "express herself best when cursing. She drinks the cheap whisky which is sold in the neighborhood, carries a knife, and fights the boys with whom she has promiscuous sex relations." The girl's delinquency was clearly the fault of a poor family dynamic; Frazier reassured readers that "it is needless to say that this case is not typical of this class."[67]

Frazier's example showed an aggressive and promiscuous young woman burdened by poverty, ignorance, family disorganization, and dark skin. When prodded further, the girl revealed animosity toward light-skinned women and her desire for "clothes and jewelry."[68] She rebelled in unrespectable ways when unable to access the fineries associated with being feminine and female. Consumerism's growing power and its shaping of the desires, behaviors, and responses of youth emerge here as a growing and problematic social force. Almost two decades later, Frazier would deliver scathing commentary on the "crass consumerism" of the burgeoning "black bourgeoisie," but in 1940, the sociologist merely observed the desire for consumption, its impact on personality, and the subject's connection between complexion and material goods.[69]

This dark-skinned young woman seemed incapable of claiming her skin color with genuine pride. Frazier blamed the family and the social environment for encouraging intraracial color discrimination. The unnamed Louisville teenager expressed acceptance of her dark skin in a defensive manner: "Well, I don't care if I am the blackest one—I'm glad I'm black. I wouldn't be yellah for nothin'. If I was born again I'd want to be just as black, if anything a little blacker. Hell, black is jest as good as any other color. I don't see why niggahs are always hollerin' about somebody bein' black, all niggahs are supposed to be black."[70] Despite the girl's rationale that "black" was the biological color for African Americans, her denigrating dialect and angry tone relay a problematic stance to her social world. Frazier pointed to her father's death, her tense relationship with her mother, and her being the darkest among her siblings as underlying reasons for the hostile attitude. This case differed from other first-person accounts due to its negative and aggressive tone. By highlighting this case as a first-person narrative, Frazier emphasized the young dark-skinned woman's dissatisfaction and anger as a window into problems within social institutions, including families. While Frazier assured readers that the examples of individuals were not typical of the class, by providing them he suggested that these attitudes were not unique, and perhaps more commonplace than the sociologist can state. He explained this case study as a culmination of social inequities: "It is presented to indicate in a way the effect upon personality, when, to the burden of family disorganization and ignorance and poverty, the handicap of race and color is added."[71] In this manner, Frazier underscored the importance of family in helping its members negotiate other powerful social forces, such as race, complexion, and class.

Negative connotations to "yellah" or "yellow," which referenced people of white and African ancestry, also appear in responses from this same dark-skinned fifteen-year-old girl. Her expression displayed a heightened vehemence toward women: "I don't like yellah niggahs, 'cause they think they're so damn cute. Mrs. ——— is one of them old yellah hussies. I hate her; she thinks she's cute because she's got that little old half white gal over there and she got a little money." Access to consumer goods fueled the subject's hostility toward light-skinned women whose "clothes and jewelry . . . the [yellow woman] can afford"; the dark-skinned girl was further aggravated by the fair girl who was "cute and had pretty hair."[72] In this discussion, as in the preceding one, consumer desire, practice, and power were tightly bound to values of physical beauty that weighed heavily on women.

The hatred expressed toward "yellah" women by the Louisville teenager was based on her perception of the woman's vanity and reinforced by the woman's "half white" daughter, and higher economic status. Notions of female beauty forged a line of demarcation between women—the result was even greater divisions within a segregated, gendered, and class-based society. *Negro Youth at the Crossways* did not report any vehement color-based, same-sex animosity among male youth, suggesting that this was a woman's problem and that concepts of beauty played a role in these color assessments. In calling attention to the problem of intraracial color discrimination, and in using the narrative of a dark-skinned woman to underscore the vehemence of such prejudices, Frazier's observations demonstrate the gendering of social values of color. It is interesting, then, that when describing the brown ideal as a popular, contemporary notion, Frazier found the most ready shorthand engendered as male. "Joe Louis, the 'Brown Bomber' . . . is a symbol of the conquest of the white man by the Negro. Although Joe Louis is a matter of fact brown in complexion, the very designation brown is not without significance as far as the Negro is concerned."[73]

In his reference to the period's famous African American boxer, Joe Louis—proudly and patriotically hailed as the "Brown Bomber"—Frazier argued that Louis personified the success, social advancement, and championing of so-called American values traditionally denied to African Americans. While Louis was indeed brown-skinned, the characterization of "Brown Bomber" was less representative of real complexion and more indicative of the symbolic value of brown. Louis represented African American success, doing so as a competitive boxer whose victories over Italian American Primo Carnera in 1935 and German Max Schmeling in 1938 celebrated masculinist precepts of democracy. A direct contrast to the threatening Jack Johnson, whose notoriety during the first decade of the twentieth century helped justify a view of African American men as animalistic, lascivious, and dangerous, Louis was celebrated as a national champion. His success, like Jesse Owens at the 1936 Berlin Olympics, marked sports as one of the few public arenas where African American men could be accorded status, privilege, and success.[74] If the new ideal of "brown" epitomized status, accomplishment, and a new racial identity predicated on social attainment, then it applied to both women and men but highlighted different gendered values. While Joe Louis represented the epitome of brown-skinned masculinity, Frazier's study also exposed perceived connections between brown complexions and female beauty.

Brownness and beauty developed as correlated values of womanhood. When asked which complexions were the most attractive, Frazier found that many young women cited brown complexions. Qualifications of "high brown" and "chocolate brown" sometimes emerged, but most often a middle-tone brown arose triumphant. When questioned on the type of African American woman who was considered pretty, one Louisville girl's responded: "My ideal woman is brown, not dark brown, has dreamy eyes, a small nose, a head that isn't too large, long thin eyebrows, a chin not too long nor too short. She should weigh about one hundred and twenty-five pounds, have a nice shape and coarse black hair."[75] Most distinctive in this description is the qualification of "not dark brown" when identifying the ideal beautiful woman. The reference to "coarse black hair" and "small nose" presents a puzzling compendium of physical features that can be read as individual preference influenced by competing ideas of race pride and dominant aesthetic values. Frazier also found that African Americans of brown complexions were least worried about the importance of color in social stratification. One Louisville girl, whose age was not given, was reported as saying: "If I were to be born over again, I would like to be the same brown color I am now. This color appeals to me simply because I have associated it with myself all these years and therefore I am quite content. Then, too, from careful observation I have concluded that color is not an asset in regard to worth-while achievements."[76]

Above all else, class structure appeared most crucial to youthful considerations of color. Frazier found this class-color connection drew on the reality that the majority of middle-class youth were brown-skinned; most wished for their same color if they could be born again. Like the dark-skinned lower-class youth who evoked the ideal of brown complexions, brown-skinned, middle-class youth also championed their self-identity as brown. From these findings, Frazier concluded that "when middle-class youth state they are satisfied with their brown complexion, it appears they are expressing their feeling of racial identification." The one group that partially rejected brown either as a racial identity or as a racial ideal was the upper class, whom Frazier found either preferred to be white or, in their acceptance of brown complexions, favored "a variation toward the lighter shade."[77]

Frazier's somewhat simplistic characterization of the lower classes as dark-skinned, the middle-classes as brown-skinned, and the upper classes as lighter-skinned evoked a color-class hierarchy typically believed true of African American communities. Certainly variations existed, but Frazier teased out these nuances by pinpointing the idealization of brown among the lower and middle classes, suggesting that class and color were at once inextricably bound and socially malleable. In his assessment of the growing ideal of brown, Frazier's optimism for a forward-moving African America becomes apparent. Through ideological rather than physical change, the discourse on brown offered a means to reconstitute the color-class divide and generate more positive representations of African Americans. Frazier's attention to social disorganization and his particular focus on the connection between class and culture were not replicated in the study of Charles S. Johnson, who also observed color-coded hierarchies. *Growing Up in the Black Belt* demonstrated regional variations in the notions of color that were shaped by ideas of gender and class.

Growing Up in the Black Belt

Growing Up in the Black Belt appeared in 1941 as the second ACE-commissioned sociological study to address intraracial color discrimination. Charles S. Johnson examined social and cultural forces influencing the social psychological development of African American youth, and in doing so helped pioneer the fusion of social psychology and sociological inquiry on race relations.[78] Focused on personality development, Johnson emphasized how social maladjustment stemmed from the "minority racial status of Negro youth." Johnson studied the adaptation of African American youth to their cultural environments, theorizing that "where there is lack of adjustment there is some incompatibility between the individual's behavior and social sanctions of the groups in which he seeks some form of recognition and status."[79]

Johnson was a graduate student at the University of Chicago when race riots exploded in the city in 1919. During the following decade, he played an active role in the Harlem Renaissance with his editorship of *Opportunity*, the official magazine of the National Urban League and his active role in fostering young talent of the Harlem Renaissance.[80] As an academic, Johnson became a master administrator. He liaised with white philanthropists, becoming the "gatekeeper for white-financed interventions into black life." With this administrative expertise, Johnson facilitated the development of the Department of Sociology at Fisk University into a powerful research center that offered important training to a new generation of African American sociologists.[81] Moving against the tide of northbound migrants, Johnson went south to Nashville, Tennessee, where he embarked on an illustrious career as a sociologist. At Fisk, Johnson began his ACE study, utilizing the institution's vast resources to research personality development in southern rural youth. Boldly characterizing the eight counties he studied as the nation's "black belt," Johnson's findings emphasized socioeconomic class as more divisive than color alone.

Johnson, like Frazier and others from the Chicago school of sociology, envisioned the role of social science as advancing racial progress.[82] St. Clair Drake, a prominent African American sociologist, introduced *Growing Up in the Black Belt* in its 1967 reprint. He distilled Johnson's agenda by explaining that Johnson "visualized the role of social science as one providing both data for the planners and human interest documents to evoke popular understanding and to help create a favorable climate of opinion for change."[83] The focus on youth personality and the problems hindering their adjustment to modern society offered fertile ground for Johnson's goal.

Less theoretically committed than Frazier, Johnson disengaged from culture as a protracted issue. He underscored the history of slavery as a causal factor for African American "maladjustments." An empirical leaning bent him away from long interpretations of his findings—*Growing Up in the Black Belt* relied on the subject, with the view that their telling of the story would reveal the most sociologically significant factors. In positioning the voices of African American youth as central throughout the text, Johnson portrayed a generation, supposedly speaking for themselves. Angry and discontented with their second-class citizenship, these youth still anticipated a better future.[84]

Johnson structured *Growing Up in the Black Belt* to explore how various social forces shaped the perceptions of youth toward themselves, toward others in their community, and toward their broader social worlds. The first chapter featured "personality profiles" of ten youth deemed "typical" due to the common problems shared by youth in the region. In the second chapter, Johnson outlined the history of the region as a causal force in the social worlds of southern African American youth. While the first two chapters provided first-person and sociohistorical contexts, the subsequent eight chapters focused on the various social institutions and forces that helped shape the youths' personalities. Johnson entitled these "Status and Society," "Youth and the School," "Youth and the Church," "Youth at Play," "Occupational Outlook and Incentives," "Attitudes Towards Sex and Marriage," "Intrarace Attitudes," "Color and Status," and "Relations with Whites." Discussions of complexion and color appeared throughout the text, but the most important evidence of brown as an emergent social ideal surfaced in "Color and Status."

Color arose as a major issue that influenced the "adjustment" of southern rural youth. Johnson expressed particular interest in "the social and aesthetic evaluation placed upon color, and the meaning of this for Negro youth."[85] Finding "little correlation between class and color in the southern rural area," Johnson underscored differences in complexion and hair as factors that affected social adjustment, but that "did not mark class lines within the rural Negro group."[86] Like his contemporaries in the Chicago school, Johnson pointed to urbanization—or rather the lack of it in the Deep South—as a central reason for limited social mobility in this region. Unlike the subjects in Frazier's study who lived in urbanized areas, rural youth in these southern counties placed little emphasis on class in connection with their assessments of color or complexion.

Influenced by the new discipline of social psychology, Johnson studied youth personality by drawing on the methodology applied in that subdiscipline. He consulted with several experts, including white psychiatrist Harry Stack Sullivan, to define and quantify personality formation. During the 1930s, social psychology discarded the formality of laboratory experimentation for projective techniques that included the use of toys and images to elicit responses from subjects. In addition, naturalistic methodologies such as interviews and observations, which were similar to those employed by sociologists, came into greater use.[87] *Growing Up in the Black Belt* employed interviews, projective techniques, and six questionnaire-type tests to glean quantitative assessments of personality. Specifically designed to measure "Personal Values," "Personal Attitudes," "Race Attitudes," "Occupation Ratings," and "Color Ratings," the questionnaire tests posed questions and statements to define attitudes on these subjects. Depending on the test administered, youth responded with either true or false answers or provided detailed explanations of their selections.[88]

Johnson already possessed a large amount of data upon which to draw and relied upon a team of skilled researchers who had assisted him in an earlier study.[89] Throughout most of his career, Johnson focused on the sociological study of the South, thereby contributing greatly to serious study of African Americans in the region. Johnson continued to study those areas that he had already investigated and published findings in *Shadow of the Plantation*, a 1934 monograph touted as one of his most important works. As a result, Johnson drew his subjects from a cross section of 2,241 youth from Mississippi, Tennessee, Alabama, Georgia, and North Carolina and explained his choice of eight counties on the basis of their diversified agricultural character. In his study of youth in these regions, Johnson highlighted the lack of education, poverty, and continued segregation as crucial social forces.[90] As Johnson allowed the voices and characters of southern rural youth to erupt throughout the text, their voices provided insight into the social values afforded to color; Johnson's descriptions of these young people were also quite revealing.

Sadie Randolph, a Mississippi youth of a sharecropper family, is described as "a placid girl of 18.[91] Her complexion is dark-brown and she has short, straightened hair. In her new gingham dress, which she made herself, she is neat and clean." Her stepfather is portrayed as a "pleasant-looking, medium-brown man" with "an honest, independent, good-humored air." Quite an opposite personality comes to the fore in the description of Sadie's mother. Compared to her common-law husband, she is "darker, with unkempt hair, a hard face, and a surly manner." The contrast between the easygoing, even-tempered brown-skinned man and the tough, darker-skinned woman is striking. Whether Sadie's stepfather was indeed brown-skinned and good-humored or her mother surly and dark-skinned seems less important than the use of these modifiers to contour these character sketches. As sociological analysis aims to be precise and direct, it is unlikely that Johnson employed this language to purposefully underscore social attitudes about color. Rather, these descriptors underscore the ubiquity of color as a semiotic and linguistic device that instilled understandings of gendered personalities.

Sadie's "placid" personality is augmented by her good needlework skills and her self-presentation that announces her as a "neat and clean" young woman. Compared to the aggressive, sexual, dark-skinned woman in Frazier's account, Sadie is classified as "dark brown"; her calm and cleanliness resonate as a success story. Nevertheless, as shown in "Attitude about Self," color also played a role in Sadie's self-perceptions: "She is sensitive about color and prefers a light-brown complexion, but adds, 'I like my color [dark brown] but would like to have long hair.' Her own hair is short. However, she thinks color is more important than hair, 'because you can fix hair and make it look pretty, but you can't change color.' She does not like white because 'it wrinkles quick.'"[92] This observation that the permanence of color—as compared to hair—heightened its importance reaffirms the relevance of both hair and complexion to assessments of raced and gendered identities. Sadie's comments also point to the widespread availability of hair products marketed as encouraging growth and taming unruly locks. And while skin-whitening products were also widely advertised in African American newspapers and magazines throughout the period, Sadie made no mention of their ability to "change color." No doubt, Sadie knew about these products, but the value she placed on them is unknown. It is also telling that Sadie rejected white complexions as undesirable due to their propensity to "wrinkle quick." From a youthful perspective, Sadie perceived visible aging as a negative development and one that was particularly problematic for women of lighter complexions. Sadie's pragmatic assessment of the importance of skin color over hair reveals the multiple forces of hair, complexion, and youth as key factors in the determinations of women's beauty.

Essie Mae Jones was the second young woman whose personality profile highlighted problems associated with color. The teenager from a tenant family in Alabama was described as "17 years old, tall and black"; she was dressed in "a plaid dress patterned in intense shades of red, yellow, green, and pink." Here, Johnson's portrait reveals much about the role of color in structuring gendered values of self-presentation. Essie Mae's dress immediately underscored her lower-class status. Unlike the "placid" Sadie, the dark-skinned girl's adornment in vibrant colors connoted a more forceful, troubled personality. This portrait of Essie Mae echoed some of the same attitudes disposed toward the aggressive, dark-skinned woman in Frazier's account, although the latter engaged a greater vehemence. Essie Mae also revealed antipathy toward mixed-race people, but vocalized a somewhat gentler explanation that their color was simply not aesthetically pleasing to her:

> Black is the best color. I'd rather be black than anything. All Negroes belong to the African race and if you are black you look more like an African, and people can tell you got pure blood. I'm glad I'm dark-skinned. I think colored people that look white is the worst. It shows they are mixed and been with white men. They call colored people bad names. I don't like to say it but the children says white people is all bastards, and I believe it because if you belong to the black race you should be black. I like some light-skinned people, but it just don't look good to me.[93]

Much like Frazier's dark-skinned teenager who chastised "yellah" women for consorting with white men, Essie Mae placed the responsibility for this phenomenon solely on women who have "been with white men." By using the rationale of "authentic" African-descended identities, Essie Mae affirmed biologized notions of race to claim her dark skin with pride. Her allusion to "colored people who look white" spoke to mixed-race or biracial people. Johnson found that this group—small among his sample in the rural South—faced their own particular issues.

Burdened by the taint of illegitimacy and white paternity, the color values attached to "yellow" women were far from celebratory. Very light-skinned women faced censure, but dark-skinned women were judged with equal harshness. Frazier and Johnson's sociological studies demonstrated that judgments of "pale," "light-colored," and "yellow" women were largely negative or suspicious in nature. In these same studies, Johnson and Frazier found that dark skin and Africanized features also generated negative stereotypes. While both sociologists identified these social valuations, neither fully explored how such stereotyping shaped ideas of African American identity.

Johnson found a brown-skin ideal developing as a counterpoint to negative stereotyping. In a chapter entitled "Color and Status," he described the southern rural population as largely unmixed and in which darker skin tones characterized the majority of the population. To the 2,214 youth in this region, a "simple test" was administered to seek their responses to thirty "value judgments" concerning skin color. These judgments included such declarations as "The ugliest girl you know," "The best woman you know," and "The smartest girl you know." Offering assessments of both women and men, the respondents were asked to circle one of the six color groupings that included black, dark brown, brown, light brown, yellow, and white. Johnson found that brown and light brown consistently ranked the highest in positive value statements and lowest in negative assessments. Of the 2,214 youth polled using this method, Johnson interviewed five hundred "for further information and insights into the status problems associated with color."[94] When asked for responses to "pleasant and unpleasant stimuli in terms of color associations," southern rural youth consistently reiterated the association of brown skin with beauty, socioeconomic status, and moral standing.[95]

In Johnson's testing, light brown ranked higher than brown. When polled for the "best color to be," 46.5 percent of girls and 38.3 percent of boys elected "light brown." Second was "brown" as 20.1 percent of girls and 23.5 percent of boys elected this complexion as the "best color to be." While boys and girls claimed light brown and brown as the most desirable, more girls than boys made this decision. Physical beauty was also most equated with light brown and brown complexions. A greater percentage of male and female respondents declared light brown (44.4 percent of girls and 43.8 percent of boys) when asked to assess "the most beautiful girl you know" than did the percentage answering "light brown" when asked about "the most handsome boy you know" (41.7 percent of girls and 34.9 percent of boys). When it came to aesthetic evaluations, light brown still prevailed as the most popular selection, but the looks of brown men fared better than that of women: 16.7 percent of girls and 20 percent of boys considered the brown man's looks to be most appealing, compared to 16.1 percent of girls and 14.1 percent of boys making the same statement about the brown woman's aesthetic appeal.

It appears that young men and boys were more likely to opt for darker skin tones when assessing the beauty of the other sex. Even more telling is the assessment of dark brown. Only 13.1 percent of girls and 11.2 percent of boys agreed that dark-brown girls and women were among the most beautiful, but dark-brown boys and men garnered 18.7 percent of the female votes and 19.8 percent of males when asked about the most handsome. Johnson's findings show that despite the privileging of light brown and brown as an aesthetic ideal among rural youth, African American girls and women cited dark-brown men as more handsome than men who were the lighter color of brown. While darkness of skin appears more accepted by women when assessing the other sex, the reverse does not prove true of men's views of female beauty. Boy's responses show a privileging of light brown, brown, and yellow, as compared to that of girls, who positioned light brown, dark brown, and brown as the most attractive.[96]

Johnson qualified these quantitative assessments by providing for readers a selection of statements that addressed the ideal of brown. Solicited from respondents, these included: "I'd rather be light brown, but I wouldn't want to be yellow"; "It's better to be brown or light-brown, because one is too conspicuous when he is all black or yellow"; "If I could be any color I'd be light-brown, it looks the best"; "I like light-brown first, because it's pretty and you are able to wear any color when you are that color"; and "Black people can't use make-up, but light-brown people can; that's my color." No provision of age, class, or gender appears to contextualize these statements. Somewhat more telling are the few individual voices of African American rural girls and young women who address matters of color. Elsie Carter, a fifteen year old from a poor family, is described as "very dark, with hair about an inch long and straightened." Self-aware about her complexion, Elsie stated that she would be happier if brown-skinned as "this . . . is a prettier color and you can look nice in different colors of clothes."[97] Elsie was not the only respondent in Johnson's or Frazier's study to find access to a wider variety of clothes as a reason for desiring a brown complexion. These responses underscore the continued, heightened importance of consumer goods in constructing ideas and images of African American womanhood. In these instances, complexion appears as an important factor in the choice of dressing oneself in a fashionable and acceptable manner. The concern over the color of clothing adorning bodies of different complexions heaped additional burdens on women and girls, especially those of limited economic means who would not have had the luxury to be selective about their wardrobe. "Laundered Denims" appeared as the title of one review of Johnson's *Growing Up in the Black Belt*, capturing the importance, the limitations, and the creative ways southern rural youth found to fashion this new consumer-based respectability.[98]

Johnson also found discrepancies in self-assessments of complexion. Repeatedly, the sociologist found that African American youth claimed themselves to be "a shade or more lighter" than their "true" complexions. To determine the true complexions of the subjects, Johnson relied on the "consensus of the group of interviewers and testers, and comparison made with the aid of the color top." But Johnson did not provide any breakdown of the color composition of the testers and interviewers themselves; nor did he provide information on how and when the "color top" was used to assess differentiations in color. Recognizing the limitations of this methodology, Johnson asserted that while "an objective index was impossible, . . . the results of the estimate seem fairly significant."[99] Of the 721 cases where estimates of the subject's complexion was made, Johnson concluded that self-estimates were most accurate for dark-brown youths and most erroneous when youth designated themselves black and light-brown. The subjectivity of the sociological team complicates this reading as judgments on color were at best relative and at worst entangled with stereotyped notions. Only 2.4 percent of girls and young women qualified their own skin tones as black, compared to the 23.3 percent who, according to the testers, fell into this category. In addition, 40.2 percent of girls presented themselves as light brown, as compared to the estimates that only 9.9 percent truly fit this profile. This was a consistent finding for both genders, but girls and young women more frequently classified themselves as lighter in complexion. Johnson also found that appraisals of parents reflected a similar gendering of color values; 46.7 percent of girls and 43.2 percent of boys classified their mothers as not only light brown but also as lighter complexioned than their fathers.[100]

The gendering of color becomes evident in Johnson's findings, although the sociologist did not directly interpret its meaning. African American female youth, faced with idealized notions of female beauty as light brown or brown-skinned, envisioned themselves as being lighter complexioned than their "real" skin tones. Consistent descriptions of mothers as light brown and lighter complexioned than fathers inscribed a hierarchy of color values. Heterosexual marital partnership defined lighter women with darker men as an order to be maintained; in a region largely characterized by dark-skinned African Americans, 43.2 percent of girls and 46.7 percent of boys claimed to have light-brown-skinned mothers. Johnson's assertion that the majority of youth claimed themselves to be lighter-skinned than their true complexions suggests that this was also true about the descriptions of the complexions of their parents. Most important, the consistent assessment of mothers as light brown and as lighter-skinned than fathers suggests a gendered hierarchy of color that idealized African American womanhood as brown-skinned and fairer than the other sex.[101]

Johnson's testing of the "color factor in the personality development of Negro youth" revealed the growing importance of brown as a social and aesthetic ideal to both observer and subject. In a region where the majority of African Americans were dark-skinned, Johnson found little connection between class and color. Johnson argued that color did not create class divisions in the rural South but generated "problems of [personality] adjustment." The omissions and the observations of *Growing Up in the Black Belt* demonstrate how these youthful subjects judged women and girls more harshly against the color scale, especially in terms of values of female beauty. While Frazier and Johnson classified brown as a generally desirable complexion among youth, Parrish investigated the meaning of brown more closely and confirmed its growing importance. Brown's relative freedom from overly positive or negative assessments arose in Parrish's study and underscored the malleability of brown as a complexion as tenable for the rearticulation of gendered racial identities.

"Color Names and Color Notions"

Published in 1946 in the *Journal of Negro Education*, Parrish's "Color Names and Color Notions" explored the social values attached to a diversely complexioned African America and introduced the subject as a complex and taboo social phenomenon. "Although few Negroes are willing to concede the validity of the assertion that color plays any significant role in the organization of Negro society," Parrish declared, "there is ample evidence that differences in skin color receive at least verbal recognition in the Negro community."[102] Parrish went further than simply describing, naming, or identifying the problems associated with color. Through systematic study, he excised cryptic meanings behind the "verbal recognition" and identification of color by testing social understandings and values accorded to women and men of varying complexions. The article was based on research Parrish conducted for his 1944 doctoral dissertation, "The Significance of Color in the Negro Community," which proposed to "discover the nature of color differentiation and discrimination in Negro society" and "to ascertain as far as possible the significance or role of such differentiation."[103] Parrish found that dark- and light-skinned individuals, and women in particular, generated more incisive and negative social judgments.[104]

Far less is known about Parrish, who like Frazier and Johnson was also trained in the Chicago school of sociology, but his accomplishments are noteworthy. Born in 1899 in Louisville, Kentucky, Parrish was the only child of ex-slaves. His father, Charles H. Parrish Sr., was a renowned member of the African American Louisville community and made impressive contributions to the community through his work as an educator, Baptist minister, and president of the NAACP Louisville chapter. His family's emphasis on education steered the younger Parrish to follow in his father's footsteps, and in 1951 he became the first African American faculty member at the University of Louisville in Kentucky. Parrish later headed the university's Department of Sociology, remaining at the institution until his retirement in 1969.[105] It is no coincidence that Frazier's *Negro Youth at the Crossways* drew on Louisville, Kentucky—Parrish's hometown—as one of the towns in his study. Between 1931 and 1951, Parrish taught sociology and education at the Louisville Municipal College for Negroes, and while there he supervised the fieldwork for Frazier's study. Frazier and Parrish acknowledged each other in their respective works Frazier for Parrish's work on his study, and Parrish for Frazier's permission to utilize research gathered in his dissertation.

Despite drawing on much of the same evidence, Parrish disagreed with Frazier's analysis of the connection between color, class, and culture. Rather, Parrish argued that "roughly speaking, the social stratification follows occupational lines. But it would be a mistake to assume that distinctions are inevitably made on an occupational basis. Class demarcations are not clearly defined." Parrish found "little evidence of class consciousness except on the part of the very few who base their contentions upon other considerations than income or occupational status." Parrish debated Frazier's designation of certain groups as "lower class," stating that "popularly the term 'low class' is reserved for those who, in addition to their poverty and ignorance, exhibit a callous indifference to the accepted values." Finally, Parrish underscored the importance of social mobility in this community, arguing that "the mark of respectability, even, perhaps, to a greater extent than occupation or income, distinguishes middle-class people from the masses below them."[106] Parrish concluded that skin color played a particularly important role in the social mobility of dark-skinned African Americans: "Moving up the social scale or from poorer to better residential areas one encounters fewer dark persons and relatively greater numbers of light and medium brown persons. Dark skin color is a greater handicap to status advancement for women than it is for men."[107] Parrish's view of class theorized the limited importance of occupation and wealth in structuring Louisville's African American community. The more crucial determinant of color appeared in creating, sustaining, and advancing "accepted values" that helped define "the mark of respectability."

Parrish tested his view that ideas about color were popularly understood, accepted, and endowed with corresponding stereotypes of behavior and personality. A list of more than 143 "color names" from approximately thirty people was collected, and these names, though not exhaustive, "probably included the more commonly used terms." Parrish then presented the list to sixty students at Louisville Municipal College and asked the subjects to indicate which terms they heard being used by African Americans to refer to others of their race. The most readily recognizable included "bright," "half-white," "high brown," "light brown," "brownskin," "dark brown," and "ink spot." Among the more unusual ones were "clinker," "come-on-tan," "blackout," "jungle yellow," "tease-em-brown," "honest black," and "won't stop-Black." When asked to supply names that did not appear on the list, the responses of young people included "teakettle blond," "stove pipe blonde," "high yaller," "pink toe," and "chocolate drop."[108]

In his methodological approach to the quantification of color names, Parrish rejected projective devices such as the Milton Bradley color top employed by others, including Johnson in *Growing Up in the Black Belt*.[109] Parrish found these readings unsatisfactory in defining "the status implications of various shades of color," and searched for "a more elastic and less complicated measuring procedure." This resulted in a "psychological color rating technique" that took the form of a color scale. Using the twenty-five most readily recognizable color names, Parrish asked the sixty subjects to quantify the color names by assigning them a numerical value along a scale ranging from zero to fifty. With zero being the lightest and fifty being the darkest, these names were then grouped into clusters. In grouping the color terms, four clusters proved dominant and were labeled with a color name popular in each grouping, namely "High Yellow," "High Brown," "Brownskin," and "Black." While the elaborate grouping of color suggested a wide range of color differentiation among African Americans, Parrish pointed out that the "actual color distribution of the Negro community appears to be skewed toward the darker shades—'Brownskin' and 'Chocolate Brown.'" Parrish argued that if these terms represented color "stereotypes," then they referenced only a "few individuals who exhibit conspicuous differences in other physical traits that distinguish them from the many other people of the same or nearly the same color." Indeed, the terms spoke to real complexion only peripherally; the terms more accurately captured perceptions of behavior attached to stereotypical views of personality types.[110]

Parrish also elicited "spontaneous responses to the presentation of color names" to uncover stereotyped associations with color names. The respondents included an unspecified number of subjects ranging from twelve to eighteen years of age, and Parrish ensured as much anonymity as possible by constructing a rather complex seating and response arrangement. The subjects were asked to provide descriptions of both physical and personality traits for the following color clusters: "high yellow," "African," "chocolate brown," "light," "high brown," "black," and "fair." Consistently, Parrish found light and dark shades most often depicted in negative ways. Such unfavorable responses included those pertaining to "high yellow," "light" and "fair." One comment, "I'd rather see a light boy than a girl," made explicit the more negative judgment applied to mixed-race women. While providing no explanation for this statement, it is reasonable to assume that light-skinned women continued to represent a more problematic social identity. In the continued close censorship of social intercourse between white women and African American men, it appears that lighter-skinned women presented the greater problem. Perhaps lighter-skinned women represented the threat of continued interracial sexual encounters and reproduction, and in that manner women of this color group evoked the shame and, at times, the betrayal of the race. Parrish reminded the reader that much disfavor toward this group emerged from their "dominant influence" or status.[111] Like Johnson and Frazier, Parrish connected the history of a mixed-race elite to negative associations with lighter-skinned women. This historicizing of the connection between light-skin and dominant class status helped create the psychic space for new racialized identities. From the negative stereotyping of light-skinned women and men, the creation of positive depictions of African Americans who achieved social and economic success became tenable and even necessary.

Little distinction along gender lines emerge in Parrish's findings on dark-skinned youth; rather, fairly general negative stereotypes evolved. Perceived as quarrelsome, difficult to get along with, and riddled with inferiority, dark-skinned African Americans were seen as the least attractive, even prompting such aspersions as "evil" and "ugly." Other descriptions were kinder, though no less condescending, simply stating that only a few in this group were attractive and that close attention to dress was necessary. Parrish concluded that the two extremes—black and high yellow—were the groups most often stereotyped and the ones to whom the most intense emotion was directed.[112] His findings on the values accorded to light- and dark-skinned individuals demonstrated the growing space for a mediating color.

Brown skin emerges as a malleable typology. Brown-skin women (and men) appeared in a positive light, but Parrish found that this classification held no firm stereotype of personality. This pliability—combined with its positive assessment—allowed for the development of brown skin to shape an ideal of racialized womanhood. Like Frazier and Johnson, Parrish confirmed the aesthetic idealization of brown-skinned complexion was reinforced through the relative freedom of brown skin from disparaging stereotyping: hence, the brown-skin body appeared to be the physical and intellectual one most suitable for the reconstitution of gender, class, and racial values.

Like Frazier and Johnson, Parrish also found that in terms of physical appearance and personality, brown-skinned women and men were most often associated with positive attributes. The majority of responses depicted this grouping to be "sweet and affectionate," "aggressive about rights," and of "very beautiful color provided the hair is well groomed and the other features aren't too Negroid." According to Parrish, the phrase "aggressive about rights" was a deliberately vague description. This suggests that the growing racial consciousness and political awareness among African American communities may or may not have been perceived as acceptable.[113] Within the category of brown, Parrish identified three separate subcategories: "High Brown," "Brownskin," and "Chocolate Brown." The brown-skin woman emerged as the most beautiful of these three categories, and the least stereotyped, allowing for greater variation in appearance when applied to women.

"Almost invariably," Parrish found the classification High Brown addressed to women. "Good hair and nice features" defined High Browns, and although comely, this group was prone to the same problems, and hence similar social disfavor as "High Yellows." Discrimination against darker-skinned African Americans and feelings of superiority plagued judgment of this group; despite their beauty, High Brown women were not viewed as the most socially acceptable representation of race. Chocolate Browns were also most often women. "Chocolate" or "Chocolate Drop" implied maleness, suggesting that "Brown" and not "Chocolate" was the gender modifier. Parrish did not delve into this differentiation, but the qualifier suggests that skin color continued to play a more important role in defining female beauty and gendered identities. Defined by "regular features" and "well kept, if not 'good' hair," Chocolate Browns were second only to High Browns in assessments of the "most beautiful color to be." Women of this group also faced problems specific to their complexions. According to one of his study's respondents, this group "lurks between inferiority complex and superiority complex." Parrish speculated that for this group of women, "good" hair and features overrode color as a determinant of beauty.[114]

So what then of the brown-skin group? Unlike the other two factions of people designated as Brown, "Brownskin" accrued less definite assessments. Parrish incorporated a task that asked junior high school students to respond to given color names. "Brownskin" was not provided, but two other categories of brown appeared in the test. Parrish did not explain the reason for the omission, suggesting that "Brownskin" may have appeared redundant to him when classifications of High Brown and Chocolate Brown were offered. On the dilemma of categorizing Brown, Parrish shed some light: "These shades are so typical of the Negro group as a whole that it is difficult to understand how a person in this segment of the color scale could ever be picked out for special consideration on the basis of color alone. It seems almost certain that 'Chocolate Brown' and, to a lesser degree, 'Brownskin,' if they actually designate color classes at all, denote a few individuals who exhibit conspicuous differences in other physical traits which distinguish them from many other people of the same or nearly the same color."[115]

In this ordering of brown skin tones, Brownskin and Chocolate Brown referenced distinctive descriptors that were tied to physical characteristics. Parrish also presented views on the Brownskin group as "the more reserved descriptions and characterizations given by older people." Unlike the association of High Browns and Chocolate Browns with women, the designation of "Brownskin" could be applied to both women and men. Darker in skin tone than the High Browns, but lighter than the Chocolate Browns, this group had more "Negroid features" and a "poor grade of hair." Descriptions of Brownskin women showed the view of an affable, pretty girl who lacked pretension. One young female respondent helps clarify: "Brownskin gives me a picture of a cute girl, with not good hair, but has it well kept, who is plump, dresses nicely and is full of fun and has personality plus."[116] Certainly not the most glamorous presentation, this image conjures a pretty—but not beautiful—woman who uses good sense in grooming and dress; unlike others who were assailed by inferiority or superiority, the Brownskin girl appeared as a well-adjusted and upbeat person.

The middle-of-the-road presentation of Brownskin appeared as an attainable gender ideal within reach of ordinary African American girls and women. Neither light nor dark brown in complexion, neither fine-featured nor straight-haired, the Brownskin was visibly African American in complexion and in facial features. The everydayness of the brown skin rendered this color as an ideal. Free from stereotyping, the brown-skinned woman wielded a powerful privilege to attend to her hair and features without denying her racial identity as African American or belying her respectability since performance of these duties reflected cultural values and practices associated with middle-class status. Parrish's findings showed the potent embodiment of beauty, respectability, and race pride in brown-skin womanhood as chief factors underlying an integrationist ideal.

Conclusion

By the late 1930s, ideas on color, sex, class, and gender converged to emphasize those complexions perceived as brown were not solely equalizers of social status among African Americans; the discourse on brown complexions equated these complexions with physical preparedness for racial integration and social mobility in postwar society that was made manifest in multiple ways. Scholarly findings on disorganization, youth, personality development, and color values showed a broad celebration of brown-skin women among interwar African American youth. At times, the sociological discourses produced by these three scholars proffered "brown" as a new vision of a homogenized and classless African America; at other moments, a competing view surfaced that equated middle-class status with brown complexions. By the late 1930s, Frazier, Johnson, and Parrish found that notions of brown-skin womanhood emphasized consumerist values as a path to social mobility, and this understanding surfaced among a cross section of urban and rural youth. Ultimately directed toward integration, the role of the individual appeared at center; for women, the performance of respectable brown beauty presented one strategy for moving along a moderate, middle-class, interracial movement for civil rights. Participation in the consumer economy emerged as an accessible and powerful venue to respectability: it was clearly connected to greater individual economic, social, and sexual security; it signaled race progress during a period of great uncertainty, and it appeared as one strand of a racial liberal discourse that was geared toward integration on particularly gendered terms.

Views on brownness and beauty reflected the optimistic and hopeful view of elite and middle-class African American racial liberals. They offered key contributions and assessments on race relations to the public discourse, media imagery, and intellectualizing on race between the Great Depression and World War II. Reporting on the views of those coming of age "at the crossways"—and at the dawning of the modern civil rights movement—these sociologists identified the cultivation of brown beauty as one clear avenue to attain respectability. As they commented on an ideology that had been developing over three decades, these scholars observed the final shift from social assessments of women's respectability based on "moral character" to an open endorsement of brown beauty as a modern value and timely strategic response to the broader struggle of interwar African Americans for racial equality and freedom. The media-based discourse on brown beauty identified consumerist means for women's individual social, sexual, and economic well-being. Certainly, brown beauty shored up the value of men, but it attested to the prideful representation of African American women as modern, urban, and middle-class citizens whose consuming power evidenced their rights to protections under the law.

Noting the sharp and difficult edges that formed the discourse of brown beauty during the interwar years, and pointing to its growing marketability and its expanded display in the years to follow, this book finds that brown beauty is best understood as intended by those who crafted it: a positive protest. By understanding brown beauty in this way and by exploring its construction, dissemination, significance, and silences more fully, we uncover yet another way that African Americans theorized was integral to crafting their own visuals of self and one another. In looking closely at the images and texts on brown beauty, we encounter women at the center of the interwar effort to declare their beauty, with pride.

Epilogue

Brown beauty made its most dynamic appearance during the post–World War II years when another generation of African American cultural producers, seized by an entrepreneurial spirit, and buoyed by racial liberalism and beliefs in postwar capitalism, turned to commercial modeling as a profitable enterprise and respectable profession for African American women. In 1946, the first agency to represent African American women in the field of professional modeling opened in Manhattan. The Harlem newspaper the *New York Age* hailed the moment as "another step up" in the quest for racial equality, noting that the launch of Brandford Models signaled "a new era in the advertising field."[1] Indeed, the Manhattan-based firm formed as an anticipatory response to the needs of advertisers, particularly those seeking to appeal to the "Negro market," a consumer demographic that met new recognition in the postwar years. Sales analysts offered clear prescriptions to companies wishing to appeal to the African American consumer, and of particular importance was the use of color. One analyst, David J. Sullivan, advised, "By no means color them black. Use brown-skinned girls for illustrations; then you satisfy all."[2] Throughout the late 1940s and into the mid-1950s, the representation of models as "brown-skinned" was clearly established as a happy medium and media ideal.[3]

Brown-skin models (as these models came to be described in postwar popular press) were African American women trained in the skills of modeling. Many models might well be considered brown in skin tone, but complexion and other markers of racial background varied widely, with a preference toward lighter hues. Their image dominated the covers of glossy photographic magazines like *Ebony* (1945) and *Our World* (1946), new mass-market consumer magazines produced by African Americans and geared toward everyday people. Between 1945 and 1954, a dynamic stream of photographic and consumer images augmented the landscape of African American print and visual culture, with the brown-skin woman appearing as a central focal point. Images of professional models and everyday women alike filtered into the broad and public view to affect a consumerist idealization of womanhood that underscored beauty as an attainable mainstay.

Brandford Models was one of several pioneering enterprises in African American modeling that emerged in the aftermath of World War II at the hands of a new group of professionals who continued to underscore "race pride" and "race progress" as a mainstay rationale for business. These new professionals advocated for integration in all industries connected to beauty, fashion, and modeling; at the same time, African American modeling agencies foregrounded women's beauty and style as indices of democracy and a pleasing display of fortitude in a land of postwar promise. In addition to modeling, beauty, and charm schools, modeling agencies were fast developing beauty enterprises in the postwar years: by the 1950s, hundreds of modeling and charm schools dotted the urban landscape, picking up on the energies and industries that undergirded the second Great Migration (1941–70). In an era of continued migration, modernization, and urbanization, beauty businesses related to modeling were among the few that assumed as their exclusive domain the cultivation of African American women's beauty for personal development and professional status.

As Cold War politics intensified, images of models in democratic participation with the consumer economy abounded in African American magazines and newspapers; some publications circulated among diverse and global audiences, reaching African-diasporic people and others with outward-looking views. Forging a narrative of pleasure, prosperity, and promise that was premised on values of women's femininity, heterosexual appeal, and class-appropriate style, the postwar visual discourse on brown-skin beauty signaled a crucial juncture in the pathway development of enterprises linked to beauty, fashion, and modeling.

Brown-skin models acquired significant social status as they were featured on an expanded global stage between 1945 and 1954—a short but critical period that marked the end of World War II, the hardening lines of Cold War politics, and the significant victory of *Brown v. Board of Education*, which, in 1954, made segregation illegal in public schools. Indeed, during this short period, a powerful iconography of beautiful brown women emerged to represent African-descended people in the United States by recasting beauty as a democratic right and function. By 1954, brown beauty was formalized, both at home and abroad, as a consumerist symbol of women's successful negotiation of the trials of race, sex, and womanhood in the postwar nation, still half-segregated.

ACKNOWLEDGMENTS

It is long work to write a book. Writers often describe the process to completion as a journey; in my case, this book journeyed with me—it became something other than what it started out to be, and it did so as I moved from Canada to Cleveland to the United Kingdom, my own life and academic knowledge growing and intersecting with divergent black (and white, and "other") histories and national narratives. Though this book has come a long way from when I first started my research, my first acknowledgment is to those who taught me.

I owe my biggest debt of gratitude to Molly Ladd-Taylor at York University in Toronto. As an advisor, Molly nurtured, encouraged, questioned, and pushed me to think about the complex histories around race, class, and womanhood. In particular, I thank her for many hours spent at Second Cup talking through drafts and comments, trying to work through some really critical issues in this history. My second debt of intellectual thanks goes to Marc Stein, from whom I learned a great deal. As a committee member, Marc's comments were always sharp, helpful, or funny—or, best of all worlds, all three. I also thank Marlene Shore for her fantastic graduate class on U.S. cultural history and her participation as a committee member on my thesis. Marlene's comments on my social science chapter guided me to fruitful ways at a crucial time of my thesis writing. Thanks also go to Marc Egnal for ongoing support and encouragement and for providing me with the early forum support in presenting my work as a graduate student to the Americanist meetings at York University. I will also remember kindly my other professor in U.S. history at York. I thank the belated, Bob Cuff in memory. With a smile, I will always recall his class and his comments on my paper on black lesbian consumerism (He loved it!) Other faculty members made my years at York a true training ground for the work of a historian and feminist scholar. Thank you to Kathryn McPherson, Stephen Brooke, Michele Johnson, and Jerry Ginsburg. And to Bettina Bradbury—thank you for everything! The York Women's History Reading Group also played a vital part of my graduate years, and I thank members of this group for reading and commenting on my very first paper on "the brownskin." I am also happy to have befriended fine people and scholars during those years, including Felicity, Ariel, and Galen Wright, who opened their home to me, and to those who have championed me during these last years—namely, Audrey Pyeé, and Katherine Purdue.

At Case Western Reserve University in Cleveland, Ohio, where I was honored to hold the Inaugural Postdoctoral Fellowship in African-American Studies, I am thankful to my hosts for the genuine warmth and support shown by the Department of History. Most significantly, I thank Rhonda Y. Williams, whose mentorship was nothing short of a blessing! Rhonda's encouragement, support, sharp intellect, and tireless commitment to social justice provided an invaluable blueprint for the type of academic I strive to be. I thank other faculty members, including Jonathan Sadowsky, Renee Sentilles, and Kenneth Ledford, for their kindness and support. I am also happy to have called Cleveland home, if only for a little while. Thanks to Michele Jackson, Dawn Wylde, Calvin Rydbom, Joy Bostic, Penny T. Tucker, and Marixo Lasso for helping me to enjoy the city.

At the University of Essex in Colchester, Essex, United Kingdom, I thank colleagues in the Department of History and across the university for their general encouragement and support. I thank some especially for coffees, dinners and glasses of wine shared over my years of research and writing. Included here are John Haynes, Sanja Bahun, Cathy Crawford, Michael Goodrum, Jane Hindley, Elena Hore, Jeremy Krikler, Sandra Moog, Matthias Röhrig Assunção, Dusan Radunovic, Nadine Rossol, David Rundle, Colin Samson, Roberta Suzzi Valli, Tony Swift, and Fiona Venn. I am also thankful to Nicola Farnworth, Michael and Cheryl Philip, and Grace St. George for making my transition from Toronto to Colchester an ongoing adventure.

At New York University Press, I am thankful for working with a great editor, Clara Platter, and an amazing editorial assistant, Amy Klopfenstein. Additionally, I am very grateful for the anonymous readers of the manuscript and their insightful comments.

My family deserves my enduring and heartfelt thanks. To my mother, Anisa, and my sisters, Fanzia, Sheri, and Alia, this achievement is not mine: it is ours. I could not have done this without you, or our father, Haroon Rasheed Haidarali, who inspires me still. Thanks to my niece and nephew, Adam and Kaitie, for their sweet smiles—I can't wait to spend more time with you. I am also thankful to have gained family over the course of this work. To my in-laws, Valerie and Clifford Haynes, and to my sister-in-law, Catherine Haynes, I offer heartfelt appreciation for welcoming me into their lives and for always being happy to hear about my progress, no matter how much that work kept me away from family gatherings. I am also grateful for my extended family of aunts, uncles, and cousins, namely the Ghanys, who have been tireless in their support of my academic and creative work. In particular, I thank Margaret Lopes for her generosity with gifts, treats, and flowers, and for hosting great parties to celebrate my various milestones. Thanks to Helen and Christopher Hearn for helping to make my life in England a little more "homey." I must also thank my uncles, Stephen Ghany and, in memory, Kenneth Ghany, for their encouragement and belief in the importance of my scholarship. My grandmother, Gladys Ghany, a woman who made her own unique journey, who enjoyed one hundred years of life, deserves special mention. She inspired this big family to reach for what we believe will make us happy, while maintaining faith and gratitude for all bounties. She is missed, but I know that she is smiling, happy with this achievement.

No one has shared more of this book with me than my husband, John. So, it is with such delight that I bring this work to an end being able to acknowledge the person who, in all ways, has been my most steadfast support. Throughout the years of solitary work of this book, I have been lucky to have John Haynes's critical and ongoing engagement with my work: thank you for taking so much time to help me talk through the histories I sought to capture in this work. Thank you, John, for your love, support, generosity, kindness, humor, and patience. It is so joyful being your companion.

NOTES

INTRODUCTION

1. Hurston, "How It Feels" in *A Zora Neale Hurston Reader*, 152–55.
2. Ibid.
3. Hemenway, *Zora Neale Hurston*.
4. Hurston, "Record of Freshman Interest."
5. Hurston, *Dust Tracks on a Road*, 169.
6. Hurston, "Color Struck."
7. Washington, "Introduction," 7.
8. Gage, *Colour and Culture*.
9. Russell-Cole, Wilson, and Hall, *Color Complex*; Kerr, *Paper Bag Principle*.
10. Scholarly accounts on the first great migration provide varying estimates for the number of migrants moving between these regions and date this transformation as beginning during World War I, slowing down during the Depression era of the 1930s, and then rebounding to ignite a second great migration at the United States' entry into World War II. Localized studies include Grossman, *Land of Hope*; Kusmer, *Ghetto Takes Shape*, while more generalized or overall coverage of migration includes Trotter, *Great Migration*; E. Lewis, *In Their Own Interests*; Marks, *Farewell*; Painter, *Exodusters*. Revisionist historians complicate understandings of the Great Migration in analyses of the urban South and white migration. See Kyriakoudes, *Social Origins*.
11. Hine, "Rape and the Inner Lives."
12. Darlene Clark Hine, "Black Migration to the Urban Midwest: The Gender Dimension, 1915–1945," in Trotter, *Great Migration*, 131.
13. Logan, *Negro in American Life*.
14. For example, see Hunter, *To 'Joy My Freedom*; Wolcott, *Remaking Respectability*.
15. Kasinitz, *Caribbean New York*, 41. Also see Osofsky, *Harlem*.
16. Hine, "Black Migration," 125–46.
17. U.S. Census, 1920; U.S. Census, 1930.
18. Riis, *How the Other Half Lives*, 22–25.
19. J. W. Johnson, "Making of Harlem," 635.
20. C. S. Johnson, "Black Workers and the City," 641.
21. An estimated 102,000 African-descended Caribbean people emigrated to New York City between 1901 and 1924. The majority came from the English-speaking islands, but smaller numbers of Spanish and French-speaking African Caribbean people settled in Harlem and Brooklyn. See James, "History of Afro-Caribbean Migration."

22 Ogbar, *Harlem Renaissance Revisited*, 76.
23 Baldwin and Makalani, *Escape from New York*.
24 Johns, "Sisters under the Skin," 6.
25 Foley, *Spectres of 1919*; C. Williams, *Torchbearers of Democracy*.
26 McKay, "If We Must Die."
27 Foley, *Spectres of 1919*, 13.
28 Tuttle, *Race Riot*.
29 Helbling, *Harlem Renaissance*; Hutchinson, *Harlem Renaissance*; Watson, *Harlem Renaissance*; Baldwin and Makalani, *Escape from New York*.
30 See Lawler and Davenport, *Marcus Garvey*; Cronon, *Black Moses*.
31 Baldwin, *Chicago's New Negroes*, 9.
32 Ibid., 9; Briggs, *New Negro in the Old South*, 9.
33 D. G. White, *Too Heavy a Load*, 124.
34 Wolters, *The New Negro on Campus*, 17.
35 Myrdal, *American Dilemma*, 305, 319.
36 Giddings, *When and Where I Enter*, 68–103; on HBCUs, see Roebuck and Komanduri, *Historically Black Colleges and Universities*; Foner, *Reconstruction*; Shaw, *What a Woman*.
37 Noble, *Negro Woman's College Education*, 29–30.
38 Here, and throughout this study, I consciously employ the term "race womanhood" and/or "women of the race" to reference the late-nineteenth- and early-twentieth-century championing of African American women as ambassadors of race politics. I also consciously employ "race" as a category of mostly linguistic definition. On "race womanhood," see Evelyn Brooks Higginbotham, "The Metalanguage of Race"; Higginbotham, *Righteous Discontent*; E. B. Brown, "Negotiating and Transforming"; Gilmore, *Gender and Jim Crow*.
39 Higginbotham, *Righteous Discontent*.
40 Shaw, *What a Woman*; Gaines, *Uplifting the Race*; D. G. White, *Too Heavy a Load*.
41 Hunter, *To 'Joy My Freedom*; Wolcott, *Remaking Respectability*.
42 Utaukawa Allen, "The Woman's Era," 93; Rooks, *Ladies' Pages*.
43 Shaw, "Black Club Women," 19.
44 Wolcott, *Remaking Respectability*, 57–59, 6.
45 Ibid.
46 Gatewood, *Aristocrats of Color*, 19, 24.
47 Ibid., 152.
48 Ibid., 181.
49 Ibid., 341.
50 Williamson, *New People*, 111–39.
51 Meier, "Negro Class Structure," 258–66.
52 On the rise and changing composition of this era's middle class, see Landry, *New Black Middle Class*.
53 Ibid., 20.
54 Baldwin, *Chicago's New Negroes*, 9.

55 J. Brown, *Babylon Girls*.
56 Vogel, *Scene of the Harlem Cabaret*, 53; Mumford, *Interzones*, 74–91.
57 Bessie Smith, "Young Woman Blues" (1926).
58 Mrydal, *American Dilemma*.
59 Important works include Hall, "Long Civil Rights Movement"; Biondi, *To Stand and Fight*; Countryman, *Up South*; Gilmore, *Defying Dixie*; Sugrue, *Sweet Land of Liberty*; Theoharis and Woodward, *Freedom North*; Self, *American Babylon*. For a critique of the long civil rights movement, see Cha-Jua and Lang, "Long Movement."
60 Joseph, "Waiting till the Midnight Hour," 8.
61 Cohen, *Consumers' Republic*.
62 See Hine, *Hine Sight*.
63 Baldwin, *Chicago's New Negroes*, 237.
64 Drake and Cayton, *Black Metropolis*; Weems, *Desegregating the Dollar*, 57–58; Greenberg, "*Or Does It Explode?*," chap. 5; Meier and Rudwick, "Origins of Nonviolent Direct Action"; Martin and Sullivan, "Don't Buy Where You Can't Work"; Baldwin, *Chicago's New Negroes*, 37, 42, 237–40; Pride and Wilson, *History of the Black Press*, 142–43.
65 Greenberg, "*Or Does It Explode?*," chap. 6; Cohen, *Consumers' Republic*, 46.
66 Cohen, *Consumers' Republic*, 46.
67 Johns, "Sisters under the Skin," 6.
68 Bennett, "What's in a Name?," 46–48, 50–52, 54.
69 DuBois, "In Black," 263.
70 Gross, *What Blood Won't Tell*, 17.
71 On the historic role of the black press, see Wolseley, *Black Press, U.S.A.*; Pride and Wilson, *History of the Black Press*.
72 S. Smith, *Word, Image*, 11.
73 hooks, "In Our Glory," 46.
74 Giddings, *When and Where I Enter*, 190.
75 Gates, "Trope of the New Negro," 132, 137.
76 M. Mitchell, *Righteous Propagation*, 212–13.
77 Du Bois, "American Negro in Paris," 577. Organized into four volumes, the photographs appeared in three separate albums entitled *Types of American Negroes, Georgia, U.S.A.* (vols. 1–3) and *Negro Life in Georgia, U.S.A.* (vol. 1). The albums are presently housed in the Library of Congress, Prints and Photographs Division.
78 Willis, "Sociologist's Eye," 58.
79 S. Smith, *American Archives*, chap. 6.
80 Lewis, "Small Nation of People," 30.
81 Willis, "Sociologist's Eye," 57.
82 DuBois, *Health and Physique*.
83 Ibid., 32–33.
84 L. D. Baker, *From Savage to Negro*, 1.
85 Gross, *What Blood Won't Tell*, 296.

86 Ibid., 2–10.
87 Pascoe, *What Comes Naturally*, 1–7.
88 F. J. Davis, *Who Is Black?*; Collier-Thomas and Turner, "Race, Class and Color"; Berry and Blassingame, *Long Memory*, 389–96; Stuckey, *Slave Culture*, chap. 4.
89 Pascoe, *What Comes Naturally*, 7.
90 Ibid., 180–81.
91 *United States v. Thind*, 261 U.S. 204 (1923). For insightful discussion of the *Thind* and *Ozawa* cases, as well as excerpts of these rulings, see Haney-Lopez, *White by Law*, 56–77.
92 Haney-Lopez, *White by Law*, 56.
93 Barkin, *Retreat of Scientific Racism*, 4.
94 Gross, *What Blood Won't Tell*, 226.
95 Richards, "Race," 65–159; Jackson, *Social Scientists for Social Justice*, 17–42.
96 Degler, *In Search of Human Nature*, 71, 78–80, 82–83; Cotkin, *Reluctant Modernism*, 51–73; Kuklick, *Savage Within*, 123, 262, 292, 295; Stocking, *Franz Boas Reader*, 17–19.

CHAPTER 1. BROWN BEGINNINGS

1 McDougald, "Task of Negro Womanhood," 369.
2 Ibid., 369.
3 Ibid.
4 See Hanson, *Mary McLeod Bethune*, introduction, 1–10.
5 Locke, *New Negro*, xxv.
6 McDougald, "Task of Negro Womanhood," 369.
7 Ibid., 370.
8 Wilson, *Segregated Scholars*, 179–87.
9 Newspaper clipping, n.d., Scrapbook, vol. 1, Ayer Papers.
10 Wilson, *Segregated Scholars*, 185; Scrapbook, 1931–66, Ayer Papers.
11 Kellner, *Harlem Renaissance*, 229–30.
12 Biography on Elise Johnson McDougald, in Locke, *New Negro*, 419.
13 "McDougald (Ayer), Gertrude Elise (or Elise) Johnson, 1885–1971," in Roses and Randolph, *Harlem Renaissance and Beyond*, 232.
14 For example, see Carleton Mabee, *Black Education in New York State*, as quoted in Wilson, *Segregated Scholars*, 185.
15 See chapter 5 for further explication on companionate marriage.
16 Elise Johnson McDougald, "The Women of the White Strain." Unpublished manuscript, Ayer Papers.
17 Letter from Elise Johnson McDougald Ayer to Elizabeth J. McDougald, (Bessie), n.d., Ayer Papers, personal correspondence.
18 McDougald, "Women of the White Strain."
19 Ibid.
20 Obituary, Mrs. Mary Elizabeth Johnson (1858–1929), unnamed, n.d., Scrapbook, vol. 1, Ayer Papers. This obituary offers a conflicting view on Mary Elizabeth

Johnson's immigration to the United States, claiming her entry "as an infant" rather than as a young woman in pursuit of employment opportunities as a "lady's maid."

21 McDougald, "Women of the White Strain."
22 Newspaper clipping, circa 1935, Scrapbook, vol. 1, Ayer Papers.
23 "Human Principal," *Newsweek*, July 5, 1954, Gertrude Ayer, Schomburg Clipping File, 1925–74, Sc 000, 388–1, Schomburg Center, Ayer Papers.
24 Elise McDougald Ayer as quoted in "Why a Teacher Should Also Serve as a Social Worker: Elise McDougald Ayer in 2 Fold-Service," *New York News*, August 29, 1931, as found in Scrapbook, vol. 1, Ayer Papers.
25 Ibid.
26 "New School Principal Boasts Varied Career," *New York Amsterdam News*, circa 1935, Ayer Papers.
27 Letter from U.S. literary agency to Mrs. Ayer, March 5, 1945, Scrapbook, Ayer Papers.
28 "Who's Who of the Contributors," in Locke, *New Negro*, 419.
29 "Quadroon Girl Class President," 1903, n.d., Scrapbook, vol. 1, Ayer Papers.
30 Newspaper clipping, n.d., Scrapbook, vol. 1, Ayer Papers. The *New York News Sunday Coloroto Magazine*, a supplement of the *New York News*, was published between 1942 and 1969.
31 U.S. Census, 1900.
32 J. Jones, *Labor of Love*, 155–56.
33 Ibid., 154, 193.
34 Addie W. Hunter, "A Colored Working Girl and Race Prejudice," *Crisis* (April 1916): 32–34, as quoted in J. Jones, *Labor of Love*, 179.
35 "License Five as Principals"; "Mrs. Gertrude Elise Ayer May Become Principal of Elementary School Here," newspaper clipping, n.d., Scrapbook, vol. 1, Ayer Papers.
36 "Principals' Ratings Must Jibe," *New York Sun*, n.d., Scrapbook, vol. 1, Ayer Papers.
37 L. Johnson, "Generation of Women Activists," 225; Rousemaniere, *Principal's Office*, 71.
38 L. Johnson, "Generation of Women Activists," 225, 229.
39 "Harlem's First," in column entitled "Education," in *Time*, February 18, 1935, 56.
40 McDougald, "Negro Woman Teacher," 770.
41 U.S. Census, 1920.
42 For example, see Watkins-Owens, *Blood Relations*; Turner and Turner, *Caribbean Crusaders*.
43 Ayer, "Notes on My Native Sons," 375–83.
44 L. Anderson, "Generation of Women Activists."
45 Ayer, "Notes on My Native Sons," 375, 580–81.
46 "Mrs. Gertrude E. McDougal [sic] Leads the Season in the Blue Book Marriage," newspaper clipping, n.d., Scrapbook, vol. 1, Ayer Papers.
47 Ibid.

48 "New School Principal"; "Commencement Address Delivered by New York Educator to Class of '47," ca. 1947, newspaper clipping, n.d., Scrapbook, vol. 1, Ayer Papers.
49 "New School Principal."
50 Ibid.; Alain Locke Papers.
51 "Whole Family Likes Custard," newspaper clipping, n.d., Scrapbook, vol. 2, Ayer Papers.
52 "Why a Teacher Should also Serve as a Social Worker," *New York News*, August 29, 1931, Scrapbook, vol. 1, Ayer Papers.
53 Locke, "Harlem," 629–30.
54 Chambers, *Paul U. Kellogg*, 114.
55 Long, "Genesis," 16.
56 Kennedy, *Over Here*, 285–86.
57 J. Jones, *Labor of Love*, 162.
58 Wilson, *Segregated Scholars*, 173–87.
59 *New Day for the Colored Woman Worker*.
60 "First Negro Woman Wins Principal Post," *New York Evening Journal*, January 31, 1936, newspaper clipping, Scrapbook, vol. 1, Ayer Papers.
61 Wilson, *Segregated Scholars*, 182.
62 McDougald, "Task of Negro Womanhood," 369–70.
63 Ibid., 377.
64 Wilson, *Segregated Scholars*, 184; McDougald, "Task of Negro Womanhood," 377–78.
65 "New School Principal."
66 McDougald, "Task of Negro Womanhood," 379.
67 Ibid., 380.
68 J. Jones, *Labor of Love*, 180.
69 Amott and Matthaei, "We Specialize," 158, 165–67.
70 J. Jones, *Labor of Love*, 180–81.
71 On the feminization of clerical work, see Fine, *Souls of the Skyscraper*; Kwolek-Folland, *Engendering Business*.
72 J. Jones, *Labor of Love*, 178.
73 Ibid., 178.
74 McDougald, "Task of Negro Womanhood," 372.
75 Ibid.
76 Yellin, *Racism in the Nation's Service*, 159; Moore, *Leading the Race*, 157.
77 D. G. White, *Too Heavy a Load*, 150.
78 McDougald, "Task of Negro Womanhood," 370–72.
79 Wolcott, *Remaking Respectability*, 76–77. Susan Porter Benson, *Counter Cultures*.
80 Wolcott, *Remaking Respectability*, 76–77.
81 Terborg-Penn, "Survival Strategies," 150–51.
82 As quoted in Wolcott, *Remaking Respectability*, 78.
83 E. A. Carter to John Dancy, as quoted in ibid., 87.

84 Scott, "Letters of Negro Migrants."
85 Ibid., May 22, 1917, 315.
86 McDougald, "Task of Negro Womanhood," 382.
87 "Who's Who of the Contributors," in Locke, *The New Negro,* 419.
88 Stewart, "Looking Backward to Look Forward." I thank Jeffrey C. Stewart, the chair of Black Studies at Stanford University, for his helpful email response to my query seeking to clarify some details and to hear his impressions on Reiss's use of brown in these portraits.
89 Ibid.
90 Stewart, "Winold Reiss as a Portraitist," 5.
91 Clifford, "On Ethnographic Authority"; Clifford, "Introduction: Partial Truths," 1–26.
92 Stewart, *To Color America,* 48.
93 Ps. 68:31.
94 Rollins, "Ethiopia, African Americans," 6–9.
95 Kirschke, *Art in Crisis,* 137–46. On Ethiopia, see 146–47.
96 Stewart, *To Color America,* 50.
97 Goesser, "Transcultural Modernism."
98 Undated letter from Elise Johnson McDougald to Alain Locke, *Survey Graphic Box,* Alain Locke Papers.
99 Ibid.
100 Ibid.
101 Stewart, *To Color America,* 54.
102 McDougald to Locke, undated letter, Alain Locke Papers.
103 Locke, "To Certain Philistines," 155–56.
104 McDougald to Locke, undated letter, Alain Locke Papers.
105 Carroll, *Word, Image,* 124.
106 Boas, "Instability of Human Types," 99–103.
107 Park, "Behind Our Masks," 135–36.
108 Carroll, *Word, Image,* 124–44.
109 Hunton, "Breaking Through," 684.
110 Carroll, *Word, Image,* 147.

CHAPTER 2. BEAUTIFUL BROWN SKIN

1 Advertisement, "O.K. Colored Doll Co.," *Crisis* (December 1923): 89.
2 Weems, *Desegregating the Dollar,* 17.
3 Editorial, "Live and Let Live," *Half-Century* (February 1916): 46.
4 Edwards, *Southern Urban Negro Consumer,* 169.
5 Rooks, *Ladies' Pages,* 68–69.
6 Ibid., 69.
7 Briggs, *New Negro,* 41.
8 Ibid., 128.
9 Ingham and Feldman, *African American Business Leaders,* 107.

10 Ibid., 106–8.
11 "The Baptists Go on Record," *Nashville Globe*, October 2, 1908, 8.
12 Briggs, *New Negro*, 118.
13 Ingham and Feldman, *African American Business Leaders*, 110; J. C. Smith, *Encyclopaedia of African American Business*, 109.
14 Edwards, *Southern Urban Negro Consumer*, 172–73.
15 J. C. Smith, *Encyclopaedia of African American Business*, 109.
16 Ingham and Feldman, *African American Business Leaders*, 110.
17 DuBois, "Editorial," 10.
18 M. Mitchell, *Righteous Propagation*, 173–96; Bernstein, *Racial Innocence*, 230–31.
19 "Negroes Want Negro Dolls," *Nashville Globe*, December 18, 1908, front page.
20 J. C. Smith, *Encyclopaedia of African American Business*, 105.
21 "Negroes Want Negro Dolls," front page.
22 Ibid.
23 "The Negro or Colored Doll," *Nashville Globe*, December 31, 1909, 5; "Negroes Want Negro Dolls."
24 "Negro Dolls for Negro Babies," *Atlanta Constitution*, September 28, 1908, 4.
25 "Negro or Colored Doll," 5; advertisement, "Opening of the Negro Doll Season," *Nashville Globe*, October 27, 1911, 6.
26 "Negro or Colored Doll," 5.
27 "Duquoin Negro Doll Fair," *Nashville Globe*, October 6, 1908, 3.
28 "Thousands of Negro Dolls," *New York Age*, November 9, 1911, 5.
29 M. Mitchell, *Righteous Propagation*, 182.
30 "Negro or Colored Doll," 5.
31 Ibid.
32 Among others, university dean Kelly Miller endorsed the eugenicist argument of race suicide. See Miller, "Eugenics of the Negro Race," 57–59.
33 "Little Folks Write Santa Claus," *Nashville Globe*, December 15, 1911, sec. III.
34 "Negro or Colored Doll," 5.
35 Ibid.
36 Formanek-Brunell, *Made to Play House*, 28–29.
37 Wallace-Saunders, *Mammy*, 34–36.
38 The famous doll test conducted by sociologists Kenneth and Mamie Clarke highlighted the problematic effect of complexion on childhood development. Other scholars offer compelling analyses on the role of color, racial stereotypes, and dolls. See Wilkinson, "Doll Exhibit," 19–29; Patterson, "Color Matters," 147–65.
39 Wallace-Saunders, *Mammy*, 34.
40 Sanchez-Eppler, *Touching Liberty*, 133–34.
41 Angione, *All-Bisque and Half-Bisque Dolls*, 11, 26.
42 M. Mitchell, *Righteous Propagation*, 182.
43 Angione, *All-Bisque and Half-Bisque Dolls*, 35–36.
44 Formanek-Brunell, *Made to Play House*, 92. See chapter 4, "Marketing a Campbell Kids Culture: Engendering New Kid Dolls, 1902–1914," in *Made to Play House*, for

a detailed overview on the development of the U.S. doll-making industry in competition with Germany.
45 Formanek-Brunell, *Made to Play House*, 138.
46 Ibid., 137–39.
47 J. K. Walker, *Encyclopaedia of Black Business*, 605–6.
48 Ibid.
49 "Negroes Want Negro Dolls," 1.
50 Ibid.
51 "Damaging False Report," *Nashville Globe*, December 3, 1909, 3.
52 Ibid.
53 M. Mitchell, *Righteous Propagation*, 177.
54 Ibid., 173–96.
55 "Josephine Baker," in the *Crisis* (May 1927): 86.
56 "Negro or Colored Doll," 5.
57 Advertisement, "National Negro Doll Company," *Nashville Globe*, August 11, 1911.
58 Ibid., November 13, 1908, 3.
59 Ibid., November 22, 1912, 21.
60 Ibid., November 13, 1908, 3.
61 Ingham and Feldman, *African American Business Leaders*, 108.
62 Advertisements, "National Negro Doll Company," *Nashville Globe*, October 10, 1913, 3, and October 24, 1913, 7.
63 Ibid., October 27, 1911.
64 "Negro Dolls Free," *Nashville Globe*, October 3, 1913, 4; "Great Big Beautiful Dolls," *Nashville Globe*, October 10, 1913, 3; "Other Girls Have Gone to Work . . . ," *Nashville Globe*, October 17, 1913, 11.
65 "New Departures in Harlem Business," *New York Age*, August 7, 1920, 1.
66 Formanek-Brunell, *Made to Play House*, 150; J. K. Walker, *Encyclopaedia of Black Business*, 605–6; M. Mitchell, *Righteous Propagation*, 184.
67 Advertisement, "Colored Dolls: Berry's Famous Brown Skin Dolls," *New York Age*, December 20, 1919, 7.
68 Advertisement, "Colored Dolls, Berry and Francis," *Crisis* (January 1920): 159.
69 M. Mitchell, *Righteous Propagation*, 191–92.
70 Advertisement, "Brown Skin Dolls," Bell Manufacturing Company, *Crisis* (December 1923): 93.
71 Advertisement for Bethel Manufacturing Company, "Colored Dolls and Novelties," *Crisis* (February 1927): 222.
72 Ibid., December 1924, 222.
73 DuBois, "Postscript," 142.
74 The story of Madame C. J. Walker is well known but still inspires great discussion. For a good biography of Walker, see Bundles, *On Her Own Ground*. Also see Baldwin, *Chicago's New Negroes*; S. Walker, *Style and Status*.
75 G. B. Johnson, "Newspaper Advertisements," 706.

76 The Class C grouping included "beauty preparations, patent medicines, firearms, cheap jewelry, charms and good luck emblems."
77 G. B. Johnson, "Newspaper Advertisements," 707.
78 Peiss, *Hope in a Jar*, 210–11.
79 Craig, *Ain't I a Beauty Queen?*, 47–49.
80 "Women's Beauty Will Win Prizes," *New York Age*, July 23, 1914, 1.
81 "Ideal Type of Negro Beauty," *New York Age*, August 6, 1914, 1.
82 Ibid.
83 "Hard Task for Beauty Judges," *New York Age*, August 27, 1914.
84 Ibid.
85 M. Mitchell, *Righteous Propagation*, 213–14.
86 Peiss, *Hope in a Jar*, 117.
87 "Hallie Q. Brown Again Honored," *Pittsburgh Courier*, July 18, 1925, 9.
88 Advertisement, "The Golden Brown National Beauty Contest," *Pittsburgh Courier*, June 27, 1925, 8.
89 White and White, *Stylin*, 200.
90 Advertisement, "Miss Golden Brown of America," *Pittsburgh Courier*, October 10, 1925, 8.
91 For example, see Craig, *Ain't I a Beauty Queen?*
92 Ibid., 53.
93 Peiss, *Hope in a Jar*, 215.
94 Bogle, "Negro Womanhood's Greatest Needs," 109.
95 Ibid.
96 Ibid.
97 Editorial, "Beautiful but Dumb," *Messenger* (July 1925): 275.
98 George, "Beauty Culture and Colored People," 25–26.
99 George Schuyler, "Unnecessary Negroes," *Messenger* 8 (1926): 307.
100 G. B. Johnson, "Newspaper Advertisements," 707.
101 C. S. Johnson, "Race Pride and Cosmetics," 293.
102 Editorial, "Betrayers of the Race," *Half-Century* (February 1920): 3.
103 B. Roberts, *Pageants, Parlors*, 78.
104 Letter to the editor from Mrs. Mary Vaughan, "The People's Forum," *Half-Century* (April 1920): 17–18.
105 Ibid.
106 Advertisement for High-Brown Soap, *Half-Century* (April 1920): 18.
107 Peiss, *Hope in a Jar*, 210.
108 Blackwelder, *Stylin' Jim Crow*; Gill, *Beauty Shop Politics*, 34.
109 Gill, *Beauty Shop Politics*, 34.
110 Cunard, "Harlem Reviewed," 122.
111 Haring, "Selling to Harlem," 17.
112 Ibid., 18.
113 For example, see S. Walker, *Style and Status*, 67–68, 109–10.
114 Morris, "Harlem Beauty Shops."

115 Ibid.
116 Advertisement for India Hair Grower, *Crisis* (April 1930): 142.
117 Du Bois, "Postscript," 138, 142.
118 Advertisement for Eau Denna, *Crisis* (October 1929): 358.
119 Advertisement for Alex Marks Wigs, *Crisis* (November 1925): 45.
120 Banner, *American Beauty*; Peiss, *Hope in a Jar*.
121 Banner, *American Beauty*, 141–44.
122 Peiss, *Hope in a Jar*, 39, 277.
123 Banner, *American Beauty*, 277; Peiss, *Hope in a Jar*, 151.
124 As quoted in Russell-Cole, Wilson, and Hall, *Color Complex*, 142–43; "Josephine Baker," in Cullen, *Vaudeville, Old and New*, 55–56.
125 Claude McKay, "A Negro Extravaganza," review of *Shuffle Along*, by Eubie Blake and Noble Sissle, *Liberator*, December 21, 1921, 24–26, in Huggins, *Voices from the Harlem Renaissance*, 134.
126 Heap, *Slumming*, 199.
127 J. Brown, *Babylon Girls*, 195.
128 Russell-Cole, Wilson, and Hall, *Color Complex*, 212–13.
129 Peiss, *Hope in a Jar*, 151.
130 Gordon, "Brown-Skin Fad," 458; on Tan-Off, see Peiss, *Hope in a Jar*, 233.
131 Gordon, "Brown-Skin Fad," 458.
132 Peiss, 235.
133 B. Roberts, *Pageants, Parlors*, 77–78.
134 As quoted in Peiss, *Hope in a Jar*, 233.
135 Ibid., 109; Chambers, *Madison Avenue*, 24.
136 Advertisement for Kashmir Chemical Company, *Crisis* (December 1918 and August 1918).
137 Pamphlet for Nile Queen Preparations, n.d. Claude A. Barnett Papers, Box 262, Folder 2.
138 Ibid., Box 262, Folder 3.
139 Advertisement for Kashmir Chemical Company, *Crisis* (June 1917).
140 Ibid., December 1917.
141 Pamphlet for Nile Queen Preparations, n.d., Claude A. Barnett Papers, Box 262, Folder 2.
142 Advertisement for Kashmir Chemical Company, *Crisis* (November 1914): 44.
143 Chambers, *Madison Avenue*, 25.
144 Advertisement for Kashmir Chemical Company, *Crisis* (November 1916): 44.
145 Advertisement for East India Hair Grower, *Crisis* (January 1924): 142; (May 1924): 46; (October 1925): 309; (November 1925): 50; (March 1926): 258; (April 1926): 310; (June 1926): 102; (July 1926): 154; (April 1926): 65; (May 1927): 101; (June 1927): 42; (August 1927): 214; (September 1927): 250; (October 1927): 286; (November 1927): 322.
146 "East India Hair Grower Manufacturer Dies, Following Long Illness," *Black Dispatch*, April 18, 1942.

147 "Wealthy City Negro Property Owner Dies," *Daily Oklahoman*, April 16, 1942.
148 "East India Hair Grower Manufacturer Dies."
149 Ibid., 218.
150 Advertisement for East India Hair Grower, *Crisis* (January 1924): 398.
151 Advertisements for training in beauty culture include Prof. Rohrer's World Famous Beauty School, *Crisis* (April 1929): 140; Apex College, Apex System, New York City, *Crisis* (April 1931): 143; Poro College, *Crisis* (December 1924): 92.
152 Advertisement, "Learn Beauty Culture, Mme. C. J. Walker System of Beauty Culture," *Crisis* (June 1928), back cover.
153 "Social Progress," in "Along the Color Line," *Crisis* (April 1928): 272.
154 Advertisement, "Stenographers Efficiently Trained," *Crisis* (February 1928): 69; advertisement for "The Stenographers' Institute" (October 1928): 357.

CHAPTER 3. "OF THE BROWN-SKIN TYPE"

1 George S. Schuyler, "Instructions for Contributors," reprinted in Eugene Gordon, "Negro Fictionist in America," *Saturday Evening Quill* (April 1929): 20.
2 Ibid.
3 Weems, *Desegregating the Dollar*, 35.
4 Oak, "Advertising in the Negro Press," in *Negro Newspaper*, 113–16.
5 Schuyler's brief editorship of Ziff's "Illustrated Feature Section" followed the demise of the *Messenger* in 1928 and was brokered by Robert L. Vann. See Ferguson, *Sage of Sugar Hill*, 17–18, and see 259–60n32. Also see Rasmussen and Hill, "Afterword," 263–64.
6 Oak, "Advertising in the Negro Press," 111–21.
7 Hutchinson, *Harlem Renaissance*, 342–44.
8 Gross, *What Blood Won't Tell*, 225.
9 A. A. Johnson, *Propaganda and Aesthetics*, 92–94.
10 Gates, *Signifying Monkey*, 179–80.
11 Gage, *Color and Meaning*, 15.
12 Stewart, *To Color America*, 56.
13 Welter, "Cult of True Womanhood," 151–74.
14 Stavney, "Mothers of Tomorrow," 538.
15 M. Mitchell, *Righteous Propagation*, 91.
16 L. Gordon, *Woman's Body, Woman's Right*; A. Davis, *Women, Race, and Class*.
17 L. Gordon, *Woman's Body, Woman's Right*, 115.
18 M. Mitchell, *Righteous Propagation*, 91.
19 Rodrique, "Black Community and Birth Control," 139.
20 Hine, "Great Migration," 134–37.
21 Alice Dunbar-Nelson, "Woman's Most Serious Problem," *Messenger* (March 1927): 73, 86.
22 M. Mitchell, *Righteous Propagation*, 193.
23 Douglas, *Terrible Honesty*.
24 J. A. Rogers, "The Critic," *Messenger* (April 1925): 165.

25 Hart, "Who Should Have Children?"
26 Gaines, *Uplifting the Race*, 231.
27 Bogle, "Negro Womanhood's Greatest Needs," 109.
28 Du Bois, "Damnation of Women," 164–65.
29 See D. Roberts, *Killing the Black Body*; Rodrique, "Black Community and Birth Control"; Hart, "Who Should Have Children?"
30 Blanche Schrack, "Editorial Comment," *Birth Control Review* 3, no. 9 (September 1919): 3–4.
31 Ibid., 4.
32 "A Word from Dr. Du Bois," *Birth Control Review* (September 1919): 15. Although the letter addressed to Mrs. Charles E. Knoblauch is undated, the short poem appearing below the letter is dated July 15. In 1932, Du Bois clearly articulated his advocacy for birth control. See W. E. B. Du Bois, "Black Folk and Birth Control," *Birth Control Review* 16 (June 1932): 166–67.
33 Advertisement for birth control clinics, Standard Handbook and Directory, *Crisis* (November 1931).
34 Chandler Owen, "Women and Children of the South," *Birth Control Review* 3, no. 9 (September 1919): 9.
35 Ibid.
36 Angelina Weld Grimké, "The Closing Door," *Birth Control Review* 3, no. 9 (September 1919): 10–14, and no. 10 (October 1919): 8–12.
37 Ibid. (September 1919): 10.
38 Ibid. (October 1919): 10.
39 N. Brown, *Private Politics and Public Voices*, 109.
40 Clare Corbould, "Africa the Motherland," in *Becoming African Americans*, 50.
41 First introduced in 1918 and eventually defeated in 1922, the Dyer Bill was propelled by the NAACP and moved for federal legislation against lynching. African American women were important campaigners against lynching and for the Dyer Bill. See Hall, *Revolt Against Chivalry*.
42 Carby, *Reconstructing Womanhood*; T. Davis, *Nella Larsen*; Du Cille, *Coupling Convention*; Wall, *Women of the Harlem Renaissance*.
43 A. Davis, *Blues Legacies and Black Feminism*.
44 "Newsome, Mary Effie Lee," in Roses and Randolph, *Harlem Renaissance and Beyond*, 254–57; "Effie Lee Newsome," in Patton and Honey, *Double-Take*, 243.
45 Effie Lee Newsome, "The Bronze Legacy (To a Brown Boy)," *Crisis* (October 1922), 265.
46 Ibid.
47 Georgia Douglas Johnson, "Motherhood," *Crisis* (October 1922), 265.
48 For more on Douglas Johnson, see Gloria T. Hull, "Georgia Douglas Johnson," in Hull, *Color, Sex, Poetry*, 155–211. On her role as literary hostess, see McHenry, *Forgotten Readers*.
49 Anita Scott Coleman, "Black Baby," *Opportunity* (February 1929): 53.
50 "Anita Scott Coleman," in Patton and Honey, *Double-Take*, 314.

51 Carby, *Reconstructing Womanhood*, 88–91.
52 Ibid. For scholarly interpretations on the trope of the "tragic mulatta" and the mulatta figure in late-nineteenth- and early-twentieth-century literature, see S. Brown, "Negro Character"; Carby, "Introduction"; Christian, "Images of Black Women," in Black Feminist Criticism; Sollors, *Neither Black nor White*; Christian, *Black Women Novelists*; McLendon, *Politics of Color*; Zackodnik, *Mulatta*; Raimon, *Tragic Mulatta Revisited*.
53 Wallace-Saunders, *Mammy*, 9.
54 D. G. White, *Too Heavy a Load*, 46–61; Christian, *Black Feminist Criticism*, 11–12; Carby, *Reconstructing Womanhood*, 39; Collins, *Black Feminist Thought*.
55 Sherrard-Johnson, *Portraits*, xix.
56 For example, see Larsen, *Quicksand* and *Passing*; Fauset, *Plum Bun*; Fauset, *Comedy: American Style*; Hurston, *Their Eyes*.
57 For example, see Haidarali, "Weird, Faded Glory."
58 Wallace, "Black Women in Popular Culture," 270–71.
59 The octoroon is one-eighth African American, but like the mulatto no longer existed in legal terms by 1920.
60 Georgia Douglas Johnson, "The Octoroon," *Bronze* (1922); reprinted in Patton and Honey, *Double-Take*, 154.
61 Hemenway, *Zora Neale Hurston*, 9.
62 Fauset, *Comedy: American Style*, 30.
63 Ibid., 15.
64 Ibid., 106.
65 Fauset, *Comedy: American Style,* 46.
66 Berzon, *Neither White nor Black*, 63. Also see Sollors, *Neither Black nor White*; Zackodnik, *Mulatta*.
67 Cullen, *One Way to Heaven*.
68 Thurman, *Blacker the Berry*, 128–29.
69 Ibid., 125.
70 See my longer discussion of Thurman's *The Blacker the Berry* in "The Vampingest Vamp."
71 Thurman, *Blacker the Berry,* 217.
72 White and White, *Stylin*, 191.
73 "Exalting Negro Womanhood," *Messenger* 6 (January 1924): 7.
74 N. Miller, *Making Love Modern*, 182–84, 144–45.
75 Ibid.
76 Ibid., 148.
77 Ibid., 147–55.
78 Bontemps, *Harlem Renaissance Remembered*, 12. Also see Whitmire, *Regina Anderson Andrews*.
79 Huggins, *Voices from the Harlem Renaissance*, 25.
80 Bontemps, *Harlem Renaissance Remembered*, 12.

81 Letter from W. E. B. Du Bois to Irene Baker, November 15, 1925, Du Bois Papers (MS 312).
82 Letter from W. E. B. Du Bois to Lucille Winston, January 5, 1926, Du Bois Papers.
83 Letter from the *Crisis* to Lucille Winston, September 29, 1926, Du Bois Papers.
84 Aaron Douglas is perhaps the best known of these artists. Douglas also helped illustrate *The New Negro*, though not on the same scale as Reiss, whom he admired, respected, and learned from while developing his own distinct modernist style. On Douglas, see Kirschke, *Aaron Douglas*.
85 Letter from W. E. B. Du Bois to Laura Wheeler, October 31, 1919, Du Bois Papers.
86 Letter from W. E. B. Du Bois to Winold Reiss, December 19, 1925, Du Bois Papers.
87 See S. M. Smith, *Photography on the Color Line*.
88 W. E. B. DuBois, "Opinion: Photography," *Crisis* (October 1923): 249–50.
89 *Crisis*, cover (September 1923).
90 Cherene Sherrard-Johnson, introduction to Fauset, *Comedy: American Style*, xvii.
91 Dorr and Logan, "Quality, not Mere Quantity," 69–71.
92 Du Bois as quoted in English, *Unnatural Selections*.
93 English, *Unnatural Selections*, 49–50.
94 Dorr and Logan, "Quality, not Mere Quantity," 81.
95 Molly Ladd-Taylor, "Fitter Family Contests," April 29, 2014, www.eugenicsarchive.ca.
96 Dorr and Logan, "Quality, not Mere Quantity," 69–71, 81–85.
97 "Benefits Baby Contests," 1924 and 1926, NAACP administrative file.
98 English, *Unnatural Selections*, 48.
99 White and White, *Stylin*, 195.
100 "Opinion," *Crisis* (October 1923): 247.
101 "My Picture Did Not Appear," *Crisis* (February 1930): 65.
102 "Photograph of Misses Dents," *Crisis*, cover (March 1921).
103 Preliminary research on the artist, D. Norman Tillman, shows him to be an African American commercial artist. Tillman also contributed another cover to the March 1927 issue of the *Crisis*. Entitled "Harlem Girl," the image approximates nothing of the edgy vibe as does "Drawing from Life," the image that appeared several months later.
104 "Drawing from Life," *Crisis* cover (July 1927).
105 DuBois, *Souls of Black Folk*, 13.
106 Nuyda, "30 Years," 21–22; Roces, "Gender, Nation"; Hawkins, *Co-producing the Postcolonial*, 64–65.
107 "Queen of Carnival, Manila, Philippine Island," *Crisis* (March 1925), cover.
108 Roces, "Women, Citizenship," 21.
109 Ibid., 16. On education as imperialist strategy, see Viola, "DuBois and Filipino/a American Exposure."
110 "Colored Students and Graduates of 1923," *Crisis* (July 1923): 112.
111 Schuyler, *Black No More*, 179.

CHAPTER 4. TO A BROWN GIRL

1. Bennett, "To a Dark Girl," 157. As Maureen Honey notes, this anthology "included the most comprehensive array of female poets assembled to that date." See Honey, introduction to *Shadowed Dream*, lii.
2. Bennett, "To a Dark Girl."
3. Arna Bontemps, "The Awakening: A Memoir," in *Harlem Renaissance Remembered*, 17.
4. Hughes, *Big Sea*, 216. Also see A. A. Johnson, "Literary Midwife," 149–53.
5. T. M. Davis, foreword, xiii-xxiv.
6. "Men of the Month," *Crisis* 19, no. 1 (November 1919): 341–42.
7. See Ula Yvette Taylor, *The Veiled Garvey*.
8. For the *Woman's Era* magazine, see womenwriters.digitalscholarship.emory.edu.
9. Ruggles and Robbins, "Gendered Literacy," 653, 660.
10. Ibid., 648.
11. Luckie, "The Poet," lines 1–4, 22–28.
12. T. M. Davis, foreword, xxiv.
13. Patton and Honey, *Double-Take*, xx.
14. Patton and Honey identify the key works of Cheryl Wall, Gloria T. Hull, Deborah McDowell, and Claudia Tate in pinpointing this gender privilege. See Patton and Honey, *Double-Take*, xxiv.
15. Hull, *Color, Sex, and Poetry*, 14.
16. Ibid.
17. Ibid.
18. McHenry, *Forgotten Readers*, 279–80.
19. Patton and Honey, *Double-Take*, xix, xxiii.
20. Honey, *Shadowed Dreams*, xxxviii–xxxvix.
21. Hull, *Color, Sex, and Poetry*, 34.
22. Hull, introduction to *Works of Alice Dunbar Nelson*, 1:xxxv–xxvi.
23. Alice Dunbar-Nelson, "Brass Ankle Speaks," in Hull, *Works of Alice Dunbar Nelson*, 2:311–21.
24. Ibid., 312.
25. Hull, introduction to *Works of Alice Dunbar Nelson*, xxxv.
26. Gaines, *Uplifting the Race*, 221.
27. Hull, *Works of Alice Dunbar Nelson*, 2:227, 430, as quoted in Gaines, *Uplifting the Race*, 220–21.
28. "Gwendolyn Bennett," in Roses and Randolph, *Harlem Renaissance and Beyond*, 11.
29. "Mae V. Cowdrey," in Roses and Randolph, *Harlem Renaissance and Beyond*, 69; "Clarissa Scott Delaney," in ibid., 80–81.
30. "Anne Spencer," in ibid., 299–300.
31. Ibid., 298.
32. Ibid., 299–301.

33 Ibid., 301.
34 "Anita Scott Coleman," in ibid., 59.
35 V. D. Mitchell, "Introduction" to *This Waiting for Love*, 8.
36 "Georgia Douglas Johnson," in Patton and Honey, *Double-Take*, 152.
37 Letter from W. E. B. Du Bois to the Harmon Awards, recommendation to the Harmon Foundation, June 21, 1927, Du Bois Papers, Series 1A, General Correspondence.
38 Letter from W. E. B. Du Bois to the Guggenheim Memorial Foundation, November 16, 1927, Du Bois Papers, Series 1A, General Correspondence.
39 Georgia Douglas Johnson, "Contest Spotlight," *Opportunity* (July 1927): 204.
40 Hull, *Works of Alice Dunbar Nelson*, 7–11; McHenry, *Forgotten Readers*, 276–77.
41 Patton and Honey, introduction to *Shadowed Dreams*, lix.
42 Letter to Dorothy West and Helene Johnson from Zora Neale Hurston, May 22, 1927, as reprinted in V. D. Mitchell, *This Waiting for Love*, 97.
43 Letter to Dorothy West from Helene Johnson, October 23, 1930, as reprinted in V. D. Mitchell, *This Waiting for Love*, 110.
44 "Georgia Douglas Johnson," in Patton and Honey, *Double-Take*, 152.
45 Hull, *Works of Alice Dunbar Nelson*, 175.
46 Honey, introduction to *Shadowed Dreams*, lviii.
47 Ibid.
48 Alice Dunbar-Nelson, October 1, 1921, in *Give Us Each Day*, 87–88.
49 Letter from Helene Johnson to Dorothy West, March 2, 1931, in Mitchell, *This Waiting for Love*, 112–13.
50 Ibid.
51 Hull, *Works of Alice Dunbar Nelson*, 19, 160.
52 H. Johnson, "I Am Not Proud," 75.
53 Anita Scott Coleman, "The Colorist," *Crisis* (September 1925): 75.
54 Ibid.
55 Ibid.
56 Gwendolyn Bennett, "Advice," in Cullen, *Caroling Dusk*, 157.
57 See Honey's note to "Advice" for brief consideration of Alain Locke. Honey, *Shadowed Dreams*, 8.
58 Mae V. Cowdery, "Lamps," *Crisis* (December 1927): 377.
59 Ibid.
60 Georgia Douglas Johnson, "True American," *Crisis* (April 1927): 48.
61 Ibid.
62 Ibid.
63 Nash, "Hidden History," 941–64.
64 Douglas Johnson, "Ordeal," 146.
65 Ibid.
66 Clarissa Scott Delaney, "The Mask," in Cullen, *Caroling Dusk*, 143.
67 Ibid.
68 Jessie Fauset, "Touché," in Cullen, *Caroling Dusk*, 66–67.

69 Angelina Weld Grimké, "At April," *Opportunity* (March 1925). Originally found in Angelina Weld Grimké Papers, Box 38-10, Folder 162, Undated Poems.
70 Angelina Weld Grimké, "Brown Girl," Angelina Weld Grimké Papers, Box 38-10, Folder 162, Undated Poems.
71 Certainly this is a crucial matter that demands fuller treatment. The relationship of masculinity, modern sexuality, and the gendering of the male body as brown deserves the sort of in-depth study that falls outside the scope of this work on women.
72 Helene Johnson, "Poem," in Cullen, *Caroling Dusk*, 218–19; Honey, *Shadowed Dreams*, 181, 183; V. D. Mitchell, *This Waiting for Love*, 38–39. Although not included in the original *Book of American Negro Poetry* (1922), five of Johnson's poems, including this poem, appeared in the anthology's second edition. See J. W. Johnson, *Book of American Negro Poetry*, 279–81.
73 Ibid.
74 Virginia Houston, "Troubadour," *Crisis* (July 1930).
75 Anne Spencer, "White Things," *Crisis* (March 1923), 204.
76 Anne Spencer, "Black Man o' Mine," unpublished, in Patton and Honey, *Double-Take*, 231.
77 Ibid.
78 Helene Johnson, "Futility," *Opportunity* (August 1926): 259.
79 Alice Dunbar-Nelson, "I Sit and Sew," in Cullen, *Caroling Dusk*, 73.
80 Helene Johnson, "Widow with a Moral Obligation," *Challenge* (March 1934). Also reprinted in Huggins, *Voices from the Harlem Renaissance*, 416–17; V. D. Mitchell, *This Waiting for Love*, 59–60.
81 Bradbury, *Wife to Widow*, 192–94.
82 Helene Johnson, "Widow with a Moral Obligation."
83 Helene Johnson, "Sonnet 1," *Opportunity*, (December 1931).
84 Ibid.
85 On the contested white patronage of Harlem Renaissance art, literature, theatrical works, and/or poetry, see Kellner, "Refined Racism"; Singh, *Novels of the Harlem Renaissance*.
86 Anne Spencer, "Questing," in Cullen, *Caroling Dusk*, 48–49.
87 Ibid.
88 Mae V. Cowdery, "I Sit and Wait for Beauty," *Challenge* (May 1935). On *Challenge* and its subsequent incarnation, *New Challenge*, a journal published and edited by Dorothy West between 1930 and 1937, see Hutchinson, *Cambridge Companion*, 49; Daniel, "Challenge Magazine."
89 Anita Scott Coleman, "Black Faces," *Opportunity* (October 1929): 320.
90 Anita Scott Coleman, "Impressions from a Family Album," *Crisis* (February 1930): 56.
91 One of the most powerful expressions of the influence of the aesthetic idealization of "white beauty" through blue eyes appears in Toni Morrison's Pulitzer-prize-winning novel, *The Bluest Eye* (1970).
92 Ibid.

93 Hull, *Works of Alice Dunbar Nelson*, 12–13.
94 Gaines, *Uplifting the Race*, 211.
95 Hull, *Give Us Each Day*, 95, as quoted in Gaines, *Uplifting the Race*, 211.
96 Dunbar-Nelson's diary entries reveal this delight at the ages of fifty-two, fifty-three, and fifty-four (Chudacoff, *How Old Are You?*, 132).
97 Wall, *Women of the Harlem Renaissance*, 12.
98 Georgia Douglas Johnson, "Welt," in J. W. Johnson, *Book of American Negro Poetry*, 132.
99 Georgia Douglas Johnson, "To a Young Wife," *Crisis* (May 1931): 15.
100 Alice Dunbar-Nelson, "The Proletariat Speaks," *Crisis* (November 1929): 149.
101 Ibid.
102 Ibid.
103 Ibid.
104 Anne Spencer, "Letter to My Sister," *Ebony and Topaz*, reprinted in Patton and Honey, *Double-Take*, 229. The editors note that this poem is also known as "Sybil Warns Her Sister." "Letter to My Sister" was a revised version of "Sybil Warns Her Sister." See "Spencer, Anne Bethel Bannister Scales," in Roses and Randolph, *Harlem Renaissance and Beyond*, 298–303.
105 Spencer, "Letter to My Sister."
106 Hine, "Rape and the Inner Lives."
107 Ibid.
108 Blanche Taylor Dickinson, "Revelation," in Cullen, *Caroling Dusk*, 107–9.
109 Ibid., 108.
110 Ibid.
111 Ibid., 109.

CHAPTER 5. BROWNING THE *DARK PRINCESS*

1 Du Bois, *Dark Princess*. Epigraph is on page 8.
2 Ibid., 7–8.
3 Ibid., 14.
4 Ibid., 22.
5 Ibid., 34.
6 Quoted in Tate, *Psychoanalysis and Black Novels*, 54.
7 Ibid.
8 Singh, *Novels of the Harlem Renaissance*, 122.
9 Rampersad, *Art and Imagination*, 204.
10 For example, see Larsen, *Quicksand* and *Passing*; Fauset, *Plum Bun*.
11 Said, *Orientalism*, 73.
12 Ibid.
13 Ibid., 5.
14 V. Kennedy, *Edward Said*, 38.
15 Said, *Orientalism*, 207.
16 Bhabha, *Location of Culture*.

17 Spivak, "Can the Subaltern Speak?," 4, 93.
18 R. Lewis, *Gendering Orientalism*, 4.
19 Ibid.; V. Kennedy, *Edward Said*; L. Lowe, *Critical Terrains*.
20 Said, *Orientalism*, 45.
21 Kennedy, *Edward Said*, 43–46.
22 Singh, *Novels of the Harlem Renaissance*, 57.
23 Prashad, *Karma of Brown Folk*, 39.
24 Ibid.
25 Fauset, *Plum Bun*, 218.
26 Prashad, *Karma of Brown Folk*, 39.
27 Martia O. Bonner, "On Being Young—a Woman—and Colored," *Crisis* 31, no. 2 (December 1925): 112.
28 Du Bois, *Dark Princess*, 218.
29 Ibid.
30 Ibid., 219.
31 Ibid.
32 Mullen and Watson, "Introduction: Crossing the World Color Line," in *Du Bois on Asia*, xiv.
33 Mullen, *Afro-Orientalism*, xx, 4.
34 Sinha, introduction to *Mother India*, 2.
35 Ibid., 20–24.
36 Genovese, *Roll, Jordan, Roll*.
37 Disparaging overviews of Indian culture, religion, and bodies include Mayo's assessment: "The whole pyramid of the Indian's woes, material and spiritual poverty, sickness, ignorance, political minority, ineffectiveness, not forgetting that subconscious conviction of inferiority which he ever bares and advertises by his gnawing and imaginative alertness for social affronts rests upon a rock-bottom physical base. This base is, simply, his manner of getting into the world and his sex-life thenceforward" (*Mother India*, 29–30).
38 Sinha, introduction to *Mother India*, 39–49.
39 Ibid., 25.
40 Ibid.
41 Tate, introduction to Du Bois, *Dark Princess*, xiv.
42 Tate, "Race and Desire," 160.
43 Tate, introduction to Du Bois, *Dark Princess*, ix.
44 Tate, "Race and Desire," 180.
45 On the rise of modern sexuality, see D'Emilio and Freedman, *Intimate Matters*, chap. 11; Bailey, *Front Porch to Back Seat*; K. White, *Sexual Liberation*; Simmons, "Modern Sexuality."
46 Simmons, *Making Marriage Modern*, 150–64.
47 Curwood, *Stormy Weather*, 4, 167.
48 D. L. Lewis, *W. E. B. DuBois*, 267.
49 Ibid., 187.

50 Lemons, "Womanism."
51 Orchestrated by Du Bois, the ill-fated marriage of Yolande Du Bois and Cullen was widely covered in the African American press. Jacqueline C. Jones teases out the gender and class implications of Cullen's darker complexion (as a man) compared to Du Bois's lighter tone (as a woman) in her essay, "'So the Girl Marries': Class, the Black Press, and the Du Bois-Cullen Wedding of 1928," in Ogbar, *Harlem Renaissance Revisited*, 45–62.
52 Lemons, "Womanism," 200.
53 W. E. B. Du Bois, "So the Girl Marries," *Crisis* (June 1928).
54 W. E. B. Du Bois, "I Bury My Wife," *Negro Digest* (October 1950), 38.
55 Carby, "Souls of Black Men," 10–14.
56 Hodes, "Fractions and Fictions," 240–41.
57 Ibid., 241.
58 Ibid., 241–42.
59 Ibid., 244.
60 Ronald Takaki, "The Tide of Turbans," in *Strangers from a Different Shore*, 62–65; Leonard, *Making Ethnic Choices*, 24–30.
61 Takaki, "Tide of Turbans," 294–97.
62 Incisive histories that both synthesize and complicate the histories of Asian Americans include Daniels, *Asian America*; Chan, *Asian Americans*; Hing, *Making and Remaking*.
63 Leonard, *Making Ethnic Choices*, 2.
64 Ibid., 68–71.
65 Ibid., 68.
66 Du Bois, *Dusk of Dawn*.
67 Appiah, "Uncompleted Argument," 36.
68 Olson, "Du Bois and Race Concept," 214–30.
69 Du Bois, "Conservation of Races," 21.
70 Ibid., 21.
71 Ibid.
72 Dickson, "Dilemma of 'Race,'" 340.
73 Appiah, "Conservation of 'Race,'" 38.
74 Joel Olson, "Du Bois and Race Concept," in *Racially Writing the Republic*, 214–30.
75 Du Bois, *Souls of Black Folk*, 213–21.
76 Ibid., 221.
77 Du Bois, "World Problem," 36.
78 Ibid.
79 Keisha N. Blain studies the rise of black international feminism among working-class women during the 1930s, focusing on Pearl Sherrod as an important antiracist activist who led the Detroit-based organization The Development of Our Own. Blain argues for recognizing Sherrod's role as a "non-state female actor" who helped shape black internationalist movements during global crisis, government repression, and censorship. See Blain, "Rights of Dark People."

80 M. M. Washington, "Colored Women's International Council," 7–10.
81 Terrell, "What It Means," 383–84.
82 See Rief, "Banded Close Together"; Matterson, "African American Women's Global Journeys."
83 Matterson, "African American Women's Global Journeys," 36.
84 Mullen and Watson, "Introduction," viii.
85 Du Bois, "Clash of Color," in Mullen and Watson, *Du Bois on Asia*, 73.
86 Mullen and Watson, "Introduction," viii; Mullen, "Afro-Asian International," 221.
87 Mullen, "Afro-Asian International," 221.
88 Horne, *End of Empires*, 80–81.
89 Ibid., 201.
90 Slate, *Colored Cosmopolitanism*, 2.
91 Kapur, *Raising Up a Prophet*.
92 Slate, *Colored Cosmopolitanism*, 1–5, 65–92.
93 Kapur, *Raising Up a Prophet*.
94 Slate., 9.
95 Horne, *End of Empires*, 9.
96 Ibid., 4, 56.
97 Mullen and Watson, *Du Bois on Asia*, xviii.
98 Letter from Lala Lajpat Rai to W. E. B. Du Bois, October 6, 1927, Du Bois Papers, Series 1A, General Correspondence.
99 Letter to *People* editor from W. E. B. Du Bois, January 10, 1929, Du Bois Papers, Series 1A, General Correspondence.
100 Marable, *Malcolm X*, 2.
101 Du Bois, "India," 3.
102 Wright, *Color Curtain*, 11–14.
103 Horne, *End of Empires*, 2.
104 Du Bois, *American Negro*, 49.
105 Du Bois, *World and Africa*, 176–78.
106 Ibid.
107 Du Bois, *Dark Princess*, 19.
108 Ibid.
109 Ibid., 20, 227.
110 Du Bois, *Dusk of Dawn*, 638. Other important African American writers queried the relevance of this "racial feeling," especially by the middle decades of the twentieth century. Of particular importance is Richard Wright, whose 1953 journey to the Gold Coast (now Ghana) led him to question: "Africa! Being of African descent, would I be able to feel and know something about Africa on the basis of a 'common' racial heritage? . . . According to some popular notions of 'race,' they ought to be something of me down there in Africa. . . . But I could not feel anything African about myself and I wondered, 'What does being African mean?'" (*Black Power*, 3–4).
111 Du Bois, "Clash of Color," quoted in Mullen and Watson, *Du Bois on Asia*, 70–73.

112 Du Bois, *Dark Princess*, 14.
113 Ibid., 223. Following emancipation and well into the 1960s, domestic work proved the mainstay of African American women's employment, especially in the rural South. The service position of waitressing can be viewed as an extension of women being tied to domestic and service-oriented work. The tobacco industry also had been an important employer of African American women since the early nineteenth century, offering women employment outside of agriculture or domestic service. However, African American women in this industry performed the dirtiest and most arduous job working as stemmers. This pattern of being relegated to the toughest and most menial labor continued as employment in factories and other industrial spaces opened to African American women. For discussions of women's labor, see J. Jones, *Labor of Love*; Clark-Lewis, *Living In*.
114 Du Bois, *Dark Princess*, 223.
115 Ibid., 222.
116 On the history of sexual violence endured by African American women and their efforts at coping and resisting, see Hine, "Rape and the Inner Lives," 912–20; Hall, "'Mind That Burns,'" 329–49; G. Jones, *Corregidora*.
117 Du Bois, *Dark Princess*, 222.
118 Ibid., 9, 10, 17.
119 Ibid., 17.
120 Ibid., 4.
121 Ibid., 7. For a compelling look at the role of stylized masculine presentation in both Du Bois's fictional work as well as in his own life, see M. L. Miller, "Du Bois and the Dandy."
122 Du Bois, *Dark Princess*, 307.
123 The representation of Kautilya as an Indian princess is consistent with the general historic production of exoticized presentations of women of color. For example, Native American women endured this stereotyping that has been named the "Pocahontas Perplex." See R. Green, "Pocahontas Perplex"; Barman, "Taming Aboriginal Sexuality."
124 Du Bois, *Dark Princess*, 8.
125 Ibid., 17.
126 Ibid., 209.
127 Ibid., 14–15.
128 Ibid., 29.
129 Ibid, 28–29.
130 Ibid., 16.
131 As quoted in Shaw, *What a Woman*, 90.
132 Du Bois, *Dark Princess*, 8.
133 Ibid., 208.
134 Ibid., 219.
135 Ibid., 268.
136 Ibid., 272.

137 Ibid., 267.
138 Ibid., 264.

CHAPTER 6. SOCIOLOGICAL DISCOURSES ON COLOR, CLASS, AND GENDER, FROM DEPRESSION TO WORLD WAR II

1 Frazier, *Negro Youth*, 194.
2 "Ophelia Settle Egypt," in J. C. Smith, *Notable Black American Women*, vol. 1.
3 Suggs, *Black Press*, 40.
4 Farrar, *Baltimore Afro-America*, 19; Chester Higgins, Sr., "Is the Black Press Dying?," *Crisis* (August–September 1980): 240–41, www.blackpressresearchcollective.org.
5 Oak, *Negro Newspaper*, "Appendix II, Directory of Negro Newspapers," 151–65.
6 Blain, "We Want to Set."
7 On the role of the black press, see Wolseley, *Black Press, U.S.A.*; Washburn, *African American Newspaper*; Finkle, *Forum for Protest*.
8 W. Baker, *Jesse Owens*.
9 Thompson, "Should I Sacrifice," 3.
10 Washburn, "Courier's Double V Campaign."
11 "The Courier Picks Two 'Double V' Girls of the Week," *Pittsburgh Courier*, August 22, 1942, 4.
12 Washburn, *Question of Sedition*.
13 Sitkoff, *Struggle for Black Equality*.
14 Finkle, "Conservative Aims."
15 Henry Lee Moon, "History of the Crisis," *Crisis*, 60th Anniversary Edition (November 1970): 385.
16 Rampersad, *Art and Imagination*, 162–63.
17 Du Bois, "Postscript," 149.
18 Moon, "History of the *Crisis*," 385.
19 Wilkins and Mathews, *Standing Fast*, 118.
20 Roy Wilkins, "The Roosevelt Record," *Crisis* 47, no. 11 (November 1940): 343.
21 Pencak, "*Crisis*," 518.
22 Brinkley, introduction to *End of Reform*.
23 Kellogg, "Civil Rights Consciousness," 18.
24 E. Williams, "Crossroads of the Caribbean," 510–14.
25 Kirby, *Black Americans*.
26 Lindquist, *Race, Social Science*, 4.
27 Holloway, *Confronting the Veil*, 34–48.
28 Ruth Feldstein, *Motherhood in Black and White*, 1–11.
29 M. E. Williams, "*Crisis* Cover Girl," 203–4.
30 The *Crisis* circulation figures from 1942 to 1946 were 20,000–59,540.
31 Korsta and Lichtenstein, "Opportunities Found and Lost," 811.
32 Kelley, *Race Rebels*, 164.
33 "Oldest and Boldest," NAACP, www.naacp.org, and www.naacp.3cdn.net.

34 Sitkoff, *Struggle for Black Equality*, 18.
35 Bracey, Meir, and Rudwick, *Black Sociologist*; Young and Deskins, "Early Traditions."
36 Young and Deskins, "Early Traditions," 445–77.
37 Park and Burgess, *Introduction*; Park, "Conflict and Fusion."
38 Scott, *Contempt and Pity*, 58–59.
39 Matthews, *Quest for American Sociology*, 101.
40 Scott, *Contempt and Pity*, 63–68.
41 Richards, "Race," 65–72; L. D. Baker, *From Savage to Negro*, 125–26; Jackson, *Social Scientists*, 7–8; Silverberg, *Gender and American Social Science*, 17.
42 Scott, *Contempt and Pity*, 20.
43 Farris, review of *Color, Class*, 139.
44 Ibid.
45 James W. Ivy, "Laundered Denims," review of *Growing Up in the Black Belt*, in *Crisis* (1941): 203.
46 Lindsay, Review of *Color, Class*, 362.
47 Ibid.
48 Fowler, Review of *Color, Class*, 708.
49 Davis and Dollard, *Children of Bondage*; Warner, Junker, and Adams, *Color and Human Nature*.
50 Warner, *Color and Human Nature*.
51 Lindsay, *Social Service Review* 361.
52 Frazier, *Negro Youth at the Crossways*, 261.
53 Ibid., 3–17.
54 Ibid., xxxv, n. 4.
55 Jessie Carney Smith, ed., "E. Franklin Frazier," in *Notable Black American Men*, 428.
56 The debate over culture between Herskovits and Frazier was longstanding. On Herskovits's celebration of African cultural retention among African Americans, see his *Myth of the Negro Past*.
57 Frazier quoted in Holloway, *Confronting the Veil*, 134.
58 Holloway, *Confronting the Veil*, 123–56.
59 Frazier, *Negro Youth at the Crossways*, 273.
60 In Washington, D.C., 112 girls and 94 boys were interviewed; in Louisville, Kentucky, 33 girls and 29 boys were interviewed (Frazier, *Negro Youth at the Crossways*, xxxv, n. 4).
61 Frazier, *Negro Youth at the Crossways*, 273.
62 Matthews, *Quest for American Sociology*, 94–105. On the connections between sociology and social service work and the moral reform efforts within the disciplines, see Shore, *Science of Social Redemption*, chap. 2.
63 Matthews, *Quest for American Sociology*, 100.
64 Ibid., 94–105; Shore, *Science of Social Redemption*, chap. 2; Young and Deskins, "Early Traditions," 451.

65 Frazier, *Negro Youth at the Crossways*, 290.
66 Ibid., 25.
67 While the body of Frazier's sociological work focused on patterns of social organization, the family proved to be his main empirical focus. These works include Frazier, "Family Disorganization," 204–7; Frazier, *Negro Family in Chicago*; Frazier, "Traditions and Patterns." For a discussion of Frazier's sociological contribution to the study of the African American family, see Young and Deskins, "Early Traditions," 464.
68 Frazier, *Negro Youth at the Crossways*, 51–52.
69 In 1957, Frazier delivered his now-famous castigation of the African American middle class. This account differs greatly in tone and vision from *Negro Youth at the Crossways*. In many ways, the latter work was more hopeful and optimistic about the future of African American society and culture. By the late 1950s, this positive vision dissipated. See Frazier, *Black Bourgeoisie*.
70 As quoted in Frazier, *Negro Youth at the Crossways*, 53.
71 Frazier, *Negro Youth at the Crossways*, 53.
72 Ibid., 53.
73 Ibid., 180.
74 Schapp, *Triumph*; Boskin, *Jesse Owens*.
75 Frazier, *Negro Youth at the Crossways*, 181.
76 Ibid.
77 Ibid., 185, 194.
78 Young and Deskins, "Early Traditions," 465; Gilpin, *Charles S. Johnson*, 130–31.
79 C. S. Johnson, *Growing Up*, xxi–xxvi.
80 As the founding editor, Johnson anthologized selected work from *Opportunity* to appear in the anthology *Ebony and Topaz*. This anthology appeared in 1927; this year also marked the end of Johnson's tenure as the magazine's editor.
81 Holloway, *Confronting the Veil*, 143.
82 "Charles S. Johnson," in *Notable Black Men*, 616–19.
83 Drake, introduction to *Growing Up*, xi.
84 Holloway, *Confronting the Veil*, 124–25, 142–43; Gilpin, *Charles S. Johnson*, 130–31.
85 C. S. Johnson, *Growing Up*, 256.
86 Ibid., 272.
87 Jackson, *Social Scientists*, 24–30; Belgrave and Allison, *African American Psychology*, 8–12.
88 For examples and discussion of these tests, see appendix B in C. S. Johnson, *Growing Up*, 334–52.
89 Gilpin, *Charles S. Johnson*, 126–27, 130–31.
90 C. S. Johnson, *Growing Up*, ix–xi.
91 Johnson provided all of his subjects with pseudonyms.
92 C. S. Johnson, *Growing Up*, 9.
93 Ibid., 15.
94 Ibid., 258.

95 Ibid., 256–73.
96 Ibid., 256–58.
97 Ibid., 270.
98 Ivy, "Laundered Denims," 203.
99 Ibid., 265.
100 Ibid., 265–66.
101 Ibid.
102 Parrish, "Color Names and Color Notions," 13.
103 Parrish, "Significance of Color." The published article drew on the dissertation's third chapter, "Intra-Group Notions about Color Classes." Other chapters include "The Role of Color in Negro-White Relations," "Intra-Group Notions about Color Classes," "Subjective Reactions to Color Notions," "The Acquisition of Color Attitudes," "The Role of Color in the Family," "The Extreme Groups—Social Limitations and Pressures," and "The Extreme Color Groups: Personality."
104 Parrish conducted this research between 1938 and 1941. See his introduction to "Significance of Color" for his explanation of this timeframe.
105 "Charles H. Parrish, Sr.," in J. C. Smith, *Notable Black American Men*, 911–13; Biographical Sketch, Charles Henry Parrish Papers, University of Louisville Libraries, Louisville, Kentucky. Parrish's publications include "Education of Negroes in Kentucky," "Negro Higher Education," "Desegregation in Public Education," and "Desegregated Higher Education in Kentucky."
106 Parrish, "Significance of Color," 3–4.
107 Ibid., 174.
108 Parrish, "Significance of Color," 37–38; Parrish, "Color Names and Color Notions," 13–14.
109 Parrish, "Significance of Color," 40–41; Guthrie, *Even the Rat*, 22–23; C. S. Johnson, *Growing Up*, 265.
110 Parrish, "Significance of Color," 40–46; Parrish, "Color Names and Color Notions," 13–20.
111 Parrish, "Significance of Color," 46–47.
112 Ibid., 50–53.
113 Ibid., 48–51.
114 Ibid., 48–49; Parrish, "Color Names and Color Notions," 15–20.
115 Parrish, "Significance of Color," 44–45.
116 Ibid., 49.

EPILOGUE

1 "Another Step Up," newspaper clipping, July 31, 1946, Barbara Watson Collection.
2 Sullivan, "Don't Do This," 48, 50.
3 Haidarali, "Polishing Brown Diamonds."

BIBLIOGRAPHY

PRIMARY SOURCES
Manuscript and Microfilm Collections
Alain Locke Papers. Moorland Spingarn, Howard University, Washington, D.C.
Angelina Weld Grimké Papers, Moorland-Spingarn Research Center, Oral History Department, Howard University, Washington, D.C.
Barbara Watson Collection. Schomburg Center for Research in Black Culture, Manuscript Division, New York Public Library, New York City.
Charles Henry Parrish Papers. University of Louisville Libraries, Louisville, Kentucky.
Claude A. Barnett Papers. Chicago Historical Society, Chicago.
Gertrude Elise Ayers Papers, Manuscript Division, Schomburg Center for Research in Black Culture. New York: New York Public Library.
NAACP Papers. Special Subject Files, 1912-39. Library of Congress, Manuscript Division, Washington, D.C.
Schomburg Center for Research in Black Culture Clipping File. New York: New York Public Library.
W. E. B. Du Bois Papers. Special Collections and University Archives, University of Massachusetts, Amherst Libraries.
Works Progress Administration. *American Life Histories: Manuscripts from the Federal Writers' Project, 1936-1940*. Library of Congress, Manuscript Division, Washington, D.C.

Newspapers and Periodicals
Atlanta Constitution
Birth Control Review
Black Dispatch
Challenge and New Challenge
Chicago Defender
Crisis
Daily Oklahoman
Half-Century
Messenger
Nashville Globe
New York Age
New York Amsterdam News
Opportunity
Pittsburgh Courier

Saturday Evening Quill
Survey Graphic
Woman's Era

Government Publications

U.S. Bureau of the Census. *Historical Statistics of the United States: Colonial Times to 1970.* Washington, D.C.: Government Printing Office, 1975.

U.S. Department of Commerce, Bureau of the Census. *Negroes in the United States, 1920–1932.* Washington, D.C.: Government Printing Office, 1935.

U.S. Department of Commerce, Bureau of the Census. *Negro Population, 1790–1915.* 1918. Reprint, Washington, D.C.: Government Printing Office, 1969.

Books, Pamphlets, Articles, Poems, and Speeches

Ayer, Gertrude Elise. "Notes on My Native Sons—Education in Harlem." *Freedomways* 3 (Summer 1963): 375–83.

Bennett, Gwendolyn. "To a Dark Girl" and "Advice." In *Caroling Dusk: An Anthology of Verse by Black Poets of the Twenties*, ed. Countee Cullen. 1927. Reprint, New York: Carol Publishing Group, 1993.

Bennett, Lerone, Jr. "What's in a Name? Negro vs. Afro-American vs. Black." *Ebony* 23 (November 1967): 46–48, 50–52, 54.

Boas, Franz. "The Instability of Human Types." *Papers on Interracial Problems Communicated to the First Universal Race Congress Held at the University of London.* July 26–29, 1911.

Bontemps, Arna, ed. *The Harlem Renaissance Remembered.* New York: Dodd Mead, 1972.

Cullen, Countee, ed. *Caroling Dusk: An Anthology of Verse by Black Poets of the Twenties.* 1927. Reprint, New York: Carol Publishing Group, 1993.

———. *One Way to Heaven.* New York: Harper and Brothers, 1932.

Cunard, Nancy. "Harlem Reviewed." In *Negro Anthology.* 1934. Reprint, New York: Negro University Press, 1969.

Davis, Allison, and John Dollard. *Children of Bondage: The Personality Development of Negro Youth in the Urban South.* Washington, D.C.: American Council of Education, 1941.

Dickinson, Blanche Taylor. "Revelation." In *Caroling Dusk: An Anthology of Verse by Black Poets of the Twenties*, edited by Countee Cullen, 1927. Reprint, New York: Carol Publishing Group, 1993.

Douglas Johnson, Georgia. "The Ordeal." In *The New Negro*, ed. Alain Locke. New York: Albert and Charles Boni, 1925.

———. "Welt." In *Book of American Negro Poetry*, ed. James Weldon Johnson. 1931. Reprint, New York, 1983.

Drake, St. Clair, and Horace Cayton. *Black Metropolis: A Study of Negro Life in a Northern City.* 1945. Reprint, Chicago: University of Chicago Press, 2015.

Du Bois, W. E. B. *The American Negro and the Darker World.* New York: National Committee to Defend Negro Leadership, 1957.

———. "The American Negro in Paris." *American Monthly Review of Reviews* (November 1900): 577.

———. "The Clash of Color: Indians and American Negroes." *Aryan Path* 8 (March 1936): 111–15.

———. "The Conservation of Races." American Negro Academy, Occasional Papers, no. 2, 1897.

———. "Damnation of Women." In *Darkwater: Voices from within the Veil*. New York: Schocken Books, 1920.

———. *Dark Princess: A Romance*. Introduction by Claudia Tate Jackson. 1928. Reprint, Jackson: University Press of Mississippi, 1995.

———. *Dusk of Dawn: A Chapter toward an Autobiography of a Race Concept*. New York: Harcourt, Brace, 1940.

———. "India." In *Writings in the Periodicals Edited by W. E. B. Du Bois: Selections from the "Horizon: A Journal of the Color Line,"* ed. Herbert Aptheker. 1907. Reprint, New York: Kraus-Thomson, 1985.

———. *The Souls of Black Folk*. In *Three Negro Classics*. Introduction by John Hope Franklin. 1903. Reprint, New York: Avon Books, 1965.

———. *The World and Africa: An Inquiry into the Part which Africa Has Played in World History*. New York: International, 1965.

———. "The World Problem of the Color Line." *Manchester Leader*, November 16, 1914.

Du Bois, W. E. B., ed. *The Health and Physique of the Negro American. Report of a Social Study made under the direction of Atlanta University; together with the Proceedings of the Eleventh Conference for the Study of Negro Problems, held at Atlanta University, on May the 29th, 1906*. Atlanta: Atlanta University Press, 1906.

Dunbar-Nelson, Alice. "Brass Ankles Speaks." In *The Works of Alice Dunbar Nelson*, vols. 1–3, ed. Gloria T. Hull. New York: Oxford University Press, 1988.

———. *Give Us Each Day: The Diary of Alice Dunbar-Nelson*. Edited by Gloria T. Hull. New York: W. W. Norton, 1984.

———. "I Sit and Sew." In *Caroling Dusk: An Anthology of Verse by Black Poets of the Twenties*, ed. Countee Cullen. 1927. Reprint, New York: Carol Publishing Group, 1993.

Edwards, Paul K. *The Southern Urban Negro Consumer*. New York: Negro Universities Press, 1932.

Farris, Robert E. L. Review of *Color, Class, and Personality. American Journal of Sociology* 48, no. 1 (1942): 139–40.

Fauset, Jessie. *Comedy: American Style*. Introduction by Cherene Sherrard-Johnson. 1933. Reprint, New Brunswick, NJ: Rutgers University Press, 2010.

———. *Plum Bun: A Novel without a Moral*. 1928. Reprint, with an introduction by Deborah E. McDowell. London; Boston: Pandora Press, 1985.

———. *There Is Confusion*. 1924. Reprint, Boston: Northeastern University Press, 1989.

———. "Touché." In *Caroling Dusk: An Anthology of Verse by Black Poets of the Twenties*, ed. Countee Cullen, 66–67. 1927. Reprint, New York: Carol Publishing Group, 1993.

Fowler, Manet. Review of *Color, Class, and Personality*. *American Anthropologist*, n.s. 44, no. 4 part 1 (October–December 1942): 708.
Frazier, E. Franklin. *Black Bourgeoisie: The Rise of a New Middle Class in the United States*. New York: Free Press, 1957.
———. "Family Disorganization among Negroes." *Opportunity* 9 (July 1931): 204–7.
———. *The Negro Family in Chicago*. Chicago: University of Chicago Press, 1932.
———. *Negro Youth at the Crossways: Their Personality Development in the Middle States*. Washington, D.C.: American Council on Education, 1940. Reprint, New York: Schocken Books, 1967.
———. "Traditions and Patterns of Negro Family Life in the United States." In *Race and Culture Contacts*. Boston: Beacon Press, 1957.
George, Louis W. "Beauty Culture and Colored People." *Messenger* 2 (July 1918): 25–26.
Gordon, Eugene. "The Brown-Skin Fad." *Plain Talk* (October 1929): 458.
Hackley, Azalia E. *The Colored Girl Beautiful*. Kansas City, MO: Burton, 1916.
Haring, H. A. "Selling to Harlem." *Advertising and Selling* 11, no. 14 (October 31, 1928): 17–18, 50–53.
Herskovits, Melville. *The Myth of the Negro Past*. New York: Harper and Brothers, 1941.
Hughes, Langston. *The Big Sea*. New York: Alfred A. Knopf, 1940.
Hunton, Eunice Roberta. "Breaking Through." *Survey Graphic: Harlem, Mecca of the New Negro* (March 1925): 684.
Hurston, Zora Neale. "Color Struck: A Play in Four Scenes." *Fire!!* (November 1926): 7–14.
———. *Dust Tracks on a Road: An Autobiography*. 1942. Reprint, Chicago: University of Illinois Press, 1984.
———. *I Love Myself When I Am Laughing: A Zora Neale Hurston Reader*. Edited by Alice Walker. Introduction by Mary Helen Washington. New York: Feminist Press, 1979.
———. "Record of Freshman Interest." December 16, 1925. Barnard Archives. www.sfonline.barnard.edu.
———. *Their Eyes Were Watching God*. 1937. Foreword by Sherley Anne Williams. Reprint, Urbana: University of Illinois Press, 1978.
Johnson, Charles S. "Black Workers and the City." *Survey Graphic: Harlem, Mecca of the New Negro* (March 1925): 641–43.
———. *Growing Up in the Black Belt: Negro Youth in the Rural South*. 1941. Reprint, New York: Schocken Books, 1967.
———. "Race Pride and Cosmetics." *Opportunity* (October 1925): 293.
Johnson, Charles S., ed. *Ebony and Topaz*. New York: National Urban League, 1927.
Johnson, Guy B. "Newspaper Advertisements and Negro Culture." *Journal of Social Forces* 3, no. 4 (May 1925): 706–9.
Johnson, Helene. "I Am Not Proud." *Saturday Evening Quill* (April 1929): 75.
———. *This Waiting for Love: Helene Johnson, Poet of the Harlem Renaissance*. Edited by Verner D. Mitchell. Amherst: University of Massachusetts Press, 2000.
Johnson, James Weldon. "The Making of Harlem." *Survey Graphic, Harlem: Mecca of the New Negro* (March 1925): 635–39.

Johnson, James Weldon, ed. *Book of American Negro Poetry.* 1931. Reprint, New York, 1983.
Larsen, Nella. *Quicksand* and *Passing.* 1928 and 1929. Reprint. Introduction by Deborah E. McDowell. New Brunswick, NJ: Rutgers University Press, 1986.
Lindsay, Inabel Burns. Review of *Color, Class, and Personality* by Robert Sutherland. *Social Service Review* 16, no. 2 (June 1942): 361–62.
Locke, Alain. "Harlem." Introduction to "Harlem: Mecca of the New Negro." *Survey Graphic* (March 1925): 629–30.
———. "To Certain of Our Philistines." *Opportunity* (May 1925): 155–56.
Locke, Alain, ed. *The New Negro: An Interpretation.* New York: Albert and Charles Boni, 1925.
Luckie, Ida Evans. "The Poet." *Woman's Era* (July 1896): 13–14.
Mayo, Katherine. *Mother India.* 1927. Reprint edited with an introduction by Mrinalini Sihna. Ann Arbor: University of Michigan Press, 2000.
McDougald, Elise Johnson. "The Negro Woman Teacher and the Negro Student." *Messenger* (July 1923): 769–70.
McKay, Claude. "If We Must Die." *Liberator* (July 1919): 21.
———. "The Task of Negro Womanhood." In *The New Negro: An Interpretation*, ed. Alain Locke. New York: Albert and Charles Boni, 1925.
Miller, Kelly. "The Eugenics of the Negro Race." *Scientific Monthly* 5, no. 1 (July 1917): 57–59.
Mitchell, Verner D., ed. *This Waiting for Love: Helene Johnson, Poet of the Harlem Renaissance.* Amherst: University of Massachusetts Press, 2000.
Myrdal, Gunnar. *An American Dilemma: The Negro Problem and Modern Democracy.* New York: Harper and Brothers, 1944.
A New Day for the Colored Woman Worker: A Study of Colored Women in Industry in New York City. Investigators, Jessie Clark and Gertrude E. McDougald. New York: C. P. Young, 1919.
Noble, Jeanne. *The Negro Woman's College Education.* New York: Columbia University, Bureau Publications, 1956.
Oak, Vishnu. *The Negro Newspaper.* Yellow Springs, Ohio: Antioch Press, 1948.
Park, Robert E. "Behind Our Masks." *Survey* (May 1926): 135–36.
———. "The Conflict and Fusion of Cultures with Special Reference to the Negro." *Journal of Negro History* 4 (April 1919): 113–33.
Park, Robert E., and Ernest Burgess. *An Introduction to the Science of Sociology.* Chicago: University of Chicago Press, 1921.
Parrish, Charles H. "Color Names and Color Notions." *Journal of Negro Education* 15, no. 1 (Winter 1946): 13–20.
———. "Desegregated Higher Education in Kentucky." *Journal of Negro Education* 27, no. 3 (Summer 1958): 260–68.
———. "Desegregation in Public Education." *Journal of Negro Education* 24, no. 3 (Summer 1955): 382–84.
———. "The Education of Negroes in Kentucky." *Journal of Negro Education* 16, no. 3 (Summer 1947): 354–60.

———. "Negro Higher Education and Professional Education in Kentucky." *Journal of Negro Education* 17, no. 3 (Summer 1948): 289–95.
———. "The Significance of Color in the Negro Community." Ph.D. diss., University of Chicago, 1944.
Schuyler, George S. *Black No More.* New York: Modern Library, 1999.
Scott, Emmett J., ed. "Letters of Negro Migrants of 1916–1918." *Journal of Negro History* 4, no. 3 (July 1919): 290–340.
Scott Delaney, Clarissa. "The Mask." In *Caroling Dusk: An Anthology of Verse by Black Poets of the Twenties*, ed. Countee Cullen. 1927. Reprint, New York: Carol Publishing Group, 1993.
Spencer, Anne. "Questing." In *Caroling Dusk: An Anthology of Verse by Black Poets of the Twenties*, ed. Countee Cullen. 1927. Reprint, New York: Carol Publishing Group, 1993.
Sullivan, David J. "Don't Do This—If You Want to Sell Your Products to Negroes!" *Sales Management* 52 (March 1, 1943): 46–50.
Terrell, Mary Church. "What It Means to Be Colored in Capital of the U.S." Speech delivered October 10, 1906, United Women's Club, Washington, D.C. Reprinted in her autobiography, *A Colored Woman in a White World.* 1940. Reprint, Washington, D.C.: National Association of Colored Women's Clubs, 1968.
Thompson, James Q. "Should I Sacrifice to Live Half American?" *Pittsburgh Courier*, January 31, 1942.
Thurman, Wallace. *The Blacker the Berry: A Novel of Negro Life.* 1929. Reprint, New York: Simon and Shuster, 1996.
Warner, W. Lloyd. *Color and Human Nature: Negro Personality Development in a Northern City.* Washington, D.C.: American Council on Education, 1941.
Warner, Lloyd W., Buford H. Junker, and Walter A. Adams. *Color and Human Nature: Negro Personality Development in a Northern City.* Washington, D.C.: American Council of Education, 1941.
Washington, Margaret Murray. "Colored Women's International Council." *Southern Workman* 52 (January 1923), 7–10.
Williams, Eric. "Crossroads of the Caribbean." *Survey Graphic* (November 1942): 510–14.
Wright, Richard. *Black Power: A Record of Reactions to the Land of Pathos.* New York: Harper and Brothers, 1954.
———. *The Color Curtain: A Report on the Bandung Conference.* Introduction by Gunnar Myrdal. New York: World Publishing, 1956. Reprinted with afterword by Amritjit Singh. Jackson: University Press of Mississippi, 1994.

SECONDARY SOURCES

Allen, Utaukwa. "The Woman's Era: Constructing Black Women's Identity in the Late Nineteenth Century." In *Women's Magazines in Print and New Media*, ed. Noliwe Rooks, Victoria Pass, and Ayana Weekley, 93–11. New York: Routledge, 2017.

Amott, Teresa, and Julie Matthaei. "We Specialize in the Wholly Impossible: African American Women." In *Race, Gender, and Work: A Multicultural Economic History of Women in the United States*. Boston: South End Press, 1996.
Angione, Genevieve. *All-Bisque and Half-Bisque Dolls*. Exton, Pa.: Schiffer, 1969.
Appiah, Kwame Anthony. "The Conservation of 'Race.'" *Black American Literature Forum* 23, no. 1 (Spring 1989): 37–60.
———. "The Uncompleted Argument: Du Bois and the Illusion of Race." In *"Race," Writing, and Difference*, ed. Henry Louis Gates Jr., 21–37. Chicago: University of Chicago Press, 1985.
Bailey, Beth L. *From Front Porch to Back Seat: Courtship in Twentieth-Century America*. Baltimore, MD: Johns Hopkins University Press, 1988.
Baker, Houston, Jr. *Modernism and the Harlem Renaissance*. Chicago: University of Chicago Press, 1987.
Baker, Lee D. *From Savage to Negro: Anthropology and the Construction of Race, 1896–1954*. Berkeley: University of California Press, 1998.
Baker, William. *Jesse Owens: An American Way of Life*. New York: Free Press, 1988.
Baldwin, Davarian L. *Chicago's New Negroes: Modernity, the Great Migration, and Black Urban Life*. Chapel Hill: University of North Carolina Press, 2007.
Baldwin, Davarian L., and Minkah Makalani, eds. *Escape from New York: The New Negro Renaissance beyond Harlem*. Minneapolis: University of Minnesota Press, 2013.
Banner, Lois. *American Beauty*. New York: Knopf, 1983.
Barkin, Elazar. *The Retreat of Scientific Racism: Changing Concepts of Race in Britain and the United States between the World Wars*. Cambridge: Cambridge University Press, 1992.
Barman, Jean. "Taming Aboriginal Sexuality: Gender, Power and Race in British Columbia, 1850–1900." *BC Studies*, no. 111–16 (1997): 237–66.
Belgrave, Faye Z., and Kevin W. Allison. *African American Psychology: From Africa to America*. Thousand Oaks, CA: Sage, 2006.
Benson, Susan Porter. *Counter Cultures: Saleswomen, Managers, and Customers in American Department Stores, 1890–1940*. Urbana: University of Illinois Press, 1988.
Bernstein, Robin. *Racial Innocence: Performing American Childhood from Slavery to Civil Rights*. New York: New York University Press, 2011.
Berry, Mary Frances, and John W. Blassingame. *Long Memory: The Black Experience in America*. New York: Oxford University Press, 1983.
Berzon, Judith. *Neither White nor Black: The Mulatto Character in American Fiction*. New York: New York University Press, 1978.
Bhabha, Homi. *The Location of Culture*. New York: Routledge, 1994.
Biondi, Martha. *To Stand and Fight: The Struggle for Civil Rights in Postwar New York City*. Cambridge, MA: Harvard University Press, 2003.
Blackwelder, Julia Kirk. *Stylin' Jim Crow: African American Beauty Training during Segregation*. College Station: Texas A&M University, 1984.
Blackwell, Joyce. *No Peace without Freedom: Race and the Women's International League for Peace and Freedom, 1915–1975*. Carbondale: Southern Illinois University Press, 2004.

Blain, Keisha N. "[F]or the Rights of Dark People in Every Part of the World": Pearl Sherrod, Black Internationalist Feminism, and Afro-Asian Politics during the 1930s." *Souls* 17, nos. 1–2 (January–June 2015): 90–112.

———. "'We Want to Set the World on Fire': Black Nationalist Women and Diasporic Politics in the *New Negro World*, 1940–1944." *Journal of Social History* 49, no. 1 (2015): 194–212.

Bogle, Bonnie. "Negro Womanhood's Greatest Needs: A Symposium." *Messenger* 9 (April 1927): 109.

Boskin, Joseph. *Jesse Owens: An American Life.* New York: Free Press, 1986.

Bracey, John, August Meir, and Elliot Rudwick. *The Black Sociologist: The First Half Century.* Belmont, CA: Wadsworth, 1971.

Bradbury, Bettina. *Wife to Widow: Lives, Laws, and Politics in Nineteenth-Century Montreal.* Vancouver: UBC Press, 2011.

Briggs, Gabriel A. *The New Negro in the New South.* New Brunswick, NJ: Rutgers University Press, 2015.

Brinkley, Alan, *The End of Reform: New Deal Liberalism in Recession.* New York: Vintage Books, 1996.

Brown, Elsa Barkley. "Negotiating and Transforming the Public Sphere: African American Political Life in the Transition from Slavery to Freedom." *Public Culture* 7 (Fall 1994): 107–46.

Brown, Jayna. *Babylon Girls: Black Women Performers and the Shaping of the Modern.* Durham: University of North Carolina Press, 2008.

Brown, Nikki. *Private Politics and Public Voices: Black Women's Activism from World War I to the New Deal.* Bloomington: Indiana University Press, 2006.

Brown, Sterling. "Negro Character as Seen by White Authors." In *Dark Symphony: Negro Literature in America*, ed. James A. Emanuel and Theodore L. Gross, 139–71. 1933. Reprint, New York: Free Press, 1968.

Bundles, A'Lelia. *On Her Own Ground: The Life and Times of Madam C. J. Walker.* New York: Simon and Schuster, 2001.

Carby, Hazel V. Introduction to Frances E. W. Harper's *Iola LeRoy*, ix–xxvi. Boston: Beacon, 1987.

———. *Reconstructing Womanhood: The Emergence of the Afro-American Woman Novelist.* New York: Oxford University Press, 1987.

———. "The Souls of Black Men." In *Next to the Color Line: Gender, Sexuality, and W. E. B. Du Bois*, ed. Susan Gillman and Alys Eve Weinbaum, 235–37. Minneapolis: University of Minnesota Press, 2007.

Carroll, Ann Elizabeth. *Word, Image and the New Negro.* Bloomington: Indiana University Press, 2005.

Cha-Jua, Sundiata K., and Clarence E. Lang. "The 'Long Movement' as Vampire: Temporal and Spatial Fallacies in Recent Black Freedom Studies." *Journal of African American History* 92, no. 2 (2007): 265–88.

Chambers, Clark A. *Paul U. Kellogg and the Survey: Voices for Social Welfare and Social Justice.* Minneapolis: University of Minnesota Press, 1971.

Chambers, Jason. *Madison Avenue and the Color Line.* University Park: University of Pennsylvania Press, 2011.
Chan, Sucheng. *Asian Americans: An Interpretive History.* Boston: Twayne, 1991.
Christian, Barbara. *Black Feminist Criticism: Perspectives on Black Women Writers.* New York: Pergamon, 1985.
———. *Black Women Novelists: The Development of a Tradition.* Westport, Conn.: Greenwood, 1980.
Chudacoff, Howard P. *How Old Are You? Age Consciousness in American Culture.* Princeton, NJ: Princeton University Press, 1992.
Clark-Lewis, Elizabeth. *Living In. Living Out.* Washington, D.C.: Smithsonian Institution Press, 1994.
Clifford, James. "Introduction: Partial Truths." In *Writing Culture: The Poetics and Politics of Ethnography,* ed. James Clifford and George E. Marcus, 1–26. Berkeley: University of California Press, 1986.
———. "On Ethnographic Authority." In *The Predicament of Culture: Twentieth Century Ethnography, Literature and Art.* Cambridge, MA: Harvard University Press, 1988.
Cohen, Lizbeth. *A Consumers' Republic: The Politics of Mass Consumption in Postwar America.* New York: Alfred A. Knopf, 2003.
Collier-Thomas, Bettye, and James Turner. "Race, Class and Color: The African American Discourse on Identity." *Journal of American Ethnic History* 14, no. 1 (Fall 1994): 5–31.
Collins, Patricia Hill. *Black Feminist Thought: Knowledge, Consciousness and the Politics of Empowerment.* New York: Routledge, 2000.
Corbould, Clare. *Becoming African Americans: Black Public Life in Harlem, 1919–1939.* Cambridge, MA: Harvard University Press, 2009.
Cotkin, George. *Reluctant Modernism: American Thought and Culture, 1880–1900.* New York: Twayne, 1992.
Countryman, Matthew J. *Up South: Civil Rights and Black Power in Philadelphia.* Philadelphia: University of Pennsylvania Press, 2006.
Craig, Maxine. *Ain't I a Beauty Queen? Black Women, Beauty, and the Politics of Race.* Oxford: Oxford University Press, 2002.
Cronon, David E. *Black Moses: The Story of Marcus Garvey and the Universal Negro Improvement Association.* Madison: University of Wisconsin Press, 2006.
Cullen, Frank, with Florence Hackman and David McNeilly. *Vaudeville, Old and New: An Encyclopedia of Variety Performers in America.* Vol. 1. New York: Routledge, 2007.
Curwood, Anatasia. *Stormy Weather: Middle-Class African American Marriages between the Two World Wars.* Chapel Hill: University of North Carolina Press, 2010.
Daniel, Walter C. "*Challenge Magazine:* An Experiment that Failed." *CLA Journal* 19 (1976): 494–503.
Daniels, Roger. *Asian America: Chinese and Japanese in the United States since 1850.* Seattle: University of Washington Press, 1988.
Davis, Allison, and John Dollard. *Children of Bondage: The Personality Development of Negro Youth in the Urban South.* Washington, D.C.: American Council on Education, 1940.

Davis, Angela. *Blues Legacies and Black Feminism: Gertrude "Ma" Rainey, Bessie Smith and Billie Holliday.* New York: Vintage Books, 1999.
———. *Women, Race, and Class.* New York: Random House, 1971.
Davis, James F. *Who Is Black? One Nation's Definition.* University Park: Pennsylvania State University Press, 1991.
Davis, Thadious M. Foreword to Jessie Fauset, *There Is Confusion,* xiii–xxiv. Boston: Northeastern University Press, 1989.
———. *Nella Larsen: Novelist of the Harlem Renaissance.* Baton Rouge: Louisiana State University Press, 1994.
Degler, Carl N. *In Search of Human Nature: The Decline and Revival of Darwinism in American Social Thought.* New York: Oxford University Press, 1991.
D'Emilio, John, and Estelle B. Freeman. *Intimate Matters: A History of Sexuality in America.* Chicago: University of Chicago Press, 1988.
Dent, Gina, ed. *Black Popular Culture.* Seattle: Bay Press, 1992.
Dickson, Bruce J., Jr. "W. E. B. Du Bois and the Dilemma of 'Race.'" *American Literary History* 7, no. 2 (Summer 1995): 334–43.
Dorr, Gregory Michael, and Angela Logan. "Quality, Not Mere Quantity, Counts: Black Eugenics and the NAACP Baby Contests." In *A Century of Eugenics in America: From the Indiana Experiment to the Human Genome Era,* ed. Paul Lombardo. Bloomington: Indiana University Press, 2011.
Douglas, Ann. *Terrible Honesty: Mongrel Manhattan in the 1920s.* New York: Picador, 1995.
Du Cille, Anne. *The Coupling Convention: Sex, Text and Tradition in Black Women's Fiction.* New York: Oxford University Press, 1993.
English, Daylanne K. *Unnatural Selections: Eugenics in America Modernism and the Harlem Renaissance.* Chapel Hill: University of North Carolina Press, 2004.
Farrar, Hayward. *The Baltimore Afro-American, 1892–1950.* Westport, CT: Greenwood, 1998.
Feldstein, Ruth. *Motherhood in Black and White.* New York: Cornell University Press, 2000.
Ferguson, Jeffrey B. *The Sage of Sugar Hill: George S. Schuyler and the Harlem Renaissance.* New Haven, CT: Yale University Press, 2005.
Fine, Lisa. *The Souls of the Skyscraper: Female Clerical Workers in Chicago, 1870–1930.* Philadelphia: Temple University Press, 1990.
Finkle, Lee. "The Conservative Aims of Militant Rhetoric: Black Protest during World War II." *Journal of American History* 60, no. 3 (December 1973): 692–713.
———. *Forum for Protest: The Black Press during World War II.* Cranbury, NJ: Associated University Presses, 1975.
Fisher, Rebecka Rutledge. "The Anatomy of a Symbol: Reading W. E. B. Du Bois's *Dark Princess: A Romance. CR: The New Centennial Review* 6, no. 3 (Winter 2006): 91–128.
Foley, Barbara. *Spectres of 1919: Class and Nation in the Making of the New Negro.* Urbana: University of Illinois Press, 2003.
Foner, Eric. *Reconstruction: America's Unfinished Revolution, 1863–1877.* New York: Harper Collins, 1988.

Formanek-Brunell, Miriam. *Made to Play House: Dolls and the Commercialization of American Girlhood.* Baltimore: Johns Hopkins University Press, 1998.

Fredrickson, George M. *The Black Image in the White Mind: The Debate on African American Character and Destiny, 1817–1914.* New York: Harper and Row, 1971.

Gage, John. *Color and Meaning: Art, Science and Symbolism.* London: Thames and Hudson, 1999.

———. *Colour and Culture: Practice and Meaning from Antiquity to Abstraction.* 1993. Reprint, London: Thames and Hudson, 2012.

Gaines, Kevin P. *Uplifting the Race: Black Leadership, Politics, and Culture in the Twentieth Century.* Chapel Hill: University of North Carolina Press, 1996.

Gates, Henry Louis, Jr. *The Signifying Monkey: A Theory of African-American Literary Criticism.* Oxford: Oxford University Press, 1998.

———. "The Trope of the New Negro and the Reconstruction of the Image of the Black." *Representations* 24 (1988): 129–55.

Gatewood, Willard B. *Aristocrats of Color: The Black Elite, 1880–1920.* Bloomington: Indiana University Press, 1990.

Genovese, Eugene. *Roll, Jordan, Roll: The World the Slaves Made.* New York: Pantheon Books, 1975.

Gerstle, Gary. "The Crucial Decade: The 1940s and Beyond." *Journal of American History* 92, no. 4 (2006): 1292–99.

———. "The Protean Character of American Liberalism." *American Historical Review* 99, no. 4 (1994): 1043–73.

Giddings, Paula. *When and Where I Enter: The Impact of Black Women on Sex and Race in America.* New York: William Morrow, 1984.

Gill, Tiffany. *Beauty Shop Politics: African American Women's Activism in the Beauty Industry.* Chicago: University of Illinois Press, 2010.

Gilmore, Glenda Elizabeth. *Defying Dixie: The Radical Roots of Civil Rights, 1919–1950.* New York: W. W. Norton, 2008.

———. *Gender and Jim Crow: Women and the Politics of White Supremacy in North Carolina, 1896–1920.* Chapel Hill: University of North Carolina Press, 1996.

Gilpin, Patrick J. *Charles S. Johnson: Leadership beyond the Veil in the Age of Jim Crow.* Albany: State University of New York Press, 2003.

Goesser, Caroline. "Transcultural Modernism: Winold Reiss and American Print Culture." Winold Reiss Symposium, December 2011. John F. Kennedy Institute for North American Studies, Berlin.

Gordon, Linda. *Woman's Body, Woman's Right: Birth Control in America.* New York: Penguin, 1977.

Green, Rayna. "The Pocahontas Perplex: The Image of Indian Women in American Culture." *Massachusetts Review* 16, no. 4 (1975): 698–714.

Greenberg, Cheryl Lynn. *"Or Does It Explode?": Black Harlem in the Great Depression.* New York: Oxford University Press, 1991.

Gross, Ariela J. *What Blood Won't Tell: A History of Race on Trial in America.* Cambridge, MA: Harvard University Press, 2008.

Grossman, James R. *Land of Hope: Chicago, Black Southerners, and the Great Migration.* Chicago: University of Chicago Press, 1989.

Guthrie, Robert V. *Even the Rat Was White.* New York: Harper and Row, 1976.

Haidarali, Laila. "Polishing Brown Diamonds: African American Women, Popular Magazines and the Advent of Modelling in Early Postwar America." *Journal of Women's History* 17, no. 1 (Spring 2005): 10–37.

———. "The Vampingest Vamp Is a Brownskin: Sex, Color, Beauty and African American Womanhood, 1920–1954." Ph.D. diss., York University, Canada, 2007.

———. "'The Weird, Faded Glory of Black Girls': De-Constructing Black Female Sexuality in the Harlem Renaissance, 1920–1930." Master's thesis, University of Windsor, Canada, 1997.

Hall, Jacquelyn Dowd. "The Long Civil Rights Movement and the Political Uses of the Past." *Journal of American History* 91, no. 4 (March 2005): 1233–63.

———. "'The Mind That Burns in Each Body': Women, Rape and Racial Violence." In *Powers of Desire: The Politics of Sexuality,* ed. Ann Snitow, Christine Stansell, and Sharon Thompson, 329–49. New York: Monthly Review Press, 1983.

———. *Revolt against Chivalry: Jessie Daniel Ames and the Women's Campaign against Lynching.* New York: Columbia University Press, 1979.

Haney-Lopez, Ian. *White by Law: The Legal Construction of Race.* New York: New York University Press, 1997.

Hanson, Joyce Ann. *Mary McLeod Bethune and Black Women's Political Activism.* Columbia: University of Missouri Press, 2003.

Hart, Jamie. "Who Should Have Children? Discussions of Birth Control among African-American Intellectuals." *Journal of Negro History* 79, no. 1 (Winter 1994): 71–84.

Hawkins, Michael Gray. *Co-producing the Postcolonial: U.S.-Philippines Cinematic Relations, 1946–1986.* Los Angeles: University of California, ProQuest Dissertations Publishing, 2008.

Heap, Chad. *Slumming: Sexual and Racial Encounters in American Nightlife, 1885–1940.* Chicago: University of Chicago Press, 2008.

Helbling, Mark. *The Harlem Renaissance: The One and Many.* Westport, CT: Greenwood, 1999.

Hemenway, Robert E. *Zora Neale Hurston: A Literary Biography.* Urbana: University of Illinois Press, 1977.

Higginbotham, Evelyn Brooks. "African-American Women's History and the Metalanguage of Race." *Signs* 17, no. 2 (1992): 251–74.

———. *Righteous Discontent: The Women's Movement in the Black Baptist Church, 1880–1920.* Cambridge, MA: Harvard University Press, 1993.

Higgins, Chester, Sr. "Is the Black Press Dying?" *Crisis* (August–September 1980): 240–41. www.blackpressresearchcollective.org.

Hine, Darlene Clark. "Black Migration to the Urban Midwest: The Gender Dimension, 1915–1945." In *The Great Migration in Historical Perspective,* ed. Joe William Trotter Jr. Bloomington: Indiana University Press, 1991.

———. "Rape and the Inner Lives of Black Women in the Middle West: Preliminary Thoughts on the Culture of Dissemblance." *Signs* 14 (Summer 1989): 912–20.

Hing, Bill Ong. *Making and Remaking Asian America through Immigration Policy, 1850–1990.* Stanford, CA: Stanford University Press, 1993.

Hodes, Martha. "Fractions and Fictions in the United States Census of 1890." In *Haunted by Empire: Geographies of Intimacy in North American History,* ed. Ann Laura Stoler Durham, NC: Duke University Press, 2006.

Holloway, Jonathan Scott. *Confronting the Veil: Abram, Harris Jr., E. Franklin Frazier and Ralph Bunche, 1919–1941.* Chapel Hill: University of North Carolina Press, 2002.

Honey, Maureen, ed. *Shadowed Dreams: Women's Poetry of the Harlem Renaissance.* 2nd ed. New Brunswick, NJ: Rutgers University Press, 2006.

hooks, bell. "In Our Glory: Photography and Black Life." In *Picturing Us: African American Identity in Photography,* ed. Deborah Willis. New York: W. W. Norton, 1994.

Horne, Gerald. *The End of Empires: African Americans in India.* Philadelphia: Temple University Press, 2008.

Huggins, Nathan, ed. *Voices from the Harlem Renaissance.* New York: Oxford University Press, 1995.

Hull, Gloria T. *Color, Sex, and Poetry: Three Women Writers of the Harlem Renaissance.* Bloomington: Indiana University Press, 1987.

Hunter, Tera. *To 'Joy My Freedom: Southern Black Women's Lives and Labors after the Civil War.* Cambridge, MA: Harvard University Press, 1997.

Hutchinson, George. *The Harlem Renaissance in Black and White.* Cambridge, MA: Harvard University Press, 1995.

Hutchinson, George, ed. *The Cambridge Companion to the Harlem Renaissance.* New York: Cambridge University Press, 2007.

Ingham, John N., and Lynne B. Feldman. *African American Business Leaders: A Biographical Dictionary.* Westport, CT: Greenwood, 1994.

Jackson, John P. *Social Scientists for Social Justice: Making the Case against Segregation.* New York: New York University Press, 2001.

James, Winston. Columbia University, "The History of Afro-Caribbean Migration to the United States." www.inmotionaame.org.

Johnson, Abby Arthur. "Literary Midwife: Jessie Redmon Fauset and the Harlem Renaissance." *Phylon* 39 (1978): 149–53.

———. *Propaganda and Aesthetics: The Literary Politics of African-American Magazines of the Twentieth Century.* Amherst: University of Massachusetts Press, 1979.

Johnson, Lauri. "A Generation of Women Activists: African American Female Educators in Harlem, 1930–1950." *Journal of African American History* 89, no. 3 (2004): 223–40.

Jones, Gayl. *Corregidora.* Boston: Beacon Press, 1975.

Jones, Jacqueline. *Labor of Love, Labor of Sorrow: Black Women, Work, and the Family from Slavery to the Present.* New York: Vintage Books, 1985.

———. "'So the Girl Marries': Class, the Black Press, and the DuBois-Cullen Wedding of 1928." In *The Harlem Renaissance Revisited: Politics, Arts, and Letters,* ed. Jeffrey O. G. Ogbar. Baltimore, MD: Johns Hopkins University Press, 2010.

Joseph, Peniel. "Waiting till the Midnight Hour." *SOULS* (Spring 2000): 6–17.
Kasinitz, Philip. *Caribbean New York: Black Immigrants and the Politics of Race.* Ithaca, NY: Cornell University Press, 1992.
Kelley, Robin D. G. *Race Rebels: Culture, Politics, and the Black Working Class.* New York: Free Press, 1996.
Kellner, Bruce. "Refined Racism: White Patronage in the Harlem Renaissance." In *The Harlem Renaissance Re-examined: A Revised and Expanded Edition,* ed. Victor A. Kramer and Robert A. Rose, 121–32. Troy, NY: Whitson, 1997.
Kellner, Bruce, ed. *The Harlem Renaissance: A Historical Dictionary for the Era.* Westport, CT: Greenwood Press, 1984.
Kellogg, Peter J. "Civil Rights Consciousness in the 1940s." *Historian* 42, no. 1 (November 1979).
Kennedy, David M. *Over Here: The First World War and American Society.* New York: Oxford University Press, 2004.
Kennedy, Valerie. *Edward Said, a Critical Introduction.* Cambridge: Cambridge University Press, 2000.
Kerr, Audrey Elisa. *The Paper Bag Principle: Class, Colorism, and Rumor and the Case of Black Washington, D.C.* Knoxville: University of Tennessee Press, 2006.
Kirby, John B. *Black Americans in the Roosevelt Era: Liberalism and Race.* Knoxville: University of Tennessee Press, 1980.
Kirschke, Amy Helene. *Aaron Douglas: Art, Race, and the Harlem Renaissance.* Oxford: University of Mississippi Press, 1995.
———. *Art in Crisis: W. E. B. DuBois and the Struggle for African American Identity and Memory.* Bloomington: Indiana University Press, 2007.
Knupfer, Anne Meis. *Toward a Tendered Humanity and a Nobler Womanhood: African American Women's Clubs in Turn-of-the-Century Chicago.* New York: New York University Press, 1996.
Korsta, Robert, and Nelson Lichtenstein. "Opportunities Found and Lost: Labor, Radicals, and the Early Civil Rights Movement." *Journal of American History* 75, no. 3 (December 1988): 786–811.
Kuklick, Henrika. *The Savage Within: The Social History of British Anthropology, 1885–1945.* Cambridge: Cambridge University Press, 1991.
Kusmer, Kenneth. *A Ghetto Takes Shape: Black Cleveland, 1870–1930.* Urbana: University of Illinois Press, 1984.
Kwolek-Folland, Angel. *Engendering Business: Men and Women in the Corporate Office, 1870–1930.* Baltimore, MD: John Hopkins University Press, 1994.
Kyriakoudes, Louis M. *The Social Origins of the Urban South: Race, Gender, and Migration in Nashville and Middle Tennessee, 1890–1930.* Chapel Hill: University of North Carolina Press, 2003.
Landry, Bart. *The New Black Middle Class.* Berkley: University of California Press, 1987.
Lawler, Mary, and John Davenport. *Marcus Garvey: Black Nationalist Leader.* New York: Chelsea House, 2005.

Lemons, Gary L. "Womanism in the Name of 'Father': W. E. B. DuBois and the Problematics of Race, Patriarchy, and Art." *Phylon* 49, no. 3/4 (Autumn–Winter 2001): 185–202.
Leonard, Karen. *Making Ethnic Choices: California's Punjabi Mexican Americans*. Philadelphia: Temple University Press, 1992.
Lewis, David Levering. "A Small Nation of People: W. E. B. Du Bois and Black Americans at the Turn of the Twentieth Century." In *A Small Nation of People: W. E. B. Du Bois and African American Portraits of Progress*, The Library of Congress, with essays by David Levering Lewis and Deborah Willis. New York: Harper Collins, 2003.
———. *W. E. B. DuBois: The Fight for Equality and the American Century, 1919–1963*. New York: Henry Holt, 2000.
Lewis, Earl. *In Their Own Interests*. Berkeley: University of California Press, 1991.
Lewis, Reina. *Gendering Orientalism: Race, Femininity and Representation*. New York: Routledge, 1996.
Lindquist, Malinda Alaine. *Race, Social Science and the Crisis of Manhood, 1890–1970*. New York: Routledge, 2012.
Logan, Rayford. *The Negro in American Life and Thought: The Nadir, 1877–1901*. New York: Dial Press, 1954.
Long, Richard A. "The Genesis of Locke's *The New Negro*." *Black World* 25, no. 4 (February 1976): 14–20.
Lowe, Lisa. *Critical Terrains: French and British Orientalisms*. Ithaca, NY: Cornell University Press, 1991.
Lowe, Margaret A. *Looking Good*. Baltimore, MD: John Hopkins University Press, 2003.
Marable, Manning. *Malcolm X: A Life of Reinvention*. New York: Penguin, 2011.
Marks, Carole. *Farewell—We're Good and Gone: The Great Black Migration*. Bloomington: Indiana University Press, 1989.
Martin, Waldo E., Jr., and Patricia Sullivan, eds. "'Don't Buy Where You Can't Work' Campaigns." In *Civil Rights in the United States*. New York: Macmillan Reference USA, 2000.
Matterson, Lisa G. "African American Women's Global Journeys and the Construction of Cross-Racial Identity." *Women's Studies International Forum* 32 (2009): 35–42.
Matthews, Fred H. *Quest for American Sociology: Robert E. Park and the Chicago School*. Montreal: McGill-Queen's University Press, 1977.
McHenry, Elizabeth. *Forgotten Readers: Recovering the Lost History of Literary Societies*. Durham, NC: Duke University Press, 2002.
McLendon, Jacquelyn Y. *The Politics of Color in the Fiction of Jessie Fauset and Nella Larsen*. Charlottesville: University of Virginia Press, 1995.
Meier, August. "Negro Class Structure and Ideology in the Age of Booker T. Washington." *Phylon* 23 (Fall 1962): 258–66.
Meier, August, and Elliott Rudwick. "The Origins of Nonviolent Direct Action in Afro-American Protest: A Note on Historical Discontinuities." In *Along the Color Line: Explorations in the Black Experience*. Urbana: University of Illinois Press, 1976.

Miller, Monica L. "W. E. B. Du Bois and the Dandy as Diasporic Race Man." *Callaloo* 26, no. 3 (Summer 2003): 738–65.
Miller, Nina. *Making Love Modern: The Intimate Public Worlds of New York's Literary Women*. New York: Oxford University Press, 1999.
Mitchell, Michele. *Righteous Propagation: African Americans and the Politics of Racial Destiny after Reconstruction*. Chapel Hill: University of North Carolina Press, 2004.
Moore, Jacqueline M. *Leading the Race: The Transformation of the Black Elite in the Nation's Capital, 1880–1920*. Charlottesville: University of Virginia Press, 1999.
Morris, Vivian. "Harlem Beauty Shops." April 19, 1939. Works Progress Administration, *American Life Histories: Manuscripts from the Federal Writers' Project, 1936–1940*. Library of Congress, Manuscript Division, Washington, D.C.
Mullen, Bill V. *Afro-Orientalism*. Minneapolis: University of Minnesota Press, 2004.
———. "*Dark Princess*, and the Afro-Asian International." *positions* 11, no. 1 (2003): 217–39.
Mullen, Bill V., and Cathryn Watson, eds. *W. E. B. Du Bois on Asia: Crossing the World Color Line*. Jackson: University Press of Mississippi, 2005.
Mumford, Kevin. *Interzones: Black/White Sex Districts in Chicago and New York in the Early Twentieth Century*. New York: Columbia University Press, 1997.
Nash, Gary B. "The Hidden History of Mestizo America." *Journal of American History* 82, no. 3 (December 1995): 941–64.
Nuyda, Doris G. "30 Years of Manila Carnivals." *Mr. and Mrs.* (February 4, 1986): 21–22.
Ogbar, Jeffery O. G. *The Harlem Renaissance Revisited: Politics, Arts, and Letters*. Baltimore, MD: Johns Hopkins University Press, 2010.
Olson, Joel. "W. E. B. Du Bois and the Race Concept." In *Racially Writing the Republic: Racists, Race Rebels, and Transformations of American Identity*, ed. Bruce Baum, 214–30. Durham, NC: Duke University Press, 2009.
Osofsky, Gilbert. *Harlem: The Making of a Ghetto: Negro New York, 1890–1930*. New York: Harper and Row, 1966.
Painter, Nell Irvin. *Exodusters: Black Migration to Kansas after Reconstruction*. New York: Knopf, 1977.
Pascoe, Peggy. *What Comes Naturally: Miscegenation Law and the Making of Race in America*. New York: Oxford University Press, 2009.
Patterson, Gordon. "Color Matters: The Creation of the Sara Lee Doll." *Florida Historical Quarterly* 73, no. 2 (1994): 147–65.
Patton, Venetria K., and Maureen Honey, eds. *Double-Take: A Revisionist Harlem Renaissance Anthology*. New Brunswick, NJ: Rutgers University Press, 2010.
Peiss, Kathy. *Hope in a Jar: The Making of America's Beauty Culture*. New York: Henry Holt, 1999.
Pencak, William. "*Crisis, The: A Record of the Darker Races*." In *Encyclopaedia of African American History*. New York: Oxford University Press, 2009.
Prashad, Vijay. *The Karma of Brown Folk*. Minneapolis: University of Minnesota Press, 2000.
Pride, Armistead S., and Clint C. Wilson II. *A History of the Black Press*. Washington, D.C.: Moorland-Spingarn Press, 1997.

Raimon, Eva Allegra. *The Tragic Mulatta Revisited: Race and Nationalism in Nineteenth-Century Antislavery Fiction*. New Brunswick, NJ: Rutgers University Press, 2004.

Rampersad, Arnold. *The Art and Imagination of W. E. B. Du Bois*. Cambridge, MA: Harvard University Press, 1976.

Rasmussen, R. Kent, and Robert A. Hill. "Afterword." In George S. Schuyler, *Black Empire*. Reprint, Berkeley: University of California Press, 1993.

Richards, Graham. "Race." In *Race, Racism and Psychology: Towards a Reflexive History*, 65–159. London: Routledge, 1997.

Rief, Michelle M. "Banded Close Together: An Afrocentric Study of African American Women's International Activism, 1850–1940, and the International Council of Women of the Darker Races." Ph.D. diss., Temple University, Philadelphia, 2003.

Riis, Jacob. *How the Other Half Lives: Studies among the Tenements of New York*. New York: Charles Scribner's Sons, 1890.

Roberts, Blain. *Pageants, Parlors, and Pretty Women: Race and Beauty in the Twentieth Century South*. Durham: University of North Carolina Press, 2015.

Roberts, Dorothy. *Killing the Black Body: Race, Reproduction, and the Meaning of Liberty*. New York: Pantheon, 1997.

Roces, Mina. "Gender, Nation and the Politics of Dress in Twentieth Century Philippines." *Gender and History* 17, no. 2 (August 2005): 354–77.

———. "Women, Citizenship and the Politics of Dress." In *Gender, Politics in Asia: Women Manoeuvring within the Dominant Gender Orders*, ed. Wil Burghoorn, Kazuki Iwanga, Cecilia Milwertz, and Qi Wan. Copenhagen: NIAS Press, 2003.

Rodrique, Jessie M. "The Black Community and the Birth Control Movement." In *Passion and Power: Sexuality in History*, ed. Kathy Peiss and Christina Simmons. Philadelphia: Temple University Press, 1989.

Roebuck, Julian B., and Murty S. Komanduri. *Historically Black Colleges and Universities: Their Place in American Higher Education*. Westport, CT: Praeger, 1993.

Rollins, Leslie. "Ethiopia, African Americans, and African-Consciousness: The Effect of Ethiopia and African-Consciousness in Twentieth-Century America." *Journal of Religious Thought* 54–55 (Spring–Fall 1998): 1–25.

Rooks, Noliwe M. *Ladies' Pages: African American Women's Magazines and the Culture that Made Them*. New Brunswick, NJ: Rutgers University Press, 2004.

Roses, Lorraine Elena, and Ruth Elizabeth Randolph, eds. *Harlem Renaissance and Beyond: Literary Biographies of 100 Black Women Writers, 1900–1945*. Boston: G. K. Hall, 1990.

Rousemaniere, Kate. *The Principal's Office: A Social History of the American School Principal*. New York: SUNY Press, 2013.

Ruggles, Anne Gere, and Sarah R. Robbins. "Gendered Literacy in Black and White: Turn-of-the-Century African-American and European-American Club Women's Printed Texts." *Signs* 21, no. 3 (1996): 643–78.

Russell-Cole, Kathy, Midge Wilson, and Ronald E. Hall. *The Color Complex: The Politics of Color in a New Millennium*. 1992. Reprint, New York: Anchor Books, 2013.

Said, Edward. *Orientalism*. 1978. Reprint, Harmondsworth: Penguin, 1995.
Sanchez-Eppler, Karen. *Touching Liberty: Abolition, Feminism, and the Politics of the Body*. Berkeley: University of California Press, 1993.
Schapp, Jeremy. *Triumph: The Untold Story of Jesse Owens and Hitler's Olympics*. New York: Houghton Mifflin, 2007.
Scott, Daryl Michael. *Contempt and Pity: Social Policy and the Image of the Damaged Black Psyche, 1880–1996*. Chapel Hill: University of North Carolina Press, 1997.
Self, Robert. *American Babylon: Race and the Struggle for Postwar Oakland*. Princeton, NJ: Princeton University Press, 2003.
Shaw, Stephanie J. "Black Club Women and the Creation of the National Association of Colored Women." *Journal of Women's History* 3, no. 2 (Fall 1991): 11–25.
———. *What a Woman Ought to Be and Do: Black Professional Women Workers during the Jim Crow Era*. Chicago: University of Chicago Press, 1996.
Sherrard-Johnson, Cherene. *Portraits of the New Negro Woman: Visual and Literary Culture in the Harlem Renaissance*. New Brunswick, NJ: Rutgers University Press, 2007.
Shore, Marlene. *The Science of Social Redemption: McGill, the Chicago School, and the Origins of Social Research in Canada*. Toronto: University of Toronto Press, 1987.
Silverberg, Helene. *Gender and American Social Science: The Formative Years*. Princeton, NJ: Princeton University Press, 1998.
Simmons, Christina. *Making Marriage Modern: Women's Sexuality from the Progressive Era to World War I*. New York: Oxford University Press, 2009.
———. "Modern Sexuality and the Myth of Victorian Repression." In *Passion and Power: Sexuality in History*, ed. Kathy Peiss and Christina Simmons. Philadelphia: Temple University Press, 1989.
Singh, Amritjit. *Novels of the Harlem Renaissance: Twelve Black Writers, 1923–1933*. University Park: Pennsylvania State University Press, 1976.
Sinha, Mrinalini. Introduction to *Mother India: Selections from the Controversial 1927 Text*. Ann Arbor: University of Michigan Press, 2000.
Sitkoff, Harvard. *A New Deal for Blacks: The Emergence of Civil Rights as a National Issue: The Depression Decade*. New York: Oxford University Press, 1978.
———. *The Struggle for Black Equality, 1954–1981*. New York: Hill and Wang, 1981.
Slate, Nico. *Colored Cosmopolitanism: The Shared Struggle for Freedom in the United States and India*. Cambridge, MA: Harvard University Press, 2012.
Smith, Jessie Carney, ed. *Encyclopaedia of African American Business*. Vol. 1. Westport, CT: Greenwood, 2006.
———. *Notable Black American Men*. Detroit, MI: Gale, 1999.
———. *Notable Black American Men*. Book 2. Detroit, MI: Thomson Gale, 2007.
———. *Notable Black American Women*. Vols. 1 and 2. New York: Gale Research, 1992, 1996.
Smith, Shawn Michelle. *American Archives: Gender, Race, and Class in Visual Culture*. Princeton, NJ: Princeton University Press, 1999.
———. *Photography on the Color Line: W. E. B. Du Bois, Race, and Visual Culture*. Durham, NC: Duke University Press, 2004.

———. *Word, Image, and the New Negro: Representation and Identity in the Harlem Renaissance*. Bloomington: Indiana University Press, 2005.

Sollors, Werner. *Neither Black nor White Yet Both: Thematic Exploration of Interracial Literature*. New York: Oxford University Press, 1997.

Spivak, Gayarti Chakravorty. "Can the Subaltern Speak?" In *Colonial Discourse and Postcolonial Theory: A Reader*, ed. Patrick Williams and Laura Chisman. New York: Columbia University Press, 1994.

Stavney, Barbara Anne. "Mothers of Tomorrow: The New Negro Renaissance and the Politics of Maternal Representation." *African American Review* 32, no. 4 (Winter 1998): 533–61.

Stewart, Jeffrey C. "Looking Backward to Look Forward: Winold Reiss in Context." Keynote address, Winold Reiss Symposium. December 2011. John F. Kennedy Institute for North American Studies, Berlin, Germany.

———. *To Color America: Portraits by Winold Reiss*. Washington, D.C.: Smithsonian Institution Press, 1989.

———. "Winold Reiss as a Portraitist." In *Cincinnati Union Terminal and the Artistry of Winold Reiss*, ed. Dottie L. Lewis. Cincinnati, OH: Cincinnati Historical Society, 1993.

Stocking, George W., Jr., ed. *A Franz Boas Reader: The Shaping of American Anthropology, 1883–1911*. Chicago: University of Chicago Press, 1974.

Stuckey, Sterling. *Slave Culture: Nationalist Theory and the Foundations of Black America*. New York: Oxford University Press, 1987.

Suggs, Henry Lewis. *The Black Press in the Middle West*. Westport, CT: Greenwood, 1996.

Sugrue, Thomas. *Sweet Land of Liberty: The Forgotten Struggle for Civil Rights in the North*. New York: Random House, 2008.

Takaki, Ronald. *Strangers from a Different Shore: A History of Asian Americans*. Boston: Little, Brown, 1989.

Tate, Claudia. *Psychoanalysis and Black Novels: Desire and the Protocols of Race*. New York: Oxford University Press, 1998.

———. "Race and Desire: *Dark Princess: A Romance*." In *Next to the Color Line: Gender, Sexuality, and W. E. B. Du Bois*, ed. Susan Gilman and Alys Eve Weinbaum. Minneapolis: University of Minnesota Press, 2007.

Taylor, Ula Yvette. *The Veiled Garvey: The Life and Times of Amy Jacques Garvey*. Chapel Hill: University of North Carolina Press, 2003.

Terborg-Penn, Rosalyn. "Survival Strategies among African-American Workers." In *Women, Work and Protest: A Century of U.S. Women's Labor History*, ed. Ruth Milkman. Boston: Routledge and Kegan Paul, 1985.

Theoharis, Jeanne F., and Komozi Woodward, eds. *Freedom North: Black Freedom Struggles Outside the South, 1940–1980*. New York: Palgrave Macmillan, 2003.

Trotter, Joe William, Jr., ed. *The Great Migration in Historical Perspective*. Bloomington: Indiana University Press, 1991.

Turner, Joyce Moore, and W. Burghardt Turner. *Caribbean Crusaders and the Harlem Renaissance*. Champaign: University of Illinois Press, 2005.

Tuttle, William J., Jr. *Race Riot: Chicago in the Red Summer of 1919*. New York: Atheneum, 1970.

Viola, Michael Joseph. "W. E. B. DuBois and Filipino/a American Exposure Programs to the Philippines: Race Class Analysis in an Epoch of 'Global Apartheid.'" *Race Ethnicity and* Education. Taylor and Francis Online, May 23, 2014. https://doi.org/10.1080/13613324.2014.911165.

Vogel, Shane. *The Scene of the Harlem Cabaret: Race, Sexuality, Performance*. Chicago: University of Chicago Press, 2009.

Walker, Juliet K. *Encyclopaedia of Black Business*. Westport, CT: Greenwood, 1999.

Walker, Susannah. *Style and Status: Selling Beauty of African American Women, 1920–1975*. Lexington: University Press of Kentucky, 2007.

Wall, Cheryl A. *Women of the Harlem Renaissance*. Bloomington: Indiana University Press, 1995.

Wallace, Michelle. "Black Women in Popular Culture: From Stereotype to Heroine." In *Black Popular Culture*, ed. Gina Dent, 270–71. Seattle: Bay Press, 1992.

Wallace-Saunders, Kimberly. *Mammy: A Century of Race, Gender and Southern Memory*. Ann Arbor: University of Michigan Press, 2008.

Washburn, Patrick S. *The African American Newspaper: Voice of Freedom*. Evanston, IL: Northwestern University Press, 2006.

———. "The *Pittsburgh Courier*'s Double V Campaign in 1942." *American Journalism* 3, no. 2 (1986): 73–86.

———. *A Question of Sedition: The Federal Government Investigation of the Black Press during World War II*. New York: Oxford University Press, 1986.

Washington, Mary Helen. Introduction to *I Love Myself When I Am Laughing: A Zora Neale Hurston Reader*, ed. Alice Walker. New York: Feminist Press, 1979.

Watkins-Owens, Irma. *Blood Relations: Caribbean Immigrants and the Harlem Community, 1900–1930*. Bloomington: Indiana University Press, 1996.

Weems, Robert E., Jr. *Desegregating the Dollar: African American Consumerism in the Twentieth Century*. New York: New York University Press, 1998.

Welter, Barbara. "The Cult of True Womanhood, 1820–1860." *American Quarterly* 18 (Summer 1966): 151–74.

White, Deborah Gray. *Too Heavy a Load: Black Women in Defense of Themselves, 1894–1994*. New York: W. W. Norton, 1999.

White, Kevin. *Sexual Liberation or Sexual License? The American Revolt against Victorianism*. Chicago: Ivan R. Dee, 2000.

White, Shane, and Graham White. *Stylin: African American Expressive Culture, from Its Beginnings to the Zoot Suit*. Ithaca, NY: Cornell University Press, 1998.

Whitmire, Ethelene. *Regina Anderson Andrews, Harlem Renaissance Librarian*. Champaign: University of Illinois Press, 2014.

Wilkins, Roy, and Tom Mathews. *Standing Fast: The Autobiography of Roy Wilkins*. New York: Viking Press, 1982.

Wilkinson, Doris. "The Doll Exhibit: A Psycho-Cultural Analysis of Black Female Stereotypes." *Journal of Popular Culture* 21, no. 2 (1987): 19–29.

Williams, Chad. *Torchbearers of Democracy: African American Soldiers in the World War I Era*. Chapel Hill: University of North Carolina Press, 2010.

Williams, Megan E. "The *Crisis* Cover Girl: Lena Horne, the NAACP, and Representations of African American Femininity, 1941–1945." *American Periodicals* 16, no. 2 (2006): 203–4.

Williams, Rhonda Y. *Concrete Demands: The Search for Black Power in the 20th Century*. New York: Routledge, 2015.

Williamson, Joel. *New People: Miscegenation and Mulattoes in the United States*. Baton Rouge: Louisiana State University Press, 1980.

Willis, Deborah. "The Sociologist's Eye: W. E. B. Du Bois and the Paris Exposition." In *A Small Nation of People: W. E. B. Du Bois and African American Portraits of Progress*, with essays by David Levering Lewis and Deborah Willis. New York: Harper Collins, 2003.

Wilson, Francille Rusan. *The Segregated Scholars: Black Social Scientists and the Creation of Black Labour Studies, 1890–1950*. Charlottesville: University of Virginia Press, 2007.

Wolcott, Victoria. *Remaking Respectability: African American Women in Interwar Detroit*. Chapel Hill: University of North Carolina Press, 2001.

Wolseley, Roland E. *The Black Press, U.S.A.* 2nd ed. Ames: Iowa State University Press, 1990.

Wolters, Raymond. *The New Negro on Campus*. Princeton: Princeton University Press, 1976.

Yellin, Eric Steven. *Racism in the Nation's Service: Government Workers and the Color Line in Woodrow Wilson's America*. Chapel Hill: University of North Carolina Press, 2013.

Young, Alford A., Jr., and Donald R. Deskins Jr. "Early Traditions of African-American Sociological Thought." *Annual Review of Sociology* 27 (2001): 445–77.

Zackodnik, Teresa C. *The Mulatta and the Politics of Race*. Jackson: University of Mississippi Press, 2004.

INDEX

Note: Photo plate images are indicated by their plate numbers in italic.

ACE. *See* American Council on Education
activism: civil rights activism, 19–20, 234; consumer, 20; against lynching by African American women, 116, 279n41
advertising: in African American newspapers, 65–68, 83, 87, 88, 96, 105, 278n5; in African American press, 65–68; in African American print culture, 62–68, 63; African American women and, 30, 62–64; for beauty culture training, 100–101, 278n151; beauty products, 82–83, 87, 89, 91–92, 93, 94–97, 98, 99, 100, 276n76; brown beauty and, 61, 62, 63, 64–68, 85; brown-skin beauty and, 61, 62, 63, 64–68, 79, 97, 102, 103; of brown-skin dolls, 78, 79–80, 81; for clerical work training, 99, 101–2; color, women's beauty and, 95–96; cosmetics, 82–83, 85, 87–90, 92, 95–97, 98, 100; in *Crisis*, 62, 63, 63, 64, 67–68, 79, 80, 82, 83, 91–92, 93, 97, 99, 100, 101, 102, 114; Kashmir Chemical Company and, 95–97, 98; in magazines, 65–68, 83, 88, 91–92, 93; marketing language for Negro dolls, 73, 75, 77–80; middle class and, 64; of Negro dolls, 62, 63, 64, 75, 77–80; Negro girls and, 30, 62, 63, 64, 77, 78, 79; Negro women's beauty promoted by, 96; New Negro womanhood and, 64; New Negro women and, 61–64, 80, 82; by Walker Manufacturing Company, 82; white skin beauty and, 88; women of color and, 97

"Advice" (Bennett), 170
Africa: black Africans, 77; Ethiopia, 55; pan-Africanism, 11, 55, 210, 215, 288n10
African American culture, 238–39, 291n56. *See also* African American print culture; *specific topics*
African American men: Asian Indian princess and, 193–96, 199–200, 202, 205, 209–10, 215–22; black and, 179; brown and, 177–78, 179, 287n71; poetry of, 156–60; race suicide and, 112; sports and, 243; women's poetry and, 177–80; writers and Harlem Renaissance literary print culture, 156–57, 158, 159–60. *See also* New Negro men
African American newspapers, 228–30; advertising in, 65–68, 83, 87, 88, 96, 105, 278n5; "Illustrated Feature Section" magazine insert in, 105, 278n5. *See also* African American print culture
African American print culture: advertising in, 62–68, 63; brown beauty advertising in, 63, 64–68; photography in, 21; racial discourse on brown beauty in, 21. *See also* black press; Harlem Renaissance literary print culture; New Negro print culture
African Americans: black identifier usage by, 21; urbanization and, 9, 10; U.S. Census and categories of, 206. *See also* Negro; *specific topics*

317

African American womanhood, 29; shifting gendered ideal of, 30. *See also* brown-skin womanhood; New Negro womanhood

African American women: activism against lynching by, 116, 279n41; advertising and, 30, 62–64; in beauty industry, 82, 84–85, 89–92, 93; education and, 12, 41; Great Migration and, 8; Harlem and, 31–32; racist views of, 32–34, 35; sexual violence and, 217; social work and, 47; urban landscape and, 13; white skin beauty and, 87–88, 90. *See also* Negro women; *specific topics*

African American women, in interwar years, 12; brownness in representation of, 2, 18, 29, 30, 61. *See also specific topics*

African American women's public image, 32–34; gender conservatism and mass media imaging, 233; women's labor and, 35

African American women writers: Harlem Renaissance literary print culture and, 159–60; on motherhood, 115–16; mulatta representations and, 120–23; on womanhood, 116. *See also* women's poetry; *specific topics*

African American writers: brown-skin types and, 108; Harlem Renaissance magazines and, 107, 108; Harlem Renaissance publishers and, 105–6; "Instructions for Contributors" and, 104–6, 152; mulatta representations and, 120–23; white publishers and, 105–6; white readers and, 106. *See also* African American women writers; *specific topics*

African American youth, 30; brown-skin ideal and, 224, 225, 226, 257–58

African American youth, research on, 234; "Color Names and Color Notions," 226–27, 252–58; *Growing Up in the Black Belt*, 226, 227, 244–52; *Negro Youth at the Crossways*, 225, 226, 227, 238–44, 253, 291n60; overview, 30, 226, 258; "Studies of Negro Youth," 236–38

Afro-Asia: Afro-Asian connections, 212–16; Du Bois, W. E. B., and, 212–16

Afro-Caribbeans, 10, 267n21

Afro-Orientalism, 200

age: beauty and, 185–86; women's poetry and, 155, 184–86; women writers and, 184–86, 285n96

American Council on Education (ACE), 236, 238, 244, 245

The American Dilemma: The Negro Problem and Modern Democracy (Myrdal), 19

American imperialism, and colonization, 140, 142, 144

Anderson, Regina, 126

artists: brown-skin types and, 108; *Crisis* cover art and, 128–29, 281n84; Harlem Renaissance magazines and, 107, 108

Asian Indian princess, of *Dark Princess*, 289n123; African American men and, 193–96, 199–200, 202, 205, 209–10, 215–22; brownness and browning of, 192–96, 202–3, 209, 216–18, 221–23; brown-skin beauty of, 192–93; femininity of, 219–20; overview, 192–96; as romantic, ancient and bejeweled, 218–19. *See also Dark Princess: A Romance*

Asian Indians, 206–7

Asian Indian women: *Dark Princess* and, 194, 201, 220; representations of, 200–201. *See also* Asian Indian princess, of *Dark Princess*

Asians: as characters in Harlem Renaissance literary print culture, 198–99; Du Bois, W. E. B., and Afro-Asia, 212–16. *See also* Orientalism

"At April" (Grimké), 175, 176

Ayer, Vernon A., 36, 43

Baird, Dan W., 73–74
Baker, Josephine, 75, 76, 92, 94; doll, 75, 76;
"The Ballad of a Brown Girl" (Cullen), 155
Barnett, Claude, 95–96
beauty: age and, 185–86; black as beautiful, 183; consumerism and, 186–87, 188–90; love and, 181–82; as racial type, 84; sex, love and, 174–75, 181; women's poetry and, 174, 175, 181–90; youth and, 92, 187. *See also specific topics*
beauty contests: brown baby contests of NAACP, 132–33; Negro women's beauty and, 84–85; white womanhood and, 85
beauty culture: advertising for training in, 100–101, 278n151; African American beauty culturists, 82, 84–85, 90–92, 93; of Harlem, 90–91
beauty industry: African American women working in, 82, 84–85, 89–92, 93; black-owned businesses, 88–92, 93, 95; Harlem beauty shops, 90–91; modeling and, 261–62; white-owned businesses, 88–89, 95; youthful standards and, 92
beauty products: advertising, 82–83, 87, 89, 91–92, 93, 94–97, 98, 99, 100, 276n76; language of brown and, 95; New Negro and, 95. *See also* cosmetics
Bennett, Gwendolyn, 153–54, 163, 166, 170, 176
Berry, Victoria, 79
Berry and Ross Doll Manufacturing, 73, 78–79
Bethel Manufacturing Company, 80, *81*
Bethune, Mary McLeod, 33, 50, 53
birth: birth control, 111–15, 279n32; birth rates, 111–13; childbirth, 218
Birth Control Review, 108, 114–15, 279n32
black: African American men and, 179; African Americans identifying as, 21; as beautiful, 183; black Africans, 77; blackness in women's poetry, 118–19,
169, 170, 178, 179, 183; brown and, 6, 21; Negro as, 77
"Black Baby" (Coleman), 118–19
The Blacker the Berry (Thurman), 123–25
"Black Faces" (Coleman), 183
"Black Man o' Mine" (Spencer), 179
Black No More (Schuyler), 152
black-owned businesses, 65, 66; in beauty industry, 88–92, 93, 95
black press, 229; advertising brown beauty in, 65–68, 85; Negro women's beauty and, 83–84, 85; white-owned businesses and, 105. *See also* African American newspapers; African American print culture; magazines
blues women, 116
Boas, Franz, 27, 58
Bonner, Marita O., 199
Bontemps, Arna, 126, 156
Boyd, Richard Henry, 66–67, 68, 70, 73, 74
Brandford Models, 261
"Brass Ankles Speaks" (Dunbar-Nelson), 161–62
bronze, 117–18
"The Bronze Legacy" (Newsome), 117–18
brown: African American men and, 177–78, 179, 287n71; beauty products and language of, 95; black and, 6, 21; bronze and, 117–18; brown baby contests of NAACP, 132–33; as color of New Negro, 110; *Dark Princess: A Romance* and, 191–96, 202–3, 207, 209–10, 216–18, 221–23; Du Bois, W.E. B., usage of, 23–24, 191–96, 202–3, 207, 209–10, 216–18, 221–23; exclusionary parameters of brown as racial descriptor, 6; Harlem Renaissance poetry and, 153–55; Hurston on, 1–5; poetry and, 117–19, 153–55; as race descriptor, 24; as race signifier, 154; women's poetry and, 117–19, 153–56, 160, 161, 168, 170, 174–78, 179, 190, 191. *See also specific topics*

brown beauty, 243; advertising and, 61, 62, 63, 64–68, 85; African American print culture and racial discourse on, 21; civil rights activism and, 19; class and, 15; as cultural product, 2; Harlem and, 10; Harlem Renaissance literary print culture and, 35, 103; in interwar years, 7, 15; middle-class women and, 28; modernization and, 6–7, 10, 15, 30; New Negro cultural production and, 18; New Negro women and, 61, 103; post–World War II years, 261–62; print culture and, 21, 61; racial discourse on, 7, 21, 24, 28, 259; racist views and, 35; as respectable beauty, 13, 15, 190; women's poetry and, 154, 175, 190, 191. *See also* brown-skin beauty

"Brown Boy to a Brown Girl" (Cullen), 156

brown complexions: class and, 226, 244; Harlem and, 10; in interwar years and Great Migration, 7; middle class and, 64, 225, 226; New Negro print culture and, 17; racial discourse on, 29. *See also* African American youth, research on; brown skin

"Brown Girl" (Grimké), 175–76

brown girl representation, 126, 127

"Brown Has Mighty Things to Do" (Newsome), 118

Brown Madonna, 107, 108, 110–19

Brown Madonna (portrait by Reiss), 59, 108, 110, 129, *pl.5*

brownness, 6; of Asian Indian princess, 192–96, 202–3, 209–10, 216–18, 221–23; cultural production and, 28; New Negro women and, 3, 28; in representation of African American women in interwar years, 2, 18, 29, 30, 61. *See also* brown

brown skin, 6; tanning and brown-skin fad, 92, 94–95. *See also* brown complexions

brown-skin beauty, 190; advertising and, 61, 62, 63, 64–68, 79, 97, 102, 103; Asian Indian princess as, 192–93; as ideal type, 84–85, 100, 103, 224; modeling and, 261–62; Negro dolls and, 62, 63, 64, 79, 102, 103; overview, 102–3

brown-skin dolls, 62, 63, 64, 77; advertising of, 78, 79–80, *81*. *See also* Negro dolls

brown-skin ideal: African American youth and, 224, 225, 226, 257–58; as ideal beauty type, 84–85, 100, 224; social science and, 235–36, 257–58

brown-skin mulatta, 107; McDougald, Gertrude, as, 119–20; overview, 119–27. *See also* mulatta representations

brown-skin types: African American writers and, 108; artists and, 108; *Crisis* and, 107; Harlem Renaissance literary print culture and, 104–7, 121, 152; Harlem Renaissance magazines and, 107; as ideal beauty type, 84–85, 100, 224; Negro heroes and, 106; New Negro heroines as, 104–5; New Negro womanhood and, 127; *Opportunity* magazine and, 107; overview, 107, 152; women's poetry and, 152. *See also* Brown Madonna; brown-skin mulatta; modern brown-skin womanhood

brown-skin womanhood, 6. *See also* modern brown-skin womanhood

Bush, Ermine Casey, 133, *134*

Caroling Dusk, 153, 155, 156, 170, 177

Chicago Appeal, 83–84

Chicago Defender, 52, 63, 83, 228

civil rights: activism, 19–20, 234; New Negro movement and, 11

Clark, Jessie, 47

class: brown beauty in interwar years and, 15; brown complexions and, 226, 244; color and, 162, 236, 237, 252, 253; culture, color and, 253; elite and

upper-class light-skinned women, 125; women's poetry and, 155, 161, 162–63. *See also* middle class
clerical work, 49–50, 99, 101–2
"The Closing Door" (Grimké), 115–16
clubwomen, 13; reform and, 14, 33, 47, 86, 158; women's poetry and, 158
Coleman, Anita Scott, 118–19, 164, 169–70, 183–84
color: advertising, women's beauty and, 95–96; class and, 162, 236, 237, 252, 253; culture, class and, 253; *Dark Princess* and, 208–10, 214–17; Du Bois, W. E. B., and, 208–10, 214–17; gendering of, 179, 251; Harlem Renaissance poetry and, 155; Hurston on, 1–5; in interwar years, 6; in mulatta representations, 120–23; race, women's poetry and, 154, 169–72, 174; race and, 24, 155, 205–10, 214–16; of race and ethnicity in white America, 205–7; racial identity and, 169, 171, 228; U.S. Census usage of, 206; women's poetry and, 153–56, 160–62, 168–72, 174, 176, 177, 179, 188, 191. *See also* black; brown; *specific topics*
Color (Cullen), 155
Color, Class and Personality (Sutherland), 236, 237
Color and Human Nature (Warner), 237–38
color discrimination: Harlem Renaissance literary print culture and, 123–25. *See also* African American youth, research on; race prejudice
colored: becoming, 1–2; how it feels to be, 2; whiteness and, 3
colored dolls. *See* Negro dolls
colorism: employment and, 94; New Negro era and intraracial, 4–5
"The Colorist" (Coleman), 169–70
"Color Names and Color Notions" (Parrish), 226–27, 252–58
"Color Struck" (Hurston), 4

Comedy: American Style (Fauset), 122–23
complexion: employment and, 20; in mulatta representations, 120–23; respectability, employment and, 51–52; women's labor, respectability and, 51–52; women's poetry and, 161–62. *See also* African American youth, research on; brown complexions
consumer activism, 20
consumer culture, New Negro identity and, 17
consumerism: beauty and, 186–87, 188–90; New Negro print culture and, 16–17; urban African Americans and, 19–20; women's poetry and, 186–87, 188–90
cosmetics: advertising, 82–83, 85, 87–90, 92, 95–97, 98, 100; African American–owned cosmetic companies, 88, 89; Negro women's beauty and, 87; New Negro women and, 82, 85, 86, 87; skin whitening, 95, 124–25; Walker Manufacturing Company and, 82; white-owned cosmetic companies, 88–89, 95; white skin beauty and, 87–88
Cowdrey, Mae V., 163, 166, 170–71, 176–77, 182–83
Crisis, 16, 55, 75, 199, 237, 290n30; advertising in, 62, 63, 63, 64, 67–68, 79, 80, 82, 83, 91–92, 93, 97, 99, 100, 101, 102, 114; American imperialism, colonization and, 140, 142, 144; brown-skin types and, 107; children's issue, 127, 131–32; "Child's Number" issue, 117–18; Du Bois, W. E. B., as editor of, 54, 67, 82, 114, 127, 128–29, 133, 142, 157, 231; education issue, 129, 144, 146, *147*, 150; Fauset and, 157, 159, 166; Harlem Renaissance poetry and, 157, 158; New Negroes and, 68; New Negro men in "Men of the Month" feature, 127; Reiss and, 128–29; women's poetry in, 117–18, 171, 179, 183
Crisis Advertiser, 62, 63, 63, 68, 99

Crisis cover art, of modern brown-skin womanhood, 233–34; "After a Photograph, posed by C. M. Battey" photograph, 129, 131; artists and, 128–29, 281n84; "A Bachelor of Music from Oberlin" photograph, 146, *149*; "Bachelor of Philosophy" photograph, 146, *148*; "A Colored Graduate of the Philippine Normal School" photograph, 142, 144, *145*; "Drawing from Life" illustration, 135, *139*, 140; of educated women, 144, 146, *147*, *148*, *149*, *150*, *151*; foreign women of color and, 140, *141*, 142, *143*, 144, *145*; illustrations, 128–29, 135, *139*, 140, 281n103; light-skinned women photographs, 135, *136*, *137*, 140, *141*; "A Master of Arts" photograph, 129, *130*; New Negro photographers and, 129; "A North African Cousin of Ours" photograph, 140, *141*; overview, 127–29, 131; "Photograph from Life" photograph, 135, *137*; "Photographic Study of the Head of a Negro Woman" photograph, 135, *138*; photographs, 128, 129, *130*, 131–32, 135, *136*, *137*, *138*, 140, *141*, 142, *143*, 144, *145*, 146, *147*, *148*, *149*, *150*, *151*; "Queen of Carnival" photograph, 142, *143*; "A Salutatorian" photograph, 146, *150*; Scott, Clarissa Mae, photograph as, 146, *147*; "Study of a Negro Girl" photograph, 135, *136*; "A Western School Teacher" photograph, 146, *151*. See also *Crisis* visuals, of New Negroes

Crisis visuals, of New Negroes: of Bush, 133, *134*; "I am Black, but comely, O Ye Daughters of Jerusalem" cover graphic, 140; illustrations of children, 135, *139*, 140, 281n103; of New Negro children, 127, 131–33, *134*, 135, *136*, *139*, 140, 142, 144, *145*, 281n103; New Negro photographers and, 129, 133; "Photograph of Misses Dents," 133; photographs of children, 131–33, *134*, 135, *136*, 142, 144, *145*; photographs of New Negro women, 135; solicitations and submissions, 128–29, 133; women's sensual beauty in, 135, *138*. See also *Crisis* cover art, of modern brown-skin womanhood

Cullen, Countee, 123, 154–55, 156, 204, 287n51

cultural production: brownness and, 28. See also New Negro cultural production

cultural relativism, 27, 58

culture: color, class and, 253; popular culture and middle-class New Negro, 18; urban culture and color-inflected language, 17–18. See also African American culture; beauty culture; *specific topics*

Dancy, John, 51

dark-complexion representations: darker-skinned female characters, 202; in Harlem Renaissance literary print culture, 123–25, 202

Dark Princess: A Romance (Du Bois), 213; Asian Indian womanhood and, 194, 220; Asian Indian women and, 201; assessments of, 196; brown and, 191–96, 202–3, 207, 209–10, 216–18, 221–23; color and, 208–10, 214–17; interracial romance and, 193–97, 199–200, 202, 205, 222; marriage and, 195, 203, 205, 222; miscegenation and, 196–97, 222; modern brown-skin womanhood and, 191, 223; New Negro womanhood and, 192, 203, 223; Orientalism and, 197, 199–200, 201; overview, 191–96, 223; race and, 191–96, 205, 207, 208, 214; race womanhood and, 194, 195, 202, 203, 220; sex in, 203, 220. See also Asian Indian princess, of *Dark Princess*

Detroit Urban League, 14, 51

Dickinson, Blanche Taylor, 188–90

discrimination: employment and, 50–51. See also color discrimination

dolls: doll test, 274n38; white, 69–70, 72, 74, 183–84. *See also* Negro dolls
"The Double Task: The Struggle of Negro Women for Sex and Race Emancipation" (McDougald, G.), 45, 48, 60
Double Victory campaign, 229–30
Douglas, Aaron, 281n84
Douglas Johnson, Georgia, 118, 121, 164–65, 166, 167, 172–73, 185–87, 205
Du Bois, Nina, 204
Du Bois, W. E. B., 165; adultery of, 204, 205; Afro-Asia and, 212–16; on birth control, 114, 279n32; color and, 208–10, 214–17; as editor of *Crisis*, 54, 67, 82, 114, 127, 128–29, 133, 142, 157, 231; Exhibit of American Negroes and, 22–23, 129, 269n77; feminism and, 204–5; marriage and, 204, 205, 287n51; *The Quest of the Silver Fleece*, 202; race and, 191–96, 205, 207–11, 214–16, 234; racial identity and, 202, 207, 209, 210, 214; "So the Girl Marries," 204; *Souls of Black Folk*, 205, 210; usage of brown by, 23–24, 191–96, 202–3, 207, 209–10, 216–18, 221–23. See also *Dark Princess: A Romance*
Du Bois, Yolande Nina, 204, 287n51
Dunbar-Nelson, Alice, 112, 113, 161–62, 163, 164, 166, 167, 176, 180, 185, 186–88, 285n966
Duncan's Business School, 99, 101–2
Dyer Anti-Lynching Bill, 116, 279n41

East India Hair Grower, 91–92, 93, 97, 99, 100
education: African American women and, 12, 41; American Council on Education, 236, 238, 244, 245; *Crisis* annual issue on, 129, 144, 146, *147*, *150*; *Crisis* cover photographs of educated women, 144, 146, *147*, *148*, *149*, *150*, *151*; in Harlem, 42–43; McDougald, Gertrude, and, 39–45, 48; women in interwar years and, 12, 41. See also *Journal of Negro Education*
"Education in Harlem" (McDougald, G.), 42–43
Edwards, Paul K., 65–66
Egypt, Ophelia Settle, 227
employment: colorism and, 94; complexion and, 20; discrimination and, 50–51; respectability, complexion and, 51–52. *See also* labor
Ethiopia, 55
ethnicity, white America and color of race and, 205–7
eugenics, 27, 112, 114
Exhibit of American Negroes, 22–23, 129, 269n77

Fauset, Jessie, 116, 121, 122–23, 157, 159, 166, 174, 185, 198, 205
feminism: black, 287n79; Du Bois, W. E. B., and, 204–5
Filipinos, 142, 144
Frazier, E. Franklin, 233, 235, 236, 291n56, 292n67, 292n69; *Negro Youth at the Crossways*, 225, 226, 227, 238–44, 253, 291n60
"Futility" (Johnson, H.), 180

Gandhi, Mahatma, 212–13
Garvey, Marcus, 11, 55, 213, 228
gender: gender conservatism, 233; gendering of color, 179, 251; shifting gendered ideal of African American womanhood, 30; social science and, 227. *See also* men; New Negro womanhood, gendered tropes of; women
George, Louis W., 87
Gordon, Linda, 111
Great Migration: African American women and, 8; brown complexions in interwar years and, 7; modernization and, 7; New York City and, 8, 9; overview, 7–8, 267n10

Grimké, Angelina Weld, 115–16, 175–76, 177
Growing Up in the Black Belt (Johnson, C.), 226, 227, 244–52

hair: hair styles of New Negroes, 55–56; of Negro dolls, 71, 79, 80
hair products, 89; East India Hair Grower, 91–92, 93, 97, 99, 100; hair-straightening products, 83; youthful standards and, 92
Half-Century magazine, 65, 66, 88–89
Haring, H. A., 90
Harlem: African American population of, 42; African American women and, 31–32; beauty culture of, 90–91; beauty shops, 90–91; brown beauty and, 10; brown complexions and, 10; education in, 42–43; migration and, 9–10, 267n21; New Negro movement and, 10, 11; white observers of, 90
"Harlem Girl 1" (portrait by Reiss), 55–56, 140, *pl.3*
"Harlem: Mecca of the New Negro" (*Survey Graphic* issue), 45–46, 48, 52–60
Harlem Renaissance: Hurston and, 5; McDougald, Gertrude, and, 36, 37, 45, 119; New Negro representations and, 156
Harlem Renaissance literary print culture, 30; African American men writers and, 156–57, 158, 159–60; African American women writers and, 159–60; brown beauty and, 35, 103; brown-skin types and, 104–7, 121, 152; color discrimination and, 123–25; dark-complexion representations in, 123–25, 202; darker-skinned female characters in, 202; Indian women and, 196; masculinity and, 157; men's poetry and, 159–60; miscegenation and, 196–97; modern brown-skin womanhood and, 131, 194; mulatta representations and, 120, 121, 123, 125; New Negroes and, 104–5, 196; New Negro heroine of, 104–5; New Negro womanhood and, 125; New Negro womanhood representations and, 127; New Negro women in, 125, 127, 159; Orientalism and, 198–200; publishers, 105–6; Schuyler's "Instructions for Contributors" and, 104–6, 127, 152; women's poetry and, 157–60, 168, 190–91. *See also* African American print culture
Harlem Renaissance magazines: African American commentators and, 107; African American writers and, 107, 108; artists and, 107, 108; brown-skin types and, 107; Harlem Renaissance poetry and, 157–58; modern brown-skin womanhood visual groupings in, 131; New Negro photographers and, 108, 129; New Negro women's photographs and, 125, 126; New Negro women's portraits and, 125, 126; women's poetry and, 157–60. *See also* magazines
Harlem Renaissance poetry: brown and, 153–55; color and, 155; *Crisis* and, 157, 158; Harlem Renaissance magazines and, 157–58; men's poetry, 156–60; *Opportunity* magazine and, 156, 157, 158, 174; overview, 160. *See also* women's poetry
Hightower, Mamie, 84–85
Houston, Virginia, 178
"How It Feels to Be Colored Me" (Hurston), 1–2, 5
Hunter, Addie W., 41
Hunton, Roberta, 59
Hurston, Zora Neale, 7, 45, 116, 159, 166, 185; on brown, 1–5; "Color Struck," 4; Harlem Renaissance and, 5; "How It Feels to Be Colored Me," 1–2, 5; life of, 3–4; *Miss Hurston* portrait by Reiss, *pl.1*; "Record of Freshman Interest," 3–4; *Their Eyes Were Watching God*, 122

"I Am Not Proud" (Johnson, H.), 169
ICWDR. *See* International Council of Women of the Darker Races
illustrations: *Crisis* and, 128–29, 135, *139*, 140, 281n103; "Illustrated Feature Section" magazine insert, 105, 278n5
"Impressions from a Family Album" (Coleman), 183–84
India, 200–201, 212, 215, 218–19, 286n37. *See also* Asian Indians
Indian women, 201. *See also* Asian Indian women
individuality, racialization and loss of, 1
"Insatiate" (Cowdrey), 176–77
"Instructions for Contributors" (Schuyler), 104–6, 127, 152
intellectualizing about race: race intellectuals, 22–23; shifts during interwar years, 24–27
International Council of Women of the Darker Races (ICWDR), 210–11
interracial marriage, 197
interracial romance: *Dark Princess* and, 193–97, 199–200, 202, 205, 222. *See also* miscegenation
interwar years: race and, 7, 18–19. *See also specific topics*
"I Sit and Sew" (Dunbar-Nelson), 180
"I Sit and Wait for Beauty" (Cowdrey), 182–83

Johns, Vere, 10
Johnson, Charles S., 9, 54–55, 235, 236; *Growing Up in the Black Belt*, 226, 227, 244–52; *Opportunity* and, 87, 126, 157, 175, 226, 245, 292n80
Johnson, Elizabeth, 38
Johnson, Emma M., *99*, 101
Johnson, Guy B., 83, 87
Johnson, Helene, 164, 165–66, 167–68, 169, 178, 180–82, 287n72
Johnson, James Weldon, 9, 156
Johnson, Mary Elizabeth, 38, 270n20

Johnson, Peter Augustus, 38
Journal of Negro Education, 226–27; "Color Names and Color Notions," 252–58

Kashmir Chemical Company, 95–97, *98*
Knoblauch, Mary, 114

labor, 234; organizing of McDougald, Gertrude, 35, 39, 48. *See also* women's labor
"Lamps" (Cowdrey), 170–71
language: language of brown and beauty products, 95; Negro dolls and marketing, 73, 75, 77–80; urban culture and color-inflected, 17–18
Larsen, Nella, 116, 121, 159, 185
law: miscegenation laws, 25, 207; race and, 24–25; race descriptors and, 26
"Letter to My Sister" (Spencer), 188
Lewis, Demond, 84
liberalism: New Deal, 18–19, 231–32, 235; racial, 19, 231–33, 258
The Librarian, 60
light-skinned representations: light-brown-skinned representations, 122, 135, *136*, *137*, 140, *141*; mulatta representations, 123, 127
light-skinned women: *Crisis* cover photographs of, 135, *136*, *137*, 140, *141*; elite and upper-class, 125; New Negro womanhood representations and, 125–27
Lindsay, Inabel Burns, 237
literary works: bronze color usage in, 117–18. *See also* Harlem Renaissance literary print culture
Locke, Alain, 46, 57, 58, 110, 157; *The New Negro* magazine and, 34, 45, 46, 54, 56, 108, 112, 156
Louis, Joe, 242–43
love: beauty, sex and, 174–75, 181; beauty and, 181–82; love/sex in women's poetry, 173–75, 177, 181, 185–86; women's poetry and, 173–75, 176, 179–81

Luckie, Ida Evans, 158
lynching, 115–16, 279n41
Lyons, Sidney Daniel, 91–92, *93*, 97, 100

magazines: advertising in, 65–68, 83, 88, 91–92, *93*; "Illustrated Feature Section" magazine insert, 105, 278n5; New Negro womanhood and, 108; urban African Americans and, 65–66. *See also* African American print culture; Harlem Renaissance magazines; *specific magazines*
mammy, 120
Mammy dolls, 71–72
Manila queen of carnival, 142, *143*
marriage: *Dark Princess* and, 195, 203, 205, 222; Du Bois, W. E. B., and, 204, 205, 287n51; interracial marriages, 197; middle-class New Negroes and, 203–4
masculinity: Harlem Renaissance literary print culture and, 157; New Negroes, 11; yellow and, 178, 179
"The Mask" (Scott Delaney), *149*, 163, 173
Mayo, Katherine, 200–201, 286n37
McDougald, Elizabeth J. ("Bessie"), 37–38
McDougald, Gertrude Elise Johnson: beauty of, 43–44, 61; as brown-skin mulatta, 119–20; "The Double Task: The Struggle of Negro Women for Sex and Race Emancipation," 45, 48, 60; education and, 39–45, 48; "Education in Harlem," 42–43; Harlem Renaissance and, 36, 37, 45, 119; labor organizing of, 35, 39, 48; *A New Day for the Colored Woman Worker*, 43, 47–48; New Negro women and, 31–36, 45, 46, 48–54, 56, 59, 60, 61; news print culture and, 36, 39–40, 42–45; overview, 29–30, 34–40, 60–61; physical appearance of, 39–40, 42, 43–44, 60; Reiss's portrait of, 35, 37, 45, 52–56, 59, 60–61, 119–20, *pl.2*; representations of, 44, 60, 61; scrapbooks of, 29, 36, 39, 44; social work and, 39, 45, 47; "The Task of Negro Womanhood," 31–36, 45, 46, 48, 52–54, 56, 59, 60; unpublished memoir for daughter, 37–38; "The Women of the White Strain," 38; women's labor and, 35, 46–52, 47–52
McKay, Claude, 10, 94, 198
men: sociologists as, 227; women's poetry and, 117, 158–61, 173, 174, 177–81, 183, 186, 188, 190–91; women's reproductive rights and, 112–13. *See also* African American men; gender; masculinity
Messenger magazine, 42, 86, 87, 107–8, 112, 113, 126, 234
Meyer, Annie Nathan, 3
middle class: advertising and, 64; brown complexions and, 64, 225, 226; changing composition of, 15–21; growth of new urban, 29; New Negroes and urban, 16; urbanization and, 15
middle-class New Negroes: marriages of, 203–4; popular culture and, 18. *See also* middle class
middle-class New Negro womanhood: respectable beauty and, 87. *See also* respectable middle-class womanhood
middle-class New Negro women: women's poetry and, 155, 156, 162–63, 168. *See also* clubwomen; middle-class women
middle-class women: brown beauty and, 28; respectable middle-class womanhood, 86, 87, 159, 161, 191. *See also* middle-class New Negro women
migrant women: reform and, 14; urban sex ratios and, 40–41
migration: Harlem and, 9–10, 267n21. *See also* Great Migration
miscegenation: *Dark Princess* and, 196–97, 222; Harlem Renaissance literary print culture and, 196–97; laws about, 25, 207. *See also* interracial romance
Miss Golden Brown Contest, 84–85
modeling, 261–62

modern African American women, 12, 113, 126; women's poetry and, 160, 189, 190

modern brown-skin womanhood: *Dark Princess: A Romance* and, 191, 223; Harlem Renaissance literary print culture and, 131, 194; Harlem Renaissance magazine visual groupings of, 131; overview, 107. See also *Crisis* cover art, of modern brown-skin womanhood

modernization: brown beauty and, 6–7, 10, 15, 30; Great Migration and, 7

"A Mona Lisa" (Grimké), 177

Morris, Vivian, 90–91

motherhood: African American women writers on, 115–16; women's poetry and, 115–19

"Motherhood" (Douglas Johnson), 118

Mother India (Mayo), 200–201, 286n37

mothers: birth rates, 111–13; race suicide and, 70, 111, 274n32; white mothers, 111–13. See also Negro mothers; women's reproductive rights

mulatta, brown-skin. *See* brown-skin mulatta

mulatta representations: African American women writers and, 120–23; African American writers and, 120–23; color and complexion in, 120–23; Harlem Renaissance literary print culture and, 120, 121, 123, 125; light-brown-skinned representations, 122; light-skinned representations, 123, 127; New Negro womanhood and, 120–21; racial passing and, 122–23; whiteness and, 123; white writers and, 123

mulatto, 120, 123, 280n59

mulatto elite, 15–16, 123

Myrdal, Gunnar, 19

NAACP. *See* National Association for the Advancement of Colored People

NACW. *See* National Association of Colored Women

Nashville, 66–67, 68

Nashville Banner, 73, 74

Nashville Globe, 66–67, 69, 70, 71, 74–75, 77, 78

National Association for the Advancement of Colored People (NAACP), 10–11, 102, 132–33, 231, 234. See also *Crisis*

National Association of Colored Women (NACW), 13, 14, 33, 158

National Baptist Convention, 68

National Baptist Publishing Board, 66–67, 68

National Negro Doll Company (NNDC), 68–69, 71, 73, 74, 75, 77–78

National Urban League, 11, 33, 107. See also *Opportunity* magazine

Negro: African Americans identifying as, 21; black as, 77; brown-skin types and Negro heroes, 106. See also New Negro

Negro children: Negro dolls and, 68–72, 74, 75, 77–80; white dolls and, 69–70, 183–84. See also Negro girls; New Negro children

Negro dolls: advertising of, 62, 63, 64, 75, 77–80; Baker, J., doll, 75, 76; beauty of, 74, 75, 77, 79; Berry and Ross Doll Manufacturing, 73, 78–79; Bethel Manufacturing Company and, 80, 81; brown-skin beauty and, 62, 63, 64, 79, 102, 103; as brown-skin dolls, 62, 63, 64, 77–80; condemnations of, 71, 73–74; High Brown, 77–78; Mammy dolls, 71–72; manufacturing, 71–73, 75, 78–79; marketing language, 75, 77–80; materials used in making, 71; Negro children and, 68–72, 74, 75, 77–80; Negro girls and, 68, 70, 71, 72, 75, 77–80; Negro mothers and, 69, 73–74; NNDC and, 68–69, 71, 73, 74, 75, 77–78; O.K. Colored Doll Company and, 62, 63, 79–80; race pride and, 68, 69; racist representations, 69–71, 73, 74, 75; rag dolls, 71–72; realistic, 72–73, 75; representations, 69–71, 73–75; Topsy-Turvy dolls, 72

"Negro Fictionist in America" (Gordon, E.), 94–95, 106
Negro girls: advertising and, 30, 62, 63, 64, 77, 78, 79; brown girl representation, 126, 127; Negro dolls and, 68, 70, 71, 72, 75, 77–80; "Study of a Negro Girl" photograph, 135, 136. *See also* Negro children
Negro mothers: Negro dolls and, 69, 73–74. *See also* New Negro mothers
Negro types, of Demond Lewis, 84. *See also* brown-skin types; Reiss, type studies of
Negro women, 31. *See also* African American women; New Negro women
Negro women's beauty: advertising's promotion of, 96; beauty contests, 84–85; black press and, 83–84, 85; cosmetics and, 87. *See also* brown beauty; New Negro women's beauty
Negro youth. *See* African American youth
Negro Youth at the Crossways (Frazier), 225, 226, 227, 238–44, 253, 291n60
A New Day for the Colored Woman Worker (McDougald, G., and Clark), 43, 47–48
New Deal liberalism, 18–19, 231–33, 235
New Negro: beauty products and, 95; brown as color of, 110; *Crisis* and, 68; Harlem Renaissance literary print culture and, 104–5, 196; intraracial colorism and era of, 4–5; masculinity and, 11; photography of, 23, 269n77; race intellectuals and, 22–23; racial injustices encountered by, 10; *Survey Graphic* "Harlem: Mecca of the New Negro" issue, 45–46, 48, 52–60; urban middle class and, 16
New Negro children: *Crisis* cover art of, 127, 131, 133, *134*, 135, *136*, *139*, 140, 142, 144, *145*, 281n103; *Crisis* illustrations of, 135, *139*, 140, 281n103; *Crisis* photographs of, 131–33, *134*, 135, *136*, 142,

144, *145*; *Crisis*'s annual issue on, 127, 131–33; *Crisis* visuals of, 127, 131–33, *134*, 135, *136*, *139*, 140, 142, 144, *145*, 281n103; NAACP brown baby contests, 132–33; "Study of a Negro Girl" photograph, 135, *136*
New Negro cultural production: brown beauty and, 18. *See also* African American culture; *specific topics*
New Negro identity: consumer culture and, 17; racial identity and, 171
The New Negro magazine, 11, 110, 281n84; Locke and, 34, 45, 46, 54, 56, 108, 112, 156; "The Task of Negro Womanhood," 31–36, 45, 46, 48, 52–54, 56, 59, 60. *See also* Reiss, type studies of
New Negro men, 16; *Crisis* "Men of the Month" feature, 127; women's poetry and, 178, 179. *See also* African American men
New Negro mothers, 110; birth rates, 111–13; role of, 113–14. *See also* Brown Madonna
New Negro movement, 7, 10–11, 223
New Negro photographers: *Crisis* and, 129, 133; Harlem Renaissance magazines and, 108, 129
New Negro portraits: by Reiss, 35, 37, 45, 52–61, 119–20, 128–29. *See also* New Negro women's portraits
New Negro print culture, 16–17, 228. *See also* African American print culture; Harlem Renaissance literary print culture
New Negro representations, 22. *See also* mulatta representations; Reiss, type studies of; representations, racist
New Negro womanhood: advertising and, 64; brown-skin type and, 127; *Dark Princess: A Romance* and, 192, 194, 203, 223; Harlem Renaissance literary print culture and, 125; magazines and, 108; role as mother, 113–14; "The Task

of Negro Womanhood," 31–36, 45, 46, 48, 52–54, 56, 59, 60; women's poetry and, 116, 152, 154, 155, 156, 159, 168. *See also* African American womanhood; brown-skin womanhood; middle-class New Negro womanhood
New Negro womanhood, gendered tropes of, 107, 152. *See also* brown-skin types
New Negro womanhood representations: brown girl, 126, 127; exalted bourgeois woman, 126; Harlem Renaissance literary print culture and, 127; light-skinned women, 125–27; mulatta, 120–21; overview, 152. *See also* brown-skin types
New Negro women: advertising and, 61–64, 80, 82; brown beauty and, 61, 103; brownness and, 3, 28; cosmetics and, 82, 85, 86, 87; *Crisis* photographs of, 135; Harlem Renaissance literary print culture and, 125, 127, 159; McDougald, Gertrude, and, 31–36, 45, 46, 48–54, 56, 59, 60, 61; morality and, 86; New Negro heroines as brown-skin types, 104–5; in 1920s, 34–35; obstacles confronting, 12; respectability and, 13–14, 86, 204, 223. *See also specific topics*
New Negro women's beauty: employment and, 102; whiteness and, 183. *See also* brown beauty
New Negro women's photographs: on *Crisis* covers, 128, 129, *130*, 131–32, 135, *136*, *137*, *138*, 140, *141*, 142, *143*, 144, *145*, 146, *147*, *148*, *149*, *150*, *151*; Harlem Renaissance magazines and, 125, 126
New Negro women's portraits: Harlem Renaissance magazines and, 125, 126; of McDougald, Gertrude, 35, 37, 45, 52–56, 59, 60–61, 119–20; by Reiss, 35, 37, 45, 52–56, 59, 60–61, 119–20, 129
New Negro World, 228–29

Newsome, Effie Lee, 117–18, 166
newspapers: consumer activism by, 20; urban African Americans and, 65–67. *See also* African American newspapers; press; *specific newspapers*
news print culture: McDougald, Gertrude, and, 36, 39–40, 42–45. *See also* African American print culture
New Women: brown-skin fad and, 92; obstacles confronting, 12. *See also* New Negro women
New York Age, 10, 65, 69, 77, 78, 84, 261
New York City, Great Migration and, 8, 9
NNDC. *See* National Negro Doll Company
Noble, Jeanne, 12
"A North African Cousin of Ours" photograph, 140, *141*

octoroon, 121, 280n59
"The Octoroon" (Douglas Johnson), 121
O.K. Colored Doll Company, 62, 63, 79–80
"On Being Young—a Woman—and Colored" (Bonner), 199
Opportunity magazine, 57, 118, 180; brown-skin types and, 107; Harlem Renaissance poetry and, 156, 157, 158, 174; Johnson, Charles, and, 87, 126, 157, 175, 226, 245, 292n80
"The Ordeal" (Douglas Johnson), 172–73
Orientalism, 197–201. *See also* Asians
Owen, Chandler, 108, 114–15
Ozawa, Takao, 26

pan-Africanism, 11, 55, 210, 215, 288n10
Park, Robert Ezra, 58, 235
Parrish, Charles H., 235; "Color Names and Color Notions," 226–27, 252–58; "The Significance of Color in the Negro Community," 253, 293n103
Passing (Larsen), 121

photography: in African American print culture, 21; *Crisis* and, 128, 129, *130*, 131–33, *134*, 135, *136*, *137*, *138*, 140, *141*, 142, *143*, 144, *145*, 146, *147*, *148*, *149*; Exhibit of American Negroes, 22–23, 129, 269n77; of New Negroes, 23, 269n77. *See also Crisis* visuals, of New Negroes; New Negro photographers; New Negro women's photographs
Pittsburgh Courier, 228, 229–30
Pittsburgh Courier, 16
"Poem" (Johnson, H.), 178, 287n72
poetry: brown and, 117–19, 153–55; obligatory race poetry, 168, 169, 170, 172. *See also* Harlem Renaissance poetry; women's poetry
poetry anthologies: *Caroling Dusk*, 153, 155, 156, 170, 177; men's poetry and, 156–57, 158; women's poetry and, 160
press: racial justice and popular, 228–32. *See also* magazines; newspapers; news print culture; print culture
print culture: brown beauty and, 21, 61; McDougald, Gertrude, and news print culture, 36, 39–40, 42–45. *See also* African American print culture
"The Proletariat Speaks" (Dunbar-Nelson), 186–88

quadroon, 39–40
"Questing" (Spencer), 182
The Quest of the Silver Fleece (Du Bois, W. E. B.), 202

race, 268n38; color, women's poetry, and, 154, 169–72, 174; color and, 24, 155, 205–10, 214–16; color of race and ethnicity in white America, 205–7; *Dark Princess* and, 191–96, 205, 207, 208, 214; Du Bois, W. E. B., and, 191–96, 205, 207–11, 214–16, 234; intellectualizing about, 22–27; interwar years and, 7, 18–19; law and, 24–25; obligatory race poetry, 168, 169, 170, 172; women's poetry and, 154, 168–81. *See also* social science, on race
race concept, 208–10
race descriptors: brown as, 24; color as, 24, 155, 205–7, 210, 215; law and, 26; U.S. Census use of, 25–26, 40, 206; white as, 26
race intellectuals, New Negro and, 22–23
race prejudice, 58, 236. *See also* African American youth, research on
race pride, 5, 68, 69, 235–36
race signifier, brown as, 154
race suicide: African American men and, 112; eugenics and, 112, 114; mothers and, 70, 111, 274n32
race womanhood, 268n38; *Dark Princess* and, 194, 195, 202, 203, 220; respectable, 13, 203
racial discourse: on brown beauty, 7, 21, 24, 28, 259; on brown complexions, 29
racial identity: color and, 169, 171, 228; Du Bois, W., and, 202, 207, 209, 210, 214; New Negro identity and, 171; origin of, 2
racial injustices: New Negro and, 10; against urban African Americans, 28–29
racialization, loss of individuality and, 1
racial justice: popular press and, 228–32; racial injustices, 10, 28–29; racial liberals and, 232–33
racial liberalism, 19, 231–33, 258
racial passing, mulatta representations and, 122–23
racial type: beauty as, 84. *See also* Negro types, of Demond Lewis
racial uplift, reform and, 14
racism: against Asian Indians, 206–7; racist science, 26, 27, 227
racist representations: of African Americans, 68–71; of Negro dolls, 69–71, 73, 74, 75

racist views: of African Americans, 68–71; of African American women, 32–34, 35; brown beauty and, 35
Rai, Lala Lajput, 213
Randolph, A. Philip, 108, 234
"Record of Freshman Interest" (Hurston), 3–4
reform: clubwomen and, 14, 33, 47, 86, 158; migrant women and, 14; racial uplift and, 14. *See also* respectability
Reiss, type studies of: *Brown Madonna*, 59, 108, 110, 129, *pl.5*; *The Librarian*, 60; overview, 57, 58, 59; *Type Study I*, 59, *109*; *Type Study II* (Two Public School Teachers), 56, 57, 60, *pl.4*; *A Woman from the Virgin Islands*, 59–60
Reiss, Winold, 281n84; *Crisis* and, 128–29; "Harlem Girl 1" portrait of, 55–56, 140, *pl.3*; *Miss Hurston* portrait, *pl.1*; New Negro portraits by, 35, 37, 45, 52–61, 119–20, 128–29; overview, 54; portrait of McDougald, Gertrude, by, 35, 37, 45, 52–56, 59, 60–61, 119–20, *pl.2*
representations, racist, 68–71. *See also specific topics*
respectability: complexion, employment, 51–52; decline in 1930s of, 14–15, 28; New Negro women and, 13–14, 86, 204, 223; respectable race womanhood, 13, 203; women and, 13–15; women's labor, complexion and, 51–52
respectable beauty: brown beauty as, 13, 15, 190; middle-class New Negro womanhood and, 87
respectable middle-class womanhood, 86, 87; women's poetry and, 159, 161, 191
"Revelation" (Dickinson), 188–90
Riis, Jacob, 9
Rogers, J. A., 112
Ross, Victoria, 79
Ruffin, Josephine St. Pierre, 13, 158

Saturday Evening Quill, 106
Schrack, Blanche, 114
Schuyler, George S., 87, 107, 278n5; *Black No More*, 152; "Instructions for Contributors," 104–6, 127, 152
Scott, Clarissa Mae, 146, *147*
Scott Delaney, Clarissa, *149*, 163, 173
sex: beauty, love and, 174–75, 181; *Dark Princess* and, 203, 220; love/sex in women's poetry, 173–75, 177, 181, 185–86; women's poetry and, 168, 173–77, 180–81, 186, 188
sexual violence, 217
Shuffle Along, 92, 94
"The Significance of Color in the Negro Community" (Parrish), 253, 293n103–4
skin whitening, 95, 124–25
Smith, Bessie, 17–18
social psychology, 246
social science: brown-skin ideal and, 235–36, 257–58; gender and, 227
social science, on race, 58, 223–24, 227–28, 245. *See also* African American youth, research on
social work: African American women and, 47; McDougald, Gertrude, and, 39, 45, 47
sociologists, 223, 226, 227, 234–36, 258–59. *See also* Frazier, E. Franklin; Johnson, Charles S.; Parrish, Charles H.
"Sonnet 1" (Johnson, H.), 181–82
"So the Girl Marries" (Du Bois, W. E. B.), 204
Souls of Black Folk (Du Bois, W. E. B.), 205, 210
Spencer, Anne, 163–64, 179, 182, 188
"Studies of Negro Youth," 236–38
Survey Graphic, 108, 232; "Harlem: Mecca of the New Negro" issue, 45–46, 48, 52–60
Sutherland, Robert L., 236, 237

tanning, and brown-skin fad, 92, 94–95
"The Task of Negro Womanhood" (McDougald, G.), 31–36, 45, 46, 48, 52–54, 56, 59, 60
Terrell, Mary Church, 211
Their Eyes Were Watching God (Hurston), 122
"The Poet" (Luckie), 158
Thind, Bhagat Singh, 26
Thompson, James G., 229
Thurman, Wallace, 123–25
Tillman, D. Norman, 140, 281n103
"To a Dark Girl" (Bennett), 153–54
"To a Young Wife" (Douglas Johnson), 186
"Touché" (Fauset), 174
"Troubador" (Houston), 178
"True American" (Douglas Johnson), 171–72
Turner, Valdora, 131
type studies, of Reiss. *See* Reiss, type studies of
Type Study I, 59, 109
Type Study II (Two Public School Teachers), 56, 57, 60, *pl.4*

Universal Negro Improvement Association (UNIA), 11, 55, 79, 213, 228
upper class: brown complexions and, 226; elite and upper-class light-skinned women, 125
urban African Americans: civil rights activism by, 19–20; consumerism and, 19–20; growth of new middle-class, 29; magazines and, 65–66; New Negro movement and politicization of, 10–11; newspapers and, 65–67; racial injustices against, 28–29. *See also specific topics*
urban African American women: women's poetry, 188–90. *See also* New Negro women
urban culture, color-inflected language and, 17–18

urbanization: African Americans and, 9, 10; middle class and, 15
Urban League. *See* Detroit Urban League; National Urban League
urban middle class: growth of new, 29; New Negroes and, 16
U.S. Census: African American categories and, 206; color usage in, 206; racial descriptors in, 25–26, 40, 206

Vaughan, Mary, 88–89

Walker, C. J., 82, 90, 101, 275n74
Walker Manufacturing Company, 82, 89–90
Warner, W. Lloyd, 237–38
"Welt" (Douglas Johnson), 185–86
West, Dorothy, 166, 167–68, 284n88
Wheeler, Laura, 128
white: African American writers and white readers, 106; birth rates of white mothers, 111–13; Harlem and white observers, 90; mulatta representations and white writers, 123; as race descriptor, 26; racial liberalism and white liberals, 19, 231–33, 258; white dolls, 69–70, 72, 74, 183–84
white America: color of race and ethnicity in, 205–7; white Americans, 111
white beauty, 183; blues eyes and, 184, 284n91. *See also* white skin beauty
whiteness: citizenship and, 26; colored and, 3; mulatta representations and, 123; New Negro women's beauty and, 183; racist science and biological difference to whiteness, 26, 27; women's beauty and, 183
white-owned businesses: in beauty industry, 88–89, 95; black press and, 105
white publishers, 46; African American writers and, 105–6; Harlem Renaissance literary print culture and, 106

white skin beauty: advertising and, 88; African American women and, 87–88, 90; cosmetics and, 87–88
"White Things" (Spencer), 179
white womanhood: beauty contests and, 85; white dolls and, 184
"Widow with a Moral Obligation" (Johnson, H.), 180–81
Wilkins, Roy O., 231
William B. Ziff Company, 105, 278n5
Williams, Katherine, 65, 66
A Woman from the Virgin Islands, 59–60
womanhood: African American women writers on, 116; white, 85, 184; women's poetry and, 188. *See also* African American womanhood; New Negro womanhood; race womanhood
Woman's Era magazine, 13–14, 158
women: advertising and women of color, 97; blues women, 116; respectability and, 13–15. *See also* gender; *specific topics*
women, in interwar years, 12, 41. *See also specific topics*
"women of the race," 268n38. *See also* race womanhood
"The Women of the White Strain" (McDougald, G.), 38
women poets: biographies and overview, 160–68; dress, style, fashion and, 167–68; interactions between, 165–68
women representations: of brownness in interwar years, 2, 18, 29, 30, 61. *See also specific topics*
women's beauty: advertising, color and, 95–96; intelligence and, 86; whiteness and, 183. *See also* Negro women's beauty
women's labor, 41; African American women's public image and, 35; clerical and sales work, 49–50, 101; clerical work, 49–50, 99, 101–2; discrimination and, 50–51; domestic and service-oriented work, 216, 289n113; McDougald, Gertrude, and, 35, 46–52; New Negro women's beauty and employment, 102; respectability, complexion and, 51–52; sales work, 49–50; segregation and, 50
women's poetry: African American men in, 177–80; age and, 155, 184–86; beauty and, 174, 175, 181–90; blackness in, 118–19, 169, 170, 178, 179, 183; brown and, 117–19, 153–56, 160, 161, 168, 170, 174–78, 179, 190, 191; brown beauty and, 154, 175, 190, 191; brown-skin types and, 152; class and, 155, 161, 162–63; clubwomen and, 158; color and, 153–56, 160–62, 168–72, 174, 176, 177, 179, 188, 191; complexion and, 161–62; consumerism and, 186–87, 188–90; *Crisis* and, 117–18, 171, 179, 183; Harlem Renaissance literary print culture and, 157–60, 190–91; Harlem Renaissance magazines and, 157–60, 168; love and, 173–75, 176, 179–81; love/sex and, 173–75, 177, 181, 185–86; men and, 117, 158–61, 173, 174, 177–81, 183, 186, 188, 190–91; men's poetry and, 159–60; middle-class New Negro women and, 155, 156, 159, 162–63, 168; modern African American women and, 160, 189, 190; motherhood and, 115–19; New Negro men and, 178, 179; New Negro womanhood and, 116, 152, 154, 155, 156, 159, 168; overview, 154–56, 158–60, 190–91; poetry anthologies and, 160; race and, 154, 168–81; race and color in, 154, 169–72, 174; respectable middle-class womanhood and, 159, 161, 191; sex and, 168, 173–77, 180–81, 186, 188; urban African American women and, 188–90; womanhood and, 188; youth and, 186

women's reproductive rights: birth control, 111–15, 279n32; men and, 112–13
women writers: age and, 184–86, 285n96. *See also* African American women writers
World Tomorrow, 1
Wright, Richard, 214

"You! Inez!" (Dunbar-Nelson), 176
"Young Woman Blues," 17–18
youth: beauty and, 92, 187; beauty industry and, 92; hair products and, 92; women's poetry and, 186. *See also* African American youth

ABOUT THE AUTHOR

Laila Haidarali lectures on African American and women's history at the University of Essex in the United Kingdom.

www.ingramcontent.com/pod-product-compliance
Lightning Source LLC
Chambersburg PA
CBHW061228070526
44584CB00030B/4037